8-65

8/25

MODERN
DEVELOPMENTS
IN
AUDIOLOGY

Second Edition

MODERN DEVELOPMENTS IN AUDIOLOGY

Edited by
JAMES JERGER
Baylor College of Medicine

Second Edition

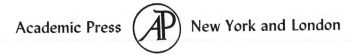

Academic Press   New York and London

A Subsidiary of Harcourt Brace Jovanovich, Publishers

ACADEMIC PRESS, INC.
111 Fifth Avenue, New York, New York 10003

United Kingdom Edition published by
ACADEMIC PRESS, INC. (LONDON) LTD.
24/28 Oval Road, London NW1

LIBRARY OF CONGRESS CATALOG CARD NUMBER: 72-82660

Second Printing, 1974

PRINTED IN THE UNITED STATES OF AMERICA

CONTENTS

1

Bone-Conduction Measurements

DONALD DIRKS

2

Speech Audiometry

TOM W. TILLMAN AND WAYNE O. OLSEN

v

3

Diagnostic Audiometry

JAMES JERGER

4

Auditory Masking

GERALD A. STUDEBAKER

5

Measurement of Hearing in Children

ROBERT FRISINA

6

Functional Hearing Loss

NORMA T. HOPKINSON

7

Aural Rehabilitation

JOHN J. O'NEILL AND HERBERT J. OYER

8

Psychoacoustic Instrumentation

WILLIAM MELNICK

9

Adaptation and Fatigue

W. DIXON WARD

10

Measurement of Acoustic Impedance at the Tympanic Membrane

DAVID J. LILLY

11

Electroencephalic Audiometry

ROBERT GOLDSTEIN

12

The Theory of Signal Detectability and the Measurement of Hearing

FRANK R. CLARKE AND ROBERT C. BILGER

13

Research Frontiers in Audiology

ROBERT C. BILGER

LIST OF CONTRIBUTORS

Numbers in parentheses indicate the pages on which the authors' contributions begin.

ROBERT C. BILGER (437,469),
Bioacoustics Laboratory, Eye and Ear Hospital, School of Medicine, University of Pittsburgh, Pittsburgh, Pennsylvania

FRANK R. CLARKE (437),
Sensory Science Research Center, Stanford Research Institute, Menlo Park, California

DONALD DIRKS (1),
Department of Surgery, Head and Neck, UCLA School of Medicine, Los Angeles, California

ROBERT FRISINA (155),
National Technical Institute for the Deaf, Rochester Institute of Technology, Rochester, New York

ROBERT GOLDSTEIN (407),
Department of Communicative Disorders, College of Letters and Science and Department of Rehabilitation Medicine, School of Medicine, The University of Wisconsin, Madison, Wisconsin

NORMA T. HOPKINSON (175),
Bioacoustics Laboratory, Eye and Ear Hospital and School of Medicine, University of Pittsburgh, Pittsburgh, Pennsylvania

JAMES JERGER (75),
Department of Otolaryngology, Division of Audiology and Speech Pathology, Baylor College of Medicine, Houston, Texas

DAVID J. LILLY (345),
Department of Speech Pathology and Audiology, University of Iowa, Iowa City, Iowa

WILLIAM MELNICK (253),
Department of Otolaryngology, Ohio State University, Columbus, Ohio

WAYNE O. OLSEN (37),
Department of Communicative Disorders, School of Speech, Northwestern University, Evanston, Illinois

JOHN J. O'NEILL (211),
Department of Speech, University of Illinois, Urbana, Illinois

HERBERT J. OYER (211),
College of Communication, Michigan State University, East Lansing, Michigan

GERALD A. STUDEBAKER (117),
Memphis Speech and Hearing Center, Memphis State University, Memphis, Tennessee

TOM W. TILLMAN (37),
Department of Communicative Disorders, School of Speech, Northwestern University, Evanston, Illinois

W. DIXON WARD (301),
Department of Otolaryngology, University of Minnesota, Minneapolis, Minnesota

PREFACE

Almost 10 years have passed since the first edition of *Modern Developments* was published in 1963.

The intervening decade has been an exciting period in audiology. We have seen the birth and first halting steps of evoked-response audiometry, the use of sophisticated signal averaging techniques to capture the brain's response to sound, increased attention to the concepts of the theory of signal detectability and its implications for auditory measurement, laterality effects during dichotic listening that have important implications not only for the evaluation of central auditory disorder but for the very nature of speech perception, the development of new and innovative techniques for the measurement of speech intelligibility, and new concepts in amplification for the hearing-impaired that have opened broad vistas in aural rehabilitation. Undoubtedly the single most significant development since the first edition appeared, however, has been the wide clinical application of impedance audiometry. The measurement techniques devised and elaborated in the Scandinavian countries during the late 1950s and early 1960s, supplemented by Zwislocki's development of an electromechanical bridge in the early 1960s, laid the groundwork for widespread clinical investigation of the diagnostic value of impedance measurements. Results are currently causing a minor revolution in audiologic practice.

Therefore, we have devoted considerable attention in the present edition, to an exposition of both basic and applied aspects of impedance measurement. In Chapter 10, *Measurement of Acoustic Impedance at the Tympanic Membrane*, Dr. David Lilly leads us through the basic concepts and definitions of impedance measurement with a firm but gentle hand. He also summarizes the wide range of applications to which impedance measures have been put. In Chapter 3, *Diagnostic Audiometry*, concrete applications of the technique are discussed in some detail.

The "impedance revolution" is, however, only one example of the rapid change characterizing so many facets of the field of audiometry. We can only hope that this small volume will not be seriously out of date before another decade passes.

xiii

PREFACE TO THE FIRST EDITION

In the family of sciences, Audiology is a young but lusty infant. Born less than two decades ago in the convergence of modern electronics and the military aural rehabilitation programs of the Second World War, this new field has already generated an extensive international literature. Inevitably, in the case of a young science, this literature has arisen from a wide variety of sources. Dedicated investigators in the allied disciplines of Psychology, Physiology, Speech Pathology, Education, and Medicine laid the scientific foundation for the field of Audiology and continue their important contributions. Within the past ten years, moreover, we have seen slow progress made in the field to produce its own core of researchers, men whose primary interest lies in hearing and hearing disorders.

The purpose of this book is to collect within a single volume the more important findings emanating from these diverse sources in recent years. The bias is frankly experimental. In each chapter, emphasis is placed on basic research findings, underlying principles, and, when appropriate, investigative technique.

Seven of the contributions bring us up to date on classical problem areas. R. F. Naunton surveys bone-conduction; J. Chaiklin and I. Ventry shed some new light on functional hearing loss; and D. R. Frisina tackles the thorny problem of measurement in children. R. Goldstein considers the various electrophysiologic indices; W. D. Ward surveys auditory fatigue and masking; and A. M. Small, Jr., covers auditory adaptation.

Five contributors address themselves to problems exciting much current interest among audiologists. O. Jepsen surveys middle ear muscle reflexes in man, and E. Bocca and C. Calearo summarize their pioneering studies of central hearing processes. Looking toward future developments in the field, W. Rudmose considers the effect of automation on audiometry, and F. Clarke and R. Bilger present a provocative discussion of the relatively new theory of signal detectability as it relates to the measurement of hearing. Finally J. D. Harris directs his verbal arsenal on what tomorrow holds for us all.

Our aim has been to present a broad coverage of the more significant research events of the past ten years and, in a few instances, to summarize where we stand on some of the perennial problems plaguing the field.

It was not our initial intent that this book cover every aspect of the field comprehensively. Nor did we visualize a handbook for the clinical practitioner, or a class textbook for the graduate student. We have sought, however, to integrate within a single volume some of the significant research events of the past decade that will be of value to researchers, teachers, and graduate students.

June, 1963

JAMES JERGER

Chapter 1

Bone-Conduction Measurements

DONALD DIRKS

University of California, Los Angeles

I. Introduction

Although the air-conduction pathway generally is considered to be the principal mode of sound transmission, the movements of a vibrating body may also be transmitted to the inner ear through direct contact with the skull. As Hood (1962) observed, no specific physiologically useful purpose has been attributed to the bone-conduction system in man. Rather, according to Bárány (1938) and Békésy (1949), the ossicular chain in man seems to be balanced to diminish bone conduction by the development of relatively substantial masses above the chain's axis of rotation. This design, while not the most optimum for air-conduc-

1

tion transmission, minimizes the effect of bone conduction so that body noises resulting from breathing, chewing, blood flow, and creaking of joints are not distractingly loud. Aside from certain theoretical considerations, the subject of bone conduction has been of primary interest to otologists and audiologists because of the diagnostic usefulness of measurements which involve this mode of excitation.

Békésy (1932) was the first investigator to demonstrate clearly that the mode of excitation of the cochlear receptors was the same for both air- and bone-conducted signals. By adjusting the amplitude and phase of an air-conducted signal, he was able to cancel a bone-conducted signal at 400 hertz (400 Hz). Békésy concluded that the vibrations of the basilar membrane from either air or bone conduction are produced by movement of the fluid near the stapes, and thus the two modes of transmission must excite the sensory receptors in the same manner.

Lowy (1942) also produced airbone cancellation of the cochlear microphonics, within the frequency range from 250 to 3000 Hz (250–3000 Hz), in guinea pigs and cats. In addition to Békésy's original conclusions, Lowy observed that when complete cancellation was achieved, the recording electrode could be moved to any new position along the cochlea without altering the cancellation. It is therefore assumed that the entire cochlear partition was at rest. Later, Wever and Lawrence (1954) verified the findings of Lowy.

II. Vibration Patterns of the Skull

Some knowledge of the vibration patterns of the skull from bone-conduction stimulation is necessary in order to understand the method by which vibrations reach the cochlea. Békésy (1932) devised an ingenious method of examining vibrations of the skull by adjusting the amplitude and phase of a vibrating probe until such vibrations were eliminated when brought into contact with various parts of the skull. This only occurs when the bony wall and the test probe are vibrating at exactly the same frequency, amplitude, and phase. Figure 1 illustrates the vibration patterns of the skull as observed by Békésy. The vibrator was applied to the forehead for these measurements. At low frequencies, primarily below 800 Hz, the skull moves as a rigid body, while the forehead and occiput move with equal amplitude in the same direction. At a frequency of approximately 800 Hz, a circular nodal line appears so that the forehead vibrates 180° out of phase with the occiput. As the frequency increases, other nodal lines occur, and the phase difference between the front and back of the head increases. In the frequency region around 1800 Hz, the skull resonates with two circular nodal lines.

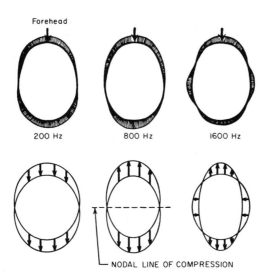

FIG. 1. Vibration pattern of the skull when the forehead is in contact with a vibrating body. Below about 200 Hz the skull behaves as a rigid body. Near 800 Hz the forehead vibrates in the opposite direction from the back of the head—a type of resonance of the skull with a nodal line of compression. Above 1500 Hz the skull vibrates in sections separated by nodal lines. Variations in the thickness of the skull produce variability in the resonance frequency. [After Békésy and Rosenblith (1951), by permission of the publishers.]

Bárány (1938) measured the vibration pattern of the skull at 435 Hz and verified Békésy's observation that the skull moves practically as a whole in this frequency area. Kirikae (1959) also conducted a detailed study of skull movement over a frequency range from 250 to 7000 Hz on a cadaver head and three dried skulls. Essentially, his results agree in the low and mid-frequencies with Békésy's observations. In addition, Kirikae established the first resonance frequency of the skulls at 1700–1800 Hz. At frequencies higher than 1800 Hz, however, the vibration patterns of the skull become very complex, the number of nodal lines increases and numerous resonance frequencies occur.

III. Theories of Bone Conduction

Most of the currently accepted concepts regarding bone conduction have evolved from the investigations and the theoretical explanations of Herzog and Krainz (1926), Békésy (1932), Bárány (1938), Kirikae (1959), Huizing (1960), Groen (1962), and Tonndorf (1966). The most widely accepted of the early theories place heavy emphasis on the mechanism of inertia and compression bone conduction which were established primarily through the investigations of Herzog and Krainz, Békésy, and Bárány.

A. Early Theory

According to Herzog and Krainz (1926), in compression bone conduction, the vibrating energy reaching the cochlea causes alternate compressions and expansions of the cochlear shell. The incompressible cochlear fluid must yield under the influence of these opposite movements in order to produce a displacement of the basilar membrane. If the elastic characteristics of the cochlear scalae were equal, then a compression of the cochlea would not produce fluid displacement. This condition is illustrated in Figure 2a. A compensatory mechanism, as shown in Figure 2b, would be required to produce the necessary volume changes in the cochlear spaces to set up a force differential on the two sides of the cochlear duct. Such a mechanism is possible since the oval window is less compliant than the round window (Kirikae, 1960). In addition, the presence of the semicircular canals and vestibule in the region of the stapes (Figure 2c) further enhances a displacement of the fluid from the scala vestibuli to the scala tympani. The contribution of compressional bone conduction is greatest at high frequencies where the skull no longer moves as a rigid body but rather is compressed and expanded segmentally in response to an alternating vibration (Békésy, 1932).

The second mode of bone-conduction stimulation is referred to as inertia bone conduction since it arises from the inertia of the ossicular chain. According to Békésy (1932) and Bárány (1938), the malleus and incus rotate around a common axis which is close to their gravitational axis. Thus, when the skull vibrates, the ossicular chain participates in this displacement but, because it is so loosely coupled to the skull, a movement of the stapes footplate is set up relative to the oval window. The inertia of the ossicles prevents them from following the skull vibration and, as a consequence, while the walls of the middle ear cavity move outward, the ossicles remain relatively motionless, exerting a force in the opposite direction. This motion leads to cochlear stimulation in the same manner as that produced by an air-conducted signal.

B. Recent Developments

Kirikae (1959) employed electrical means to measure the amplitude and phase of the skull during stimulation by a vibrator constructed of Rochelle salt crystals. As mentioned previously, he verified some of Békésy's earlier findings concerning the vibration patterns of the skull during bone-conduction stimulation. From experiments on humans, cats, and fresh human cadavers, he reported that a close relationship exists between the position of the rotary axis of the ossicular chain and the bone-conduction thresholds on the surface of the head. By loading the tympanic membrane, bone-conduction hearing was varied objectively and subjectively in the frequency region around 300 Hz. These results provide additional evidence that the inertia of the middle ear ossicles plays an important role in bone-conduction stimulation, especially in

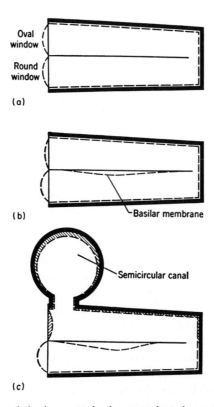

FIG. 2. Compression of the inner ear by bone-conducted sound leads to movement of the basilar membrane. The dashed lines indicate the positions of the various membranes during compression by a sound wave in the skull. (a) Hypothetical case of symmetrical compression of the cochlea and equal yielding of the membranes of the oval and round windows. No movement of the basilar membrane occurs. (b) The round window actually yields more than the oval window to equal pressures. The basilar membrane is moved slightly toward the scala tympani. (c) The semi-circular canals are also compressed, and fluid forced into the scala vestibuli causes greater movement of the membranes.

the low frequencies. Kirikae also determined the pattern of threshold distribution as the position of the vibrator was varied on different parts of the skulls of subjects with unilateral complete deafness. The differences in the threshold values become gradually equalized with increased frequency, especially above 1800 Hz. This fact demonstrated that the temporal bone vibrates in nearly the same mode independent of the position of the vibrator on the skull and the rotation axis of the ossicles. Such observations suggested that both the inertia of the ossicles and the compression of the labyrinth play a part in bone-conduction transmission in the higher frequencies. From other experiments on the stress distribution around the labyrinthine bone, he observed that even though inertia bone conduction was prevalent at both low and high frequencies, compression bone conduction still plays a major role at higher frequencies.

Huizing (1960) pointed out the inadequacy of explaining various clinical observations (Carhart notch) and experimental findings on the basis of traditional theory regarding inertia, compression, and "bone conduction by air conduction." He suggested that the mechanism of bone conduction should not be explained by presupposing that the aforementioned three methods of stimulation work in mutual cooperation. Rather, it would be better to approach the bone-conduction system as a set of complex coupled vibrating systems. When one changes the properties of these systems, clinically or experimentally, alterations take place in the mutual relationships of the impedances and couplings. Any changes in these properties not only affect the vibration of the system concerned, but also exert an influence on the vibration of the entire system.

Groen (1962), utilizing certain known structural properties of the ear, calculated several bone-conduction components. He determined that the air volume enclosed in the middle ear has a resonance around 2500 Hz. It was reasoned that stapedial fixation should eliminate that portion of the effect which acts on the inner ear while retaining the portion acting on the round window. The investigator felt that the variability in the Carhart notch was due to the variation in the frequency and magnitude of the component acting on the round window. Later Tonndorf (1966) confirmed experimentally that the compliance of the air enclosed in the middle ear spaces was an important contributor to the total bone-conduction response.

Groen also suggested that in patients with stapedial fixation, pronounced positive phase shifts would occur, causing lateralization of the tone toward the involved ear. In the region between 1000 and 2000 Hz, however, lateralization may often change from one side to another. This finding was attributed to the interaction of a phase lead with the variations in the resonance of the middle ear cavity. Such an explanation, however, was not verified by Tonndorf's (1966) investigations.

Seven basic experiments, compiled in an excellent monograph by Tonndorf (1966), are probably the most significant of the recent contributions to the theory of bone conduction. The investigator stressed the futility of accounting for all bone-conduction phenomena by a single simple mechanism. Rather, he identified three major factors and various modifying components which contribute to the total bone-conduction response. The major mechanisms were identified as (1) the reception of sound energy radiated into the external canal, (2) the inertial response of the middle-ear ossicles and inner-ear fluid, and (3) the compressional response of the inner-ear spaces. According to Tonndorf, each of these mechanisms responds actively and independently to vibrating stimulation.

Tonndorf observed that when a vibrating signal is applied to the skull, energy is produced by the walls of the external canal and transmitted to the tympanic membrane. This mode may be modified by occluding the external canal openings, by the canal resonance, and by the impedance of the tympanic membrane. An impairment of the middle ear may eliminate or reduce the transmission of the sound energy developed in the external canal.

The second identifiable bone-conduction mechanism, the inertial response, was considered to be a product of the impedance of the middle-ear ossicles and the inertia of the inner-ear fluids. The response of the ossicular chain can be modified by the air column within the external canal and by the air enclosed in the middle ear cavity.

The compressional response, the final mechanism cited, was dsecribed as a product of distortional vibration of the cochlear shell which may be independent of the cochlear openings. The response, however, is modified by the oval and round-window release as well as by the "third" window release of the cochlear aqueduct.

The normal ear integrates each of the components according to their amplitude and phase relationships. Tonndorf calculated absolute response curves individually for the various bone-conduction components as well as the total bone-conduction response curve based upon the observed amplitude and phase relationships of the bone-conduction components.

C. Summary

Even though current bone-conduction theory has a history dating back for more than 100 years, most of the important concepts and experiments have been conducted within the last 50 years. The early theories of bone conduction were often based upon little experimental evidence and even some of the more modern theorists have attempted to find a single, unifying, and simple principle underlying the very complex phenomenon of bone conduction. Of all the various concepts considered in the explanation of bone conduction, the three basic mechanisms described by Tonndorf summarize succinctly the manner in which bone-conduction excitation is brought about: (1) the reception of sound energy radiated into the external ear canal, (2) the inertial response of the middle-ear ossicles and the inner-ear fluids, and (3) the compressional response of the inner-ear spaces.

IV. Influence of the External and Middle Ear on Bone-Conduction Responses

During the past two decades, the measurement of bone-conduction thresholds has gained in clinical importance as a result of the development of new otologic surgical procedures. The usefulness of the difference between the air- and bone-conduction threshold is, in principle, established on two assumptions: first, that the threshold for air conduction reflects the function of the total auditory system, both conductive and sensorineural, and, second, that the threshold for bone-conducted stimuli is a measure of the sensorineural system. As a result of these general clinical assumptions, the discrepancy between the air- and bone-conduction threshold is often assumed to indicate the magnitude of the conductive component. Theoretically, in a purely conductive loss, the bone-conduction thresholds should be normal. However, the fact that bone-conduction sensitivity is not independent of the state of the middle ear has been repeatedly indicated from clinical observations as well as by experimentation.

Carhart (1962), in a review of the effects of stapes fixation on bone conduction, observed that conflicting opinions exist among theorists regarding the explanation of the now-familiar "Carhart notch." Other conflicts concerning the reality or unreality of enhancements in bone-conduction thresholds (prolonged bone conduction) during middle ear infections have been detailed by Naunton and Fernandez (1961). Such disputes as these are probably due to a lack of a complete understanding of the role of the outer and middle ear in bone conduction. It is instructive to review some of the literature concerning this problem.

A. Clinical Observations

Numerous examples of changes in bone-conduction thresholds in humans with various middle-ear lesions have been reported. Clinically, patients with stapes fixation due to otosclerosis often show a loss in bone-conduction thresholds in the frequency region around 2000 Hz. This notch in the bone-conduction audiogram was described originally

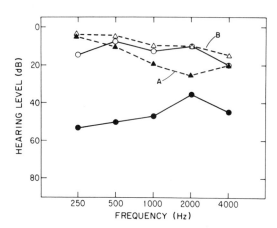

FIG. 3. Pre- and postoperative air- and bone-conduction audiogram illustrates typical configuration in a patient with otosclerosis. ●—●, Preop AC; ○—○, postop AC; ▲--▲, preop BC; △--△, postop BC. [After Békésy (1932, 1960), by permission of the publishers.]

by Carhart (1950) and now bears his name. Curve A in Figure 3 is a representative example of the bone-conduction loss resulting from stapedial fixation. The Carhart notch is present with the maximum loss at 2000 Hz. Curve B in Figure 3 shows bone-conduction levels for the same patient 8 months after successful stapedectomy with almost complete restoration of hearing. The postoperative bone-conduction levels have improved by 5 decibels (5 dB) at 500 Hz, 10 dB at 1000 Hz, 15 dB at 2000 Hz, and 5 dB at 4000 Hz. These improvements in the postoperative bone-conduction levels correspond closely to the average shifts in the bone-conduction responses due to stapedial fixation as described by Carhart. He pointed out that in cases of stapes fixation, the measurement of bone conduction cannot be considered an exact indication of the sensorineural system and suggested that allowances be made for this occurrence in estimating potential results from surgery.

Fournier (1954), Hirsh (1952), and Carhart (1962) have commented upon the incompatibility of the bone-conduction loss due to stapedial fixation with the traditional theory of inertia bone conduction. They suggested that inertia is the dominant mode of bone conduction in the low frequencies, since the head moves as a whole with no compression waves in that frequency region. In the high frequencies, however, where the movements of the skull to forced vibration become quite complex, compression bone conduction is the dominant mode. It might be anticipated from classical theory that stapedial fixation should impair inertia bone conduction with a loss primarily in the low and not the high frequencies.

Huizing (1960) discounted inertial bone conduction in explaining the Carhart notch. He suggested that in stapes fixation, the ossicular chain and cochlear fluid no longer form an entity and, thus, the influence of the chain on the cochlear fluid is practically eliminated. A shift in the bone conduction threshold would result from the elimination of such reinforcement to the cochlear oscillation, especially at the resonant frequency of the auditory ossicles. Allen and Fernandez (1960) argue that loss in bone conduction due to stapes fixation is a result of an increase in the impedance mismatch between the bone and cochlear fluid boundary. Based upon mathematical calculation, Groen (1962) determined that the air volume in the middle ear has a resonant point around 2500 Hz. He reasoned that stapes fixation would eliminate that portion of the effect which influences the inner ear while maintaining the smaller effect which acts upon the round window.

In a more recent contribution to bone-conduction theory, Tonndorf (1966) explains and demonstrates that it is essentially the missing ossicular inertial component which determines the frequency value of the maximal loss by bone conduction due to stapedial fixation. He suggests that the middle ear contribution is not confined to low frequencies as classical theory suggests. Rather, the ossicular vibrating system has a resonant frequency which varies from species to species. When responding to vibratory stimulation, the resonant frequency of the ossicular chain in man is found at 1500–2000 Hz. If the participation of the ossicular chain is eliminated or reduced due to stapedial fixation, the maximal bone-conduction loss should also correspond closely to this frequency area.

Other types of middle ear impairment which influence bone-conduction thresholds have been reported among clinical cases. Békésy (1939) and Tonndorf (1966) have each described a case in which bone-conduction thresholds were altered following radical mastoidectomy. Reduction in hearing by bone conduction was noted especially in the frequencies around 2000 Hz, the frequency area of ossicular resonance in man. Goodhill (1966) reported a Carhart-type notch extending into the higher frequencies for a patient with surgically confirmed malleal fixation. Subsequently, a patient with surgically confirmed malleal fixation was reported by Dirks and Malmquist (1969). The bone-conduction thresholds obtained at the mastoid process were severely depressed in the higher frequencies for this patient. Following operation the air-bone conduction thresholds improved by amounts substantially greater than predicted from the mastoid bone-conduction thresholds.

Hulka (1941) described a gain in the low and a loss in the high-frequency areas by bone conduction for patients with otitis media. Palva and Ojala (1955), however, did not find a shift in bone-conduction threshold in similarly diagnosed cases. Naunton and Fernandez (1961) reported results of bone-conduction tests at the frontal bone for three individuals during and following attacks of bilateral secretory otitis. When fluid was present in the middle ears of these patients, there was an improvement in bone-conduction responses at the low frequencies and a slight loss in the high frequencies. Huizing (1964) has also reported bone-conduction threshold changes in patients with otitis media, tubo-tympanitis, and chronic inflammatory processes.

Carhart (1962) reported the composite audiogram of patients with a hearing loss from chronic suppurative otitis media only (Figure 4). The bone-conduction curve was better than normal in the low frequencies but poorer than normal in high frequencies. Lierle and Reger (1946) also suggested that such configurations were not uncommon in middle ear disease. Dirks and Malmquist (1969) reported a notch in the bone-conduction curve around 2000 Hz for a group of 14 patients with otitis media. In summary, a wealth of carefully documented clinical cases have accumulated which illustrate that lesions of the middle ear may have substantial effect on bone-conduction thresholds.

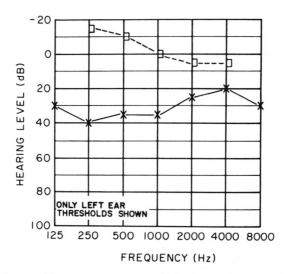

Fig. 4. Audiogram illustrates a case in which chronic suppurative otitis media in an ear free from sensorineural impairment has caused both a definite air conduction loss and a mechanical distortion of the bone-conduction threshold. The latter is clearly different from the distortion of the bone-conduction curve characteristic of stapes fixation. ×—×, air conduction; □---□, bone conduction. [After R. Carhart (1962) *In* "International Symposium: Otosclerosis." Little, Brown and Company, Boston, Massachusetts.]

B. Experimental Evidence

Bone-conduction responses have been altered experimentally in humans and animals as a result of various changes in the outer and middle ear. Four principal experimental procedures have been utilized in these experiments: (1) air pressure changes in the external auditory canal, (2) addition of a mass to the normal tympanic membrane, (3) fixation or elimination of various structures of the middle ear, and (4) occlusion of the external auditory canal.

1. Effect of Air-Pressure Changes

Producing a positive or negative change of air pressure in the external auditory canal causes a change in sensitivity for bone conduction as well as air conduction. Among the early investigations, Pohlman and Kranz (1926) and Békésy (1932) reported decreased auditory acuity in human subjects for air- and bone-conducted stimuli, especially in the low frequencies. Fowler (1920), Bárány (1938), Loch (1942), and Tarab (1958) found losses in low-frequency bone-conduction responses. In none of these studies, however, was the magnitude of the pressure change determined precisely. Clinical interest in this phenomenon has led to the so-called test of Gellé, the background of which has been described in detail by Huizing (1960).

Huizing (1960) conducted extensive experiments on the effect of air pressure change on bone-conduction thresholds. As in the earlier experiments, he observed a threshold loss for bone-conducted stimuli at frequencies lower than 4000 Hz with the greatest loss around 400 Hz. The threshold shift was greater for positive than negative pressure changes. In the experiment, a 500-Hz tone was shifted a maximum of 15 dB after a positive change of air pressure of 60–80 centimeters (60–80 cm) water.

2. Addition of a Mass to the Tympanic Membrane

Most investigators report improvements in bone-conduction responses after loading the eardrum with water, mercury, pieces of metal, or other materials (Abu-Jaudeh, 1964; Allen and Fernandez, 1960; Bárány, 1938; Brinkman et al., 1965; Kirikae, 1959; Legouix and Tarab, 1959; and Rytzner, 1954). Kirikae (1959) and Huizing (1960) have investigated changes in bone-conduction thresholds upon loading the tympanic membranes of normal listeners. In both experiments threshold gains for bone conduction averaging 20–25 decibels (20–25 dB) were observed for frequencies up to 1000 Hz. For higher frequencies, the gain diminished and no effect was seen above 1500–2000 Hz.

Tonndorf (1966) demonstrated that loading the tympanic membrane of cats caused the resonant frequency of the ossicular system to shift to a frequency lower than the normal resonant frequency. Thus, the bone conduction responses were elevated at frequencies below this resonant point.

3. ALTERATION OR ELIMINATION OF MIDDLE-EAR STRUCTURES

Changes in the amplitude and phase of cochlear microphonic responses to bone-conducted signals have been observed in animals following various alterations in the middle-ear structures. Special interest has been focused on results after stapes fixation, immobilization of the tympanic membrane, the total or partial elimination of the ossicular chain, and blockage of the oval window, round window, or both.

Smith (1943) fixated the stapes in cats by means of a thread attached to one stapedial crus. Essentially, no mass was added to the stapes by this method, although the fixation was probably not very firm. The results indicated a reduction in the bone-conduction response, especially in the frequency range around 500–1000 Hz. In other experiments of stapes fixation, amplitude losses centering around 500 Hz were reported by Tonndorf and Tabor (1962) and Tonndorf (1966). The magnitude of the loss depended on the degree of fixation.

Tonndorf further demonstrated elevation in the bone-conduction responses in various species of animals following removal of the middle-ear structures or immobilization of the tympanic membrane. In these instances, the loss was due to the total or partial elimination of the ossicular inertial component, and the frequency value of maximal loss was indicative of the ossicular resonant frequency characteristics of the particular animal species examined. A detailed explanation of the reduction in bone-conduction sensitivity following stapes fixation or immobilization of the ossicular chain has been discussed in the previous section on clinical observations.

Tonndorf has also reported changes in bone-conduction responses (as determined from changes in the amplitude and phase of cochlear microphonics) following certain alterations of the middle-ear system, such as disarticulation of the incudostapedial joint, severance of the stapedial tendon, removal of the stapes superstructure, stapedectomy, occlusion of the oval or round window, and stapes fixation. Among seven specific components which Tonndorf identified as contributing to the total bone conduction response, four (middle-ear inertia, middle-ear cavity compliance, round-window and oval-window pressure release) were directly related to the participation of the middle ear.

A diversity of opinion has existed concerning the effect of closure of the round window. Tonndorf and Tabor (1962) reported that of 25 publications reviewed, 12 authors found that closure of the round window caused the cochlear responses to alternating current signals to diminish; nine reported an improvement, and four found no change. The effects of the simultaneous closure of both windows were open to conjecture. Some authors felt that the complete blockage of both windows would impair the bone-conduction response severely because of the resultant elimination of the ossicular inertial response. Ranke (1958) suggested that the loss might be minimal since the two aqueducts and the vascular channels might have the effect of a "third window." Groen and Hoagland (1958) concluded that the cochlear aqueduct would impair high frequency more than lower frequency transmission because its frictional resistance would increase with frequency.

Subsequent experiments on the effects of window closure have been performed by Tonndorf and Tabor (1962) and Tonndorf (1966). In the latter experiment, amplitude losses averaging around 500 and 1000 Hz were observed following occlusion of the oval window. When the round window was blocked, the amplitude changes were smaller than for oval-window closure. The simultaneous blockage of both windows caused only slightly greater amplitude losses than were found when only one window was blocked. In another instance, blockage of both windows and the cochlear aqueduct produced losses of less than 10 dB for most frequencies.

These results leave one with the question of whether or not bone-conduction responses would persist if all cochlear outlets were closed. The answer to this question cannot be found in studies with experimental animals because of the impossible task of blocking all possible outlets. Tonndorf (1962), however, had performed earlier investigations with a cochlear model. Displacements of the cochlear partition occurred in the model in response to vibratory stimulation. The displacement was found to be due to distortional vibration so that the cochlear space was divided asymmetrically. This displacement was independent of any window release and solely dependent upon the differences in volume between the perilymphatic spaces. The investigator concluded that such distortional vibrations must occur, altering the space periodically. This is the basis of compression bone conduction.

4. Occlusion Effect

It is well known that when the external auditory meatus is occluded with the finger, an earphone, or a plug, an increase in the loudness of a bone-conducted signal occurs in a normal-hearing subject. This observation was originally described by Wheatstone in 1827 and constitutes one bone-conduction phenomenon which has received greater experimental attention than most others. Considerable clinical interest in this effect stems primarily from the observation by Bing (1891) that the occlusion effect is generally absent in patients with a conductive hearing loss but present in patients with a sensorineural impairment.

The effect produced by occluding the external auditory meatus consists of an improvement in low-frequency bone-conduction thresholds. Figure 5 shows the increase in loudness at threshold due to the occlusion of the external canal, according to Békésy (1939). Results of other investigators follow this same pattern of change in threshold. As a first approximation, the increase in threshold is inversely proportional to the frequency. The effect essentially disappears by 2000 Hz; however, some investigators (Huizing, 1960; Watson and Gales, 1943) reported reductions in threshold in the high-frequency regions.

The magnitude of the occlusion effect is related to the volume displacement of the cavity produced by the occluding device (Elpren and Naunton, 1963; Pholman and Kranz, 1926; Watson and Gales, 1943). However, this statement must be qualified by Zwislocki's observation (1953) that the effect may be virtually absent if the plug occludes the ear canal in the bony external meatus.

Although the magnitude of the occlusion effect has been described often, there have been relatively few acceptable explanations of the phenomenon. Rinné (1855) suggested that the effect could be explained on the basis of altered resonances in the external canal. Huizing (1960) supported this explanation based on more scientific information.

Mach (1864), in the so called *outflow theory*, reasoned that if an airborne sound could enter the cochlea via the middle ear structures, it could also leave the cochlea with equal ease. If an impairment of the middle ear occurred, less energy would escape the cochlea during bone-conduction stimulation and, thus, a larger amount of energy would

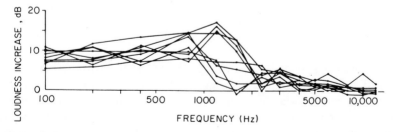

FIG. 5. Effects on loudness of closing the meatus with the finger. [From "Bone Conduction," by G. von Békésy, in *Experiments in Hearing* (E. G. Wever, ed.). Copyright 1960 by McGraw-Hill Book Company. Used with permission of McGraw-Hill Book Company.]

be utilized for reception by the cochlea. Allen and Fernandez (1960) were modern advocates of the "outflow theory."

Guild (1936) suggested that the occlusion effect was due to elimination of the airborne masking effects from ambient room noise. When the ear was covered, the ambient noise was reduced and the threshold increased. Subsequently (Huizing, 1960), the occlusion effect was found to persist even when the testing was performed in an anechoic chamber where the ambient noise level was below the masking threshold.

Békésy (1932) observed that when the skull is subject to vibrations, the lower jaw follows the displacement of the skull but moves with different amplitudes and phases since it is not directly connected with the other bones. During bone-conduction stimulation, the external auditory meatus is compressed because of the relative displacement produced by the walls of the external canal and the lagging jaw movement. When the ear canal is occluded, these resultant variations in air pressure in the canal occur and are transmitted to the cochlea via the eardrum and ossicular chain. In a later investigation, Békésy (1941) supported his concepts by the findings that a plug inserted deep in the osseous portion of the ear canal did not produce an improvement in the bone-conduction threshold.

In 1952, Franke *et al.* measured the phase relationships between the skull and lower jaw. They confirmed the importance to bone conduction of the movements of the jaw relative to the skull. Evidence contrary to Békésy's theory was presented by Allen and Fernandez (1960), who examined the occlusion effect on two patients with the lower jaw missing on one side. The occlusion effect was produced in these patients equally well in both ears.

Investigations by Goldstein and Hayes (1965), Huizing (1960), and Tonndorf (1966) have demonstrated that the occlusion effect is accompanied by an increase in the sound pressure level in the external auditory meatus. The sound pressure level in the canal was greater than the magnitude of the threshold shift due to the occluder; however, Goldstein and Hayes and Tonndorf observed a positive relationship between the two measures.

Tonndorf explains that the walls of the external meatus, when vibrating, radiate energy into the canal. Part of the energy is transmitted toward the cochlea via the middle ear. The ear canal when open constitutes a high-pass filter and, hence, when occluded, produces a low-frequency emphasis. The air contained in the external meatus creates a load on the tympanic membrane, and any changes in the length or occlusion of the canal alter this effect. Furthermore, Tonndorf reported that the relative movement between the jaw and the ear canal plays a role in the occlusion effect, although it is a minor one.

V. Physical Calibration of Bone-Conduction Testing Systems

A major problem in the measurement of bone-conduction thresholds has been the absence of a reliable and objective method for specifying the vibrational output of bone-conduction testing systems. Stable acoustic devices, such as the 2 cubic centimeter (2 cc) and 6-cc couplers, have been developed for calibration of air-conduction receivers, but no comparable instruments are available for bone vibrator calibration. Recently, the possibility for objective calibration of bone-conduction vibrators has been enhanced by the development of artificial mastoids, which are essentially immune to aging and can be manufactured within acceptable tolerance limits.

Prior to the present time, calibration of bone-conduction testing systems was performed by testing a group of normal listeners or individuals with sensorineural hearing loss, using a technique described by Carhart (1950) and Roach and Carhart (1956). The rationale for the method is based principally on the theory that air- and bone-conduction thresholds are essentially equivalent among persons with normal hearing or among patients with "pure" sensorineural losses. While this method of calibrating bone-conduction systems has been extremely valuable, variability of procedures and among listeners requires that either a large group of individuals be tested or that the measured thresholds be corrected by the amount that the air-conduction sensitivity of the group varies from audiometric zero.

Some of the difficulties encountered in using small groups of listeners for calibration purposes have been described by Wilber and Goodhill (1967). In some instances, calibration procedures have been performed with only a small number of normal listeners or by one individual with a so-called *golden ear*. As a result, values utilized for normal threshold by bone conduction have varied substantially among manufacturers, clinics, and laboratories.

In early attempts to develop an artificial mastoid, Hawley (1939), Carlisle and Mundel (1944), and Carlisle and Pearson (1951) used a viscoelastic pad to simulate the mechanical impedance of the skin and headbones. Since relatively little information concerning the impedance of the human mastoid was available at that time, these artificial mastoids represented only a first-order approximation to the human mastoid. The viscoelastic pads also varied with temperature and humidity and were susceptible to aging.

In 1955, Corliss and Koidan of the National Bureau of Standards developed a method for determining the resistive and reactive components of the impedance of the human head and mastoid. Similar data were also published by Dadson (1954), and Dadson et al. (1954) at

the National Physical Laboratory in England. These studies were a
first step leading to the design of equipment for the reliable and valid
calibration of bone vibrators.

Corliss and Koidan reported impedance parameters for the mastoid
and frontal bone under various conditions of driver size [12.5 and 20
millimeter (20 mm) diameters] and coupling force [500 and 1000 grams
(1000 gm)] over a frequency range from 40 to 10,000 Hz. In 1961,
Corliss *et al.* measured simultaneously on human subjects bone-conduction thresholds and the mechanical load presented to a driving tip 2
cm in diameter. The resultant thresholds were expressed in terms of
the least root-mean-square amplitude of the driving tip at threshold
(Figure 6), the displacement amplitude at threshold, and, by combining
the displacement amplitude and the impedance data, the least force
amplitude at threshold (Figure 7). The results in Figure 6 demonstrate
that the threshold displacement amplitude decreases with an increase
in frequency at the rate of approximately 12 dB per octave; thus, the
acceleration of the head at threshold is nearly independent of frequency.
The values of displacement amplitude at threshold for the forehead were
in general agreement with comparative results reported earlier by Watson
(1938) and Békésy (1932). The results (Figure 7) of the root-mean-
square force amplitude at threshold, in comparison with similar measurements by Békésy (1939), are also illustrated since so much of the recent
data have been reported in this manner.

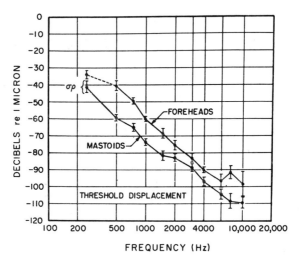

Fig. 6. Root-mean-square displacement amplitude of driving tip at threshold
of hearing, modal for 12 subjects. Bars indicate estimated standard deviations
of individual thresholds. [After Corliss *et al.* (1961), by permission of the publishers.]

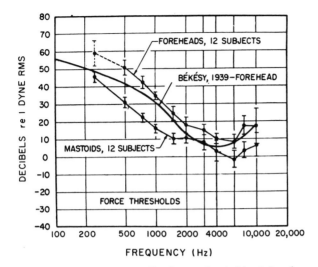

FREQUENCY (Hz)

FIG. 7. Root-mean-square force amplitude at threshold of hearing, median for 12 subjects. [After Corliss *et al.* (1961), by permission of the publishers.]

Two types of artificial mastoids have been used most frequently in recent investigations: the British artificial mastoid (British Standard 4009: 1966), which was based on data from the National Physical Laboratory; and the Beltone artificial mastoid (Weiss, 1960) which essentially incorporated impedance values reported by Corliss and Koidan (1955) of the National Bureau of Standards. The former has been used primarily in Great Britain and the latter in the United States.

The British artificial mastoid utilizes a viscoelastic pad which the developers indicate is relatively immune to aging and temperature. The Beltone artificial mastoid departs substantially from the earlier-designed artificial mastoids and uses an air-damping technique to simulate the mechanical impedance of the human mastoid. Figure 8 shows a cross-sectional view of this air-damped artificial mastoid developed by Weiss (1960). It consists of a central magnesium disk (m_1) supported by three

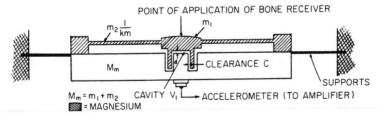

FIG. 8. Artificial mastoid construction. [After Weiss (1960), by permission of the author.]

flat magnesium springs (m_2). The central surface is flat. A plastic clip made especially for a particular type of vibrator is placed on this central surface. The plastic tip has three small projecting legs that position it securely to the central circular portion of the magnesium disk. The bone vibrator is then placed against the clip by means of a viscoelastic band across the back of the bone vibrator. The bottom portion of the central magnesium disk forms a cup which mates with a larger mass (M_m) and forms an acoustic network consisting of a cavity (V_1) and an air clearance (c). The viscous damping properties of a human mastoid are simulated by the behavior of the air in the cavity along with the clearance. The force acting on the mass (M_m) is measured by an accelerometer. The accelerometer converts the resultant acoustical vibrations to corresponding electrical signals. These signals, in turn, drive a cathode follower mounted at the base of the artificial mastoid. The output is then amplified and the result determined on a readout instrument such as a voltmeter.

The stability of the artificial mastoids developed here in the United States and in England has been determined by various investigators (Sanders and Olsen, 1964; Studebaker, 1967; Whittle, 1965; and Wilber and Goodhill, 1967). The general conclusion has been that the variability of bone-vibrator measurements made on the artificial mastoid is no larger than that observed with air-conduction receiver measurements utilizing 6-cc couplers.

Since the development of stable artificial mastoids, progress has been made toward the physical specification of the normal threshold of hearing by bone conduction. Careful study toward this goal has been undertaken on an international basis under the auspices of Technical Committee TC4 3/WG1 of the International Organization for Standardization (ISO). In 1966, an "international ring" comparison of bone-conduction threshold was instigated by this committee. The results of subjective determinations of thresholds in terms of mean excitation voltages were made for various commonly used bone vibrators. These results will afford the basic information necessary for the expression of threshold data in terms of response on an artificial mastoid. The two artificial mastoids described previously in this chapter have been considered for this purpose, and final results should appear shortly.

In 1964, the Hearing Aid Industry Conference (HAIC), through its standards committee, began to accumulate empirical results of bone-conduction thresholds for two bone vibrators commonly used in the United States. All threshold data were reported in force values obtained from calibrations performed at the front surface of the Beltone artificial mastoid. The purpose was to establish an interim norm that could be used by persons interested in bone-conduction measurements until an international standard was specified and accepted. Data from eight laboratories were used to establish the norm, and the averaged results were published by Lybarger (1966).

Figure 9 shows the HAIC threshold values when the vibrator is placed on the mastoid process. Suggested threshold values for forehead placement in a proposed American National Standard for an Artificial Head-Bone (1970) have also been included in the figure. The latter results were averaged from data on threshold differences between frontal and mastoid vibrator placements from 20 studies in which hearing-aid type vibrators were utilized. The results from Corliss *et al.* (1961) were also included in the averaged data. Further threshold data attesting to the usefulness of the HAIC norm are available in publications by Dirks *et al.* (1968), Olsen (1969), Sanders and Olsen (1964), Studebaker (1967), Weston *et al.* (1967), and Wilber and Goodhill (1967).

Robinson and Whittle (1967) in a report from the National Physical Laboratory have compared the HAIC interim threshold values to the thresholds obtained from the international ring comparison tests. The results of each group were expressed as equivalent force and acceleration values on the British artificial mastoid BS4009. The agreement between the equivalent force thresholds is surprisingly close. The authors speculate that the results may be real if one assumes that the equivalent force is independent of the artificial mastoid. When the data from both

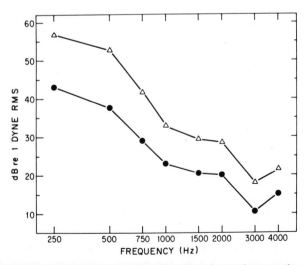

FIG. 9. Interim bone-conduction threshold calibration values at the mastoid and forehead positions, expressed in force values: decibels per 1 dyne rms. △—△, Frontal BC (ASNI, proposed); ●—●, mastoid (HAIC).

groups are expressed in equivalent threshold acceleration, the values differ, since the mechanical impedance of each artificial mastoid is not exactly the same.

In summary, the physical standardization of bone-conduction thresholds is imminent. On an international basis there are still some problems related partly to differences in the mechanical impedances of the two artificial mastoids being considered for the physical expression of the threshold data. There are also other unanswered questions raised by Dirks *et al.* (1968) and Studebaker (1967) regarding the effects of headbands, the problems of transferring the normal reference from one vibrator to another, and the appropriate application force. Further investigations in these areas may lead to modifications or additions to the currently proposed standard or to subsequent revisions in the accepted standard. During this period prior to the end of the international deliberation, it is recommended that the HAIC interim standard be utilized.

VI. Equipment and Procedure Variables

A. Bone-Conduction Vibrators

Two types of electromechanical vibrators have been utilized most often for the measurement of bone-conduction thresholds. The first is a somewhat heavy and cumbersome vibrator which was originally held by the patient or the tester's hand against the skull. In order to reduce aerial sound, the bone vibrator was enclosed in a metal or plastic case surrounded by felt with only the vibrating rod exposed to the outside. A metal ring holding a pair of rubber rings was fastened to the outside of the case. When the vibrating rod was applied to the skull, the rubber rings also made contact with the head and formed an airtight juncture.

The second type of electromechanical vibrator is the more modern hearing-aid-type vibrator. It was developed primarily for use as a hearing aid; however, it has been employed clinically because it is relatively small, lightweight, and will remain in position since it is affixed to the skull via a headband.

The hearing-aid-type vibrator, unfortunately, has numerous deficiencies as a device for testing hearing. Some of these difficulties can be appreciated from illustrations of the physical output response of such vibrators on an artificial mastoid. Figure 10 shows the frequency response of a commonly used hearing-aid-type vibrator obtained by applying a constant voltage across the vibrator. The frequency response is understandably somewhat limited to the speech frequency range since the vibrator was designed as a hearing aid. The first mechanical resonance is found near 600 Hz, and below this, the output drops rapidly. Practi-

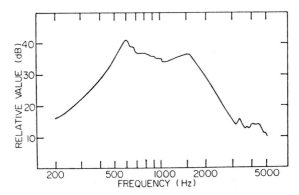

FIG. 10. Frequency response curve for the Radioear B-70-A vibrator. [After Dirks, Malmquist, and Bower (1968), by permission of the publishers.]

cally, this causes mechanical amplifications of any second harmonic component of 250 Hz, a frequency often chosen for clinical measurement. As a result, the second harmonic at 500 Hz may be amplified and nearly equal the output of the fundamental. Such waveform distortion has been measured and reported by Sanders and Olsen (1964), Weiss (1960), and Wilber and Goodhill (1967). The problem can be modified, but in doing so, the size and weight of the vibrator may have to be increased.

Above 1500 Hz the response of the vibrator again falls abruptly. It should be added here that the older and larger electromechanical units have a wider low-frequency response range with considerably less harmonic distortion than the hearing-aid-type vibrators. The output at the higher frequencies of 2000 and 4000 Hz, however, is greater for the available hearing-aid-type vibrators than for some of the older electromechanical units.

Another practical problem with the hearing-aid vibrator is that the entire case vibrates. As a result, there is always the possibility that some part of the vibrator, when located on the mastoid, might touch the pinna and set up vibrations in the external canal (Bárány, 1938) resulting in air-conducted transmission. In addition, the headband, even though damped somewhat by the contact with the head, causes the resonance peaks to shift and may even create new resonances. Weiss (1960) has demonstrated this difficulty.

The commonly used hearing-aid-type vibrator is, no doubt, more convenient to use than the older grenade-shaped bone receivers with a vibrating rod. However, the convenience may not outweigh the loss of certain desirable physical features of the older devices. The proposed ISO recommendations on bone vibrators suggest a vibrating tip with a plane circular face area of 1.75 square centimeters (1.75 cm²). Other physical changes in bone vibrators are desirable and provide a much-needed area for research and development.

B. Vibrator Placement

Traditionally, clinical bone-conduction measurements have been performed with the vibrator or the tuning fork located on the mastoid process. The preference for this site on the skull was perhaps based on the erroneous assumption that the ear under examination could be tested more or less independently of the nontest ear. Unfortunately, there is little, if any, interaural isolation by bone conduction and, hence, both cochleas may participate in the response.

Although the vertex (Bárány, 1938; Studebaker, 1962) of the skull and the teeth have been considered, the mastoid process and frontal bone have received the most attention as sites of placement. Of these two, the frontal bone has three major advantages.

First, it has been suggested that there is an increase in the test–retest reliability of bone-conduction measurements at the frontal bone. These observations were based originally on the report by Békésy (1932) that the displacement of the vibrator away from the middle of the forehead gives rise only to relatively small fluctuations in bone-conduction thresholds, whereas similar variations in placement at the mastoid process result in changes of 10 dB or more. Results by Hart and Naunton (1961) seemed to verify this observation. The comparative results of more recent investigations (Dirks, 1964; Studebaker, 1962) using hearing-aid-type vibrators with large contact areas have not demonstrated test-retest differences between mastoid and frontal bone placement that were of great practical advantage. It may be noteworthy that the observations of Békésy and Hart and Naunton were made with vibrators containing vibrating tips which covered only a small contact area.

The second advantage favoring frontal bone· placement is concerned with intersubject variability. At the frontal bone, the tissues seem to be more homogeneous over the general test area than at the mastoid process and, thus, the difference in bone-conduction thresholds among individuals should be reduced. The results of Dirks (1964) and Studebaker (1962) seem to verify this contention. The difference in intersubject variability between the two sites, however, was small.

A third advantage of forehead placement was evolved primarily from the classical investigation by Bárány in 1938. He suggested that bone-conduction tests at the frontal bone reduce the participation of the middle ear more effectively than those performed at the mastoid process. Experimental results by Link and Zwislocki (1951), Dirks and Malmquist (1969), and Studebaker (1962) on individuals with middle-ear impairments have demonstrated less hearing loss from measurements at the frontal bone than at the mastoid process. It is important to remember that in these investigations the hearing loss for subjects with middle-ear impairment is based upon normative data gathered on normal listeners at each test position. This was necessary since it requires more intensity to reach threshold at the frontal bone than at the mastoid, even on normal listeners. Although the average threshold differences were only 5 dB for the total group in the Dirks and Malmquist study, selected results suggest that in some instances this difference in threshold may be much larger. The types of physical changes which produce these large differences in threshold between the mastoid and frontal placements require investigation.

The principal disadvantage to testing bone-conduction thresholds at the frontal bone is that more intensity is required to reach threshold than for comparable mastoid measurements. The decibel differences between thresholds at the frontal bone and those at the mastoid process from various investigations are summarized in Table I. The comparisons are of current clinical interest since commercially available hearing-aid-type bone vibrators were employed in each experiment.

While the difference in thresholds at the two locations averaged approximately 10 dB, the results from six investigations cited in Table I indicate that the difference appears to be greater in the lower frequencies. These investigations were chosen since hearing-aid-type vibrators were used in each experiment. Since more energy is required to reach threshold at the frontal bone than at the mastoid process, the range of measurable hearing is reduced when testing at the frontal bone because of the power handling limitations of commercially available vibrators. This becomes a practical problem when testing patients whose bone-conduction thresholds are more than moderately reduced from normal. Except for these latter conditions, it would seem advisable to perform bone-conduction tests at the frontal bone. More clinical research would be helpful in this area.

C. Vibrator Application Force

Another source of variability in bone-conduction measurement is the force of application of the bone vibrator on the skull. In general, as vibrator application force is increased, less energy is required to reach threshold by bone conduction. There are, however, certain limitations and modifications to this general principle. Békésy (1939) and Konig (1955) investigated the variation of bone-conduction thresholds over a wide range of static forces. Their findings suggest that the largest changes in bone-conduction thresholds are observed at forces below 750 grams (750 gm). While some changes could still be observed between 1000 and 1500 gm in Konig's results, they were small. Konig suggested

TABLE I

DIFFERENCES (IN dB) BETWEEN THE MEAN THRESHOLDS MEASURED AT THE FOREHEAD AND THE MASTOID FOR SIX INVESTIGATORS IN WHICH HEARING-AID-TYPE VIBRATORS WERE USED

Investigation	Vibrator	N	Static force (gm)	Masking	Frequency (Hz)				
					250	500	1000	2000	4000
(1) Studebaker (1962)	Sonotone B-9	20	300–400	Narrow bands	15.2	16.0	10.0	12.9	9.7
(2) Dirks (1964) (Aver. of 2 studies)	Sonotone B-9	24	300–400	Narrow and wide bands	10.0	9.4	6.1	8.7	5.2
(3) Whittle (1965)	BV 11	22	350	Narrow bands	14.5	17.1	11.9	5.1	−3.0
(4) Weston et al. (1967)	Radioear B-70-A	10	400–600	Narrow bands	16.7	15.2	3.9	7.0	6.9
(5) Studebaker (1967)	Radioear B-70-A	132	300–500	White noise	13.4	16.6	12.0	10.0	8.6
(6) Dirks et al. (1968) (Aver. of 8 studies)	Radioear B-70-A	83	Varied by study	Narrow bands	14.9	13.4	10.6	13.5	7.7
				Mean [(1)–(6)]:	14.6	14.3	9.2	9.5	5.5

that it would be desirable to employ a coupling force of approximately 1000 gm in clinical audiometry so that variability would be minimal.

Harris *et al.* (1953) investigated the effects of increased application force from 100 to 500 gm at the test frequencies of 250, 1000, and 8000 Hz. The greatest change in threshold was found at 250 Hz, while little change was observed at 1000 and 8000 Hz. The authors suggested that bone-conduction receiver application force be standardized somewhere between 200 and 400 gm. In the ranges of application force where Harris *et al.* and Konig's results overlap, the results from the two experiments do not agree. In the former study the results suggest that once 400 gm is reached, thresholds for bone conduction did not change, whereas, in the latter investigation, threshold continued to change up to an application force of 1000 gm. Goodhill and Holcomb (1955), Nilo (1968), Watson (1938), and Whittle (1965) have made other contributions concerning the role of force in measuring bone conduction.

Some discrepancies concerning the role of application force are also evident in the results on measurements of the mechanical impedance of the head. Dadson (1954) observed changes in mechanical impedance by varying the force of application. Corliss and Koidan (1955), however, reported similar impedance values at coupling forces from 500 to 1000 gm. Whether or not the differences are due to the smaller number of subjects used in the latter experiments has been unresolved.

Most experimenters have observed a ceiling or limit to the magnitude of force evoking threshold variations. The evidence, however, varies on this point, and the ceiling has been placed anywhere from 400 to 1000 gm. There is a need to clarify the divergences in these results.

In the proposed international standards for bone-conduction thresholds, the suggested application force will be approximately 550 gm for a bone vibrator with a plane circular face area of 1.75 cm². Commercially available headbands exert a force of approximately 300–400 gm when the vibrator is placed on the mastoid process of adult subjects (Dirks, 1964; Studebaker, 1962). The size of the head and the tautness of the band primarily determine the application of force on a particular head. Clinically, a more flexible headband or helmet arrangement than is now used will be necessary.

VII. Masking

A. Conventional Masking

When commercially available earphones encased in the supraaural cushions are used for air-conduction measurements, the mass of the head provides an average interaural attenuation factor of approximately 40 or 50 dB. Unfortunately for bone-conduction measurements, the inter-aural attenuation factor is almost negligible regardless of the position of the vibrator on the skull. Hence, it is necessary to exclude the nontest ear by an adequate air-conducted masker when obtaining bone-conduction thresholds. There are instances, such as bilaterally symmetrical sensorineural losses, when masking may not always be necessary (Naunton, 1963), but these cases should be the exception and not the general rule. Studebaker (1963) suggests that a more efficient rule may be to apply a masker to the nontest ear whenever an airbone gap appears. Suffice it to mention in this chapter that the least complex but most accurate method for masking in bone-conduction testing has been detailed by Hood (1962). Studebaker (1967) also describes a method of masking similar to the procedure suggested by Hood. The specific procedure for masking when testing for bone-conduction thresholds will be described in detail in Chapter 4.

The common clinical problem of the unavailability of sufficient masking in the nontest ear is at least partially alleviated by the use of narrow-band masking. Although masking may theoretically be accomplished by almost any sound, it is generally accepted that narrow bands of noise centered around the test frequency provide the greatest shift in the nontest ear threshold with a minimum of sound energy (Denes and Naunton, 1952; Fletcher, 1940; Hood, 1957, 1962; Konig, 1963; Liden et al., 1959; Sanders and Rintelman, 1964; Studebaker, 1963; and Zwislocki, 1951).

The results of Littler et al. (1952), Studebaker (1962), and Zwislocki (1953) have demonstrated that the interaural attenuation factor can be increased as the area of head exposed to the transducer is decreased. This may be accomplished by introducing the masking signal via an insert receiver rather than by the standard earphone encased in either a supraaural or circumaural cushion and thus reducing the risk of cross masking. There are still some calibration problems associated with the use of insert receivers and their coupling to the ear. Nevertheless, the introduction of narrow bands of noise delivered to the nontest ear via an insert receiver should be potentially desirable when measuring bone-conduction thresholds.

B. The Rainville Technique and Its Modification

The problems of masking the nontest ear when obtaining bone-conduction threshold have led many clinicians to view the results with some uncertainty. In 1955, Rainville described a method of evaluating the status of the sensorineural system that reportedly circumvented some of the traditional problems of calibration and masking. In this method, the differential effect of air-conduction and bone-conduction masking of air-conducted pure tones was used to estimate sensorineural acuity. The original procedure described by Rainville (1955) was somewhat cumbersome, so modified procedures were devised by Jerger and Tillman (1960) and Lightfoot (1960). The Jerger and Tillman modification of the Rainville approach was called the sensorineural acuity level (SAL) test and has received considerable attention.

The SAL test is carried out by measuring the air-conduction threshold first in quiet and then in the presence of a fixed level of bone-conducted noise. The difference, in decibels, between these two measurements is then subtracted from the shift produced by the noise in normal ears which form the criterion group. The resultant totals are the estimate of sensorineural hearing loss.

Jerger and Tillman (1960) suggested two advantages of the SAL technique over conventional bone-conduction audiometry. First, the instrumentation can be easily calibrated on normal ears and, second, the same high level of masking is used in every instance. The latter of these advantages is of great practical interest to most clinicians since the question of how much masking should be used does not arise. The advantage of ease of calibration has possibly diminished due to the advent of the physical calibration of bone-conduction vibrator systems with a reliable artificial mastoid.

Serious concerns as to the validity of the SAL test as a method for quantifying sensorineural acuity have been raised by Goldstein *et al.* (1962), Martin and Bailey (1964), Naunton and Fernandez (1961), and Tillman (1963). One problem is that SAL norms are of necessity collected on normal listeners with both ears occluded, whereas bone-conduction norms and measurements are usually obtained with the test ear open. By occluding the ears of the criterion group with earphones, the sensitivity of this group is increased by the amount of the occlusion effect. In the conductive loss, however, no occlusion effect is observed and, thus, such an individual, even if his sensorineural acuity were normal, would experience less than a normal threshold shift. Dirks and Malmquist (1969), Goldstein *et al.* (1962), and Tillman (1963) have reported such findings in groups with conductive losses. The problem is exemplified in Figure 11 which shows SAL results together with other bone-conduction measurements from the Dirks and Malmquist study. Notice that SAL thresholds parallel frontal bone-conduction thresholds when the latter are obtained with the test ear occluded but are reduced by the amount of the occlusion effect when compared to open ear mastoid and frontal bone conduction thresholds. Jerger and Jerger (1965) observed that bone conduction and SAL thresholds agreed if the air-conducted signal for the SAL test was delivered via Pederson earphones, which, in general, produce no occlusion effect.

Data supplied by Tillman (1967) in Figure 12 demonstrate a second problem associated with the SAL measurements. The results in the figure show the mean hearing levels for air conduction, bone conduction, and SAL for a group of 20 subjects with pure sensorineural impairments. Notice the relatively good agreement between air- and bone-conduction thresholds while the SAL results underestimate the sensorineural acuity by 5 to 15 dB in the high test frequencies. These observations were reported recently by Tillman and Gretis (1969) but the explanation has not been fully determined. Jerger and Jerger (1965) did not observe this discrepancy on a group of ten individuals with sensorineural loss. They found that on one subject, an overshift on the SAL test was reduced by reinstructing the individual and repeating the test. Since the original findings of Tillman have been repeated, this latter explanation of the overshift does not seem sufficient. If the problems associated with the occlusion effect and overshift in the high test frequencies can be eliminated, the SAL procedure should be potentially a very useful measure of sensorineural acuity.

There are numerous instances in which masking problems leave the clinician in doubt concerning the exact sensorineural acuity level. In these cases the SAL test results may offer helpful information in assuring

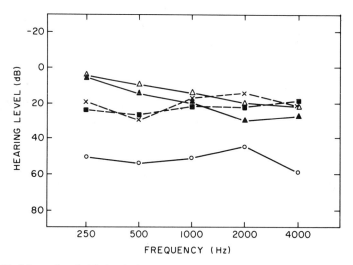

FIG. 11. Mean thresholds in decibels re: hearing level of 60 cases with conductive hearing loss for 5 frequencies and conditions. ○—○, AC; ▲—▲, BCM; △—△, BC Fu; ■--■, BC Fo; ×--×, SAL. Conductive $N = 60$. [After Dirks and Malmquist (1969), by permission of the publishers.]

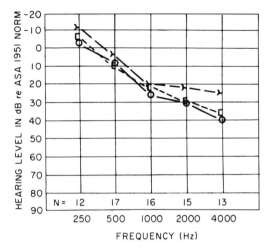

Fig. 12. Mean hearing levels by air conduction, bone conduction, and SAL for subjects with pure sensorineural hearing impairments. ◯—◯, A/C; [-- [, B/C;)— —), SAL. [After Tillman (1967).]

the diagnostician of the presence or absence of a conductive component. In this regard, the current author heartily agrees with Tillman (1967) that considering the limitations of bone-conduction audiometry in patients with conductive loss, other qualitative methods such as the SAL test must often be used to supplement the results of bone-conduction tests. For determining the presence or absence of a conductive component, the SAL test, the occlusion test, the Weber test, and the measurement of relative impedance (Jepsen, 1963) may be useful. For more precise differential diagnostic information of the type of middle ear impairment, the measurement of absolute impedance (Feldman, 1964) is most informative. The combined effects of several of these procedures together with frontal and/or mastoid bone conduction audiometry should provide a more thorough assessment of the hearing loss, especially when routine evaluation leaves the precise diagnosis in doubt.

VIII. Summary

The theoretical and clinical aspects of bone conduction have often been viewed with skepticism and justifiable concern. While our understanding of the mechanism of bone conduction remains incomplete and the clinical utility of its measurement is beset with limitations, certain very positive and productive steps have been taken during the past 5 years to solve some of these problems. Three examples deserve special mention. First, the *Revised Theory of Bone Conduction* reported by Tonndorf (1966) has introduced valuable new concepts substantiated by elaborate experimental results in addition to quantitative support for older, still valid, concepts underlying the phenomenon of bone conduction. Second, the advent of a reliable artificial mastoid has provided the investigator and clinician with the major instrument necessary for specifying the vibrational output of bone-conduction testing systems. Third, and closely related to the development of the artificial mastoid, the deliberations and experiments carried out on an international and national basis have resulted in the HAIC Interim Standard for Bone Conduction, the USA Standard for an Artificial Head-Bone, and a proposed ISO standard. These important documents have already formed the basis for the standardization and calibration of bone-conduction testing systems. We generally dwell on the limitations and problems involved in bone-conduction measurements, and so it is gratifying to end this chapter in a more positive way by recognizing three important recent contributions which have enhanced our understanding and utilization of the complex phenomenon of bone conduction.

References

Abu-Jaudeh, C. N. (1964). The effect of simultaneous loading of the tympanic membrane of the external auditory canal on bone conduction sensitivity of the normal ear. *Ann. Otol. Rhinol. Laryngol.* **73**, 934–947.

Allen, G. W., and Fernandez, C. (1960). The mechanism of bone conduction. *Ann. Otol. Rhinol. Laryngol.* **69**, 5–29.

American National Standard for an Artificial Head-Bone (proposed). Personal communication from S. F. Lybarger (1970).

Bárány, E. (1938). A contribution to the physiology of bone conduction. *Acta Oto-Laryngol. Suppl.* **26**.

von Békésy, G. (1932). Zur Theorie des Hörens bei der Schallaufnahme durch Knochenleitung. *Ann. Phys.* **13**, 111–136.

von Békésy, G. (1939). Über die Piezoelectrische Messung der absoluten Hörschwelle bei Knochenleitung. *Akust. Z.* **4**, 113–125.

von Békésy, G. (1941). Über die Schallausbreitung bei, Knochenleitung. *Z. Hals-, Nasen-, Ohrenheilk.* **47**, 430–442.

von Békésy, G. (1949). The structure of the middle ear and the hearing of one's own voice by bone conduction. *J. Acoust. Soc. Amer.* **21**, 217–232.

von Békésy, G. (1960). Bone conduction. In "Experiments in Hearing" (E. G. Wever, ed.), Ch. 6. McGraw-Hill, New York.

von Békésy, G., and Rosenblith, Walter A. (1951). The mechanical properties of the ear. In "Handbook of Experimental Psychology" (S. S. Steven, ed.), Ch. 27. Wiley, New York.

Bing, A. (1891). Ein neuer Stimmgabelversuch. Beitrag zur differential-diagnostik der Kranheiten des mechanischen Schalleitungs-und Nervosen Hörapparates. *Wien. Med. Blätter* **41**.

Brinkman, W. F. B., Marres, E. H. A. M., and Tolk, J. (1965). The mechanism of bone conduction. *Acta Oto-Laryngol.* **59**, 109–115.

British Standard 4009 (1966). An artificial mastoid for the calibration of bone vibrators. British Standards Inst., British Standards House, London.

Carhart, R. (1950). Clinical application of bone conduction. *Arch. Otolaryngol.* **51**, 798–807.

Carhart, R. (1962). Effect of stapes fixation on bone conduction response. *In* "Int. Symp. Otosclerosis" (H. F. Schuknect, ed.), Ch. 13. Little, Brown, Boston, Massachusetts.

Carlisle, R. W., and Mundel, A. B. (1944). Practical hearing aid measurements. *J. Acoust. Soc. Amer.* **16**, 45–51.

Carlisle, R. W., and Pearson, H. A. (1951). Stain-gauge type artificial mastoid. *J. Acoust. Soc. Amer.* **23**, 300–302.

Corliss, E. L. R., and Koidan, W. (1955). Mechanical impedance of the forehead and mastoid. *J. Acoust. Soc. Amer.* **27**, 1164–1172.

Corliss, E. L. R., Smith, E. L., and Magruder, J. O. (1961). Hearing by bone conduction. *In* "Proc. 3rd. Int. Congr. Acoust." (L. Cremer, ed.), Vol. 1, pp. 53–55. Elsevier, London.

Dadson, R. S. (1954). The normal threshold of hearing and other aspect of standardisation in audiometry. *Acustica* **4**, 151–154.

Dadson, R. S., Robinson, D. W., and Greig, R. G. P. (1954). The mechanical impedance of the human mastoid process. *Brit. J. Appl. Phys.* **5**, 435–442.

Denes, P., and Naunton, R. F. (1952). Masking in pure-tone audiometry. *Proc. Roy. Soc. Med.* **45**, 790–794.

Dirks, D. D. (1964). Factors related to bone conduction reliability. *Arch. Otolaryngol.* **79**, 551–558.

Dirks, D. D., and Malmquist, C. (1969). Comparison of frontal and mastoid bone-conduction thresholds in various conduction lesions. *J. Speech Hearing Res.* **12**, 725–746.

Dirks, D., Malmquist, C., and Bower, D. (1968). Toward the specification of normal bone conduction threshold. *J. Acoust. Soc. Amer.* **43**, 1237–1242.

Elpern, B. S., and Naunton, R. F. (1963). The stability of the occlusion effect. *Arch. Otolaryngol.* **77**, 376–384.

Feldman, A. S. (1964). Acoustic impedance measurements as a clinical procedure. *Int. Audiol.* **3**, 156–166.

Fletcher, H. (1940). Auditory patterns. *Rev. Mod. Phys.* **12**, 47–65.

Fournier, J. E. (1954). The false-Bing phenomenon—some remarks on the theory of bone conduction. *Laryngoscope* **64**, 29–34.

Fowler, E. P., Sr. (1920). Drum tension and middle ear pressure, their determination, significance and effect upon the hearing. *Ann. Otol. Rhinol. Laryngol.* **29**, 688–694.

Franke, E. K., von Gierke, H. E., Grossman, F. M., and von Wittern, W. W. (1952). The jaw motions relative to the skull and the influence on hearing by bone conduction. *J. Acoust. Soc. Amer.* **24**, 142–146.

Goldstein, R., and Hayes, C. (1965). The occlusion effect in bone conduction hearing. *J. Speech Hearing Res.* **8**, 137–148.

Goldstein, D. P., Hayes, C. S., and Peterson, J. L. (1962). A comparison of bone conduction thresholds by conventional and Rainville methods. *J. Speech Hearing Res.* **5**, 244–255.

Goodhill, V. (1966). The fixed malleus syndrome. *Trans. Amer. Acad. Ophthalmol. Otolaryngol.* **70**, 370–380.

Goodhill, V., and Holcomb, A. L. (1955). Cochlear potentials in the evaluation of bone conduction. *Ann. Otol. Rhinol. Laryngol.* **64,** 1213–1234.

Groen, J. J. (1962). The value of the Weber test. *In* "Int. Symp. Otosclerosis" (H. F. Schuknecht, ed.), Ch. 14. Little, Brown, Boston, Massachusetts.

Groen, J. J., and Hoagland, G. A. (1958). Bone conduction and otosclerosis of the round window. *Acta Oto-Laryngol.* **49,** 206–212.

Guild, S. R. (1936). Hearing by bone conduction: The pathways of transmission of sound. *Ann. Otol. Rhinol. Laryngol.* **45,** 736–754.

Harris, J. D., Haines, H. L., and Myers, C. K. (1953). A helmet-held bone conduction vibrator. *Laryngoscope* **63,** 998–1007.

Hart, C., and Naunton, R. F. (1961). Frontal bone conduction tests in clinical audiometry. *Laryngoscope* **71,** 24–29.

Hawley, M. S. (1939). Artificial mastoid for audiphone measurements. *Bell Lab Rec.* **18**(3), 73–75.

Herzog, H., and Krainz, W. (1926). Das kochenleitungsproblem. *Z. Hals-Nasen-Ohren Heilk.* **15,** 300–306.

Hirsh, I. J. (1952). "The Measurement of Hearing." McGraw-Hill, New York.

Hood, J. D. (1957). The principles and practice of bone conduction audiometry; a review of the present position. *Proc. Roy. Soc. Med.* **50,** 689–697.

Hood, J. D. (1962). Bone conduction: A review of the present position with especial reference to the contributions of Dr. Georg von Békésy. *J. Acoust. Soc. Amer.* **24,** 1325–1332.

Huizing, E. H. (1960). Bone conduction—the influence of the middle ear. *Acta Oto-Laryngol. Suppl.* **155.**

Huizing, E. H. (1964). Bone conduction loss due to middle ear pathology pseudoperceptive deafness. *Int. Audiol.* **3,** 89–98.

Hulka, J. (1941). Bone conduction changes in acute otitis media. *Arch. Otolaryngol.* **33,** 333–346.

Jepsen, O. (1963). Middle-ear muscle reflexes in man. *In* "Modern Developments in Audiology" (J. Jerger, ed.), Ch. 6. Academic Press, New York.

Jerger, J., and Jerger, S. (1965). Critical evaluation of SAL audiometry. *J. Speech Hearing Res.* **8,** 103–127.

Jerger, J., and Tillman, T. W. (1960). A new method for the clinical determination of sensorineural acuity level (SAL). *Arch. Otolaryngol.* **71,** 948–953.

Kirikae, I. (1959). An experimental study on the fundamental mechanism of bone conduction. *Acta Oto-Laryngol. Suppl.* **145.**

Kirikae, I. (1960). "The Structure and Function of the Middle Ear." Univ. of Tokyo Press, Tokyo, Japan.

Konig, E. (1955). Les variations de la conduction osseuse en fonction de la force de pression excerceé sur le vibrateur, 11 Congres, *Soc. Int. Audiol.,* Paris. [Cited after its English translation (1957) by the Beltone Institute for Hearing Research.]

Konig, E. (1963). The use of masking noise and its limitations in clinical audiometry. *Acta Oto-Laryngol. Suppl.* **180.**

Legouix, J. P., and Tarab, S. (1959). Experimental study of bone conduction in ears with mechanical impairment of the ossicles. *J. Acoust. Soc. Amer.* **31,** 1453–1457.

Lidén, G., Nilsson, G., and Anderson, H. (1959). Narrow band masking with white noise. *Acta Oto-Laryngol.* **50,** 116–124.

Lierle, D. M., and Reger, S. N. (1946). Correlations between bone and air conduction acuity measurements over wide frequency ranges in different types of hearing impairments. *Laryngoscope* **5**, 187–224.

Lightfoot, C. (1960). The M-R test of bone conduction. *Laryngoscope* **70**, 1552–1559.

Link, R., and Zwislocki, J. (1951). Audiometrische knochenleitungsundersuchungen. *Arch. Ohren-Nasen-Kehlkopfheilk.* **160**, 347–357.

Littler, T. S., Knight, J. J., and Strange, P. H. (1952). Hearing by bone conduction and the use of bone conduction hearing aids. *Proc. Roy. Soc. Med.* **45**, 783–790.

Loch, W. E. (1942). Effect of experimentally altered air pressure in the middle ear on hearing acuity in man. *Ann. Otol. Rhinol. Laryngol.* **51**, 995–1006.

Lowy, K. (1942). Cancellation of the electrical cochlear response with air-conducted and bone-conducted sound. *J. Acoust. Soc. Amer.* **14**, 156–158.

Lybarger, S. F. (1966). Special report—interim bone conduction thresholds for audiometry. *J. Speech Hearing Res.* **9**, 483–487.

Mach, E. (1864). Zur Theorie des Gehörorgans. *Akad. Wiss., Wien, Sitzungsher. Math.-Naturwiss. Kl.,* II. *Abth.,* **50**, 324.

Martin, F. N., and Bailey, H. A. T. (1964). Clinical comment on the sensorineural acuity level (SAL) test. *J. Speech Hearing Dis.* **29**, 326–329.

Naunton, R. F. (1963). The measurement of hearing by bone conduction. *In* "Modern Developments in Audiology" (J. F. Jerger, ed.), Ch. 1. Academic Press, New York.

Naunton, R. F., and Fernandez, C. (1961). Prolonged bone conduction: Observations on man and animals. *Laryngoscope* **71**, 306–318.

Nilo, E. R. (1968). The relation of vibrator surface area and static application force to the vibrator-to-head coupling. *J. Speech Hearing Res.* **11**, 805–810.

Olsen, W. O. (1969). Comparison of studies on bone conduction thresholds and the HAIC interim standard for bone conduction audiometry. *J. Speech Hearing Dis.* **34**, 54–57.

Palva, T., and Ojala, L. (1955). Middle ear conduction deafness and bone conduction. *Acta Oto-Laryng.* **45**, 135–142.

Pohlman, A. G., and Kranz, E. W. (1926). The influence of partial and complete occlusion of the external auditory canals on air and bone transmitted sound. *Ann. Otol. Rhinol. Laryngol.* **35**, 113–121.

Rainville, M. J. (1955). Nouvelle method d'assourdissement pour le reléve des courbes de conduction osseuse. *J. Fr. Otol-Rhino-Laryngol.* **4/8**, 851–858; also (1959). New method of masking for the determination of bone conduction curves. *Transl. Beltone Inst. Hearing Res.* No. 11.

Ranke, O. (1958). Die Schalleitung im Mittelohr im klinischer Sicht. *Z. Laryngol.* **37**, 366.

Rinné, F. H. (1855). Beiträge zur Physiologie des menschlichen Ohres. *Praegers Vierteljahresschr. Heilk.* **1**, 113.

Roach, R. E., and Carhart, R. (1956). A clinical method for calibrating the bone conduction audiometer. *Arch. Otolaryngol.* **63**, 270–279.

Robinson, D. W., and Whittle, L. S. (Oct. 1967). 2nd report on standardisation of the bone conduction threshold. NPL Aero Report AC 30, Teddington, Middlesex, England.

Rytzner, C. (1954). Sound transmission in clinical otosclerosis. *Acta Oto-Laryngol. Suppl.* **117**.

Sanders, J. W., and Olsen, W. O. (1964). An evolution of a new artificial mastoid as an instrument for the calibration of audiometer bone-conduction systems. *J. Speech Hearing Dis.* **29**, 247–263.

Sanders, J. W., and Rintelman, W. F. (1964). Masking in audiometry—a clinical evaluation of three methods. *Arch. Otolaryngol.* **80,** 541–556.

Smith, K. R. (1943). Bone conduction during experimental fixation of the stapes. *J. Exp. Psychol.* **33,** 96–107.

Studebaker, G. A. (1962). Placement of vibrator in bone-conduction testing. *J. Speech Hearing Res.* **5,** 321–331.

Studebaker, G. A. (1963). Clinical masking of air- and bone-conducted stimuli. *J. Speech Hearing Dis.* **29,** 23–35.

Studebaker, G. A. (1967). The standardization of bone-conduction thresholds. *Laryngoscope* **77,** 823–835.

Tarab, S. (1958). Le mécanisme de l'épreuve de Weber et les variations auditves en fonction de la pression d'air dans l'oreille externe et moyenne. *Rev. Laryngol. Otol. Rhinol.* **79,** 1223.

Tillman, T. W. (1963). Clinical applicability of the SAL test. *Arch. Otolaryngol.* **78,** 36–48.

Tillman, T. W. (1967). The assessment of sensorineural acuity. *In* "Sensorineural Hearing Processes and Disorders" (B. Graham, ed.), Ch. 17. Little, Brown, Boston, Massachusetts.

Tillman, T. W., and Gretis, E. S. (1969). Masking of tones by bone-conducted noise in normal and hearing-impaired listeners. *Abstr. Amer. Speech Hearing Assoc. Conv. Progr.* **79.**

Tonndorf, J. (1962). Compressional bone conduction in cochlear models. *J. Acoust. Soc. Amer.* **34,** 1127–1131.

Tonndorf, J. (1966). Bone conduction: Studies in experimental animals. *Acta Oto-Laryngol. Suppl.* **213.**

Tonndorf, J., and Tabor, J. R. (1962). Closure of the cochlear windows: Its effect upon air- and bone-conduction. *Ann. Otol. Rhinol. Laryngol.* **71,** 5–29.

Watson, N. A. (1938). Limits of audition for bone-conduction. *J. Acoust. Soc. Amer.* **9,** 294–300.

Watson, N. A., and Gales, R. S. (1943). Bone conduction threshold measurements: Effects of occlusion, enclosures, and masking devices. *J. Acoust. Soc. Amer.* **14,** 207–215.

Weiss, E. (1960). An air damped artificial mastoid. *J. Acoust. Soc. Amer.* **32,** 1582–1588.

Weston, P. B., Gengel, R. W., and Hirsh, I. J. (1967). Effects of vibrator types and their placement on bone-conduction threshold measurements. *J. Acoust. Soc. Amer.* **41,** 788–792.

Wever, E. G., and Lawrence, M. (1954). "Physiological Acoustics." Princeton Univ. Press, Princeton, New Jersey.

Wheatstone, C. (1827). Experiments on audition. *Quart. J. Sci. Arts* **67.**

Whittle, L. S. (1965). A determination of the normal threshold of hearing by bone conduction. *J. Sound Vibration* **2,** 227–248.

Wilber, L. A., and Goodhill, V. (1967). Real ear versus artificial mastoid methods of calibration of bone-conduction vibrators. *J. Speech Hearing Res.* **10,** 405–417.

Zwislocki, J. (1951). Eine verbesserte vertäubungsmethode für die audiometrie. *Acta Oto-Laryngol.* **39,** 338–356.

Zwislocki, J. (1953). Acoustic attenuation between the ears. *J. Acoust. Soc. Amer.* **25,** 752–759.

Chapter 2

Speech Audiometry

TOM W. TILLMAN

WAYNE O. OLSEN

Northwestern University

I. Introduction

Pure-tone audiometry allows quantification of hearing threshold level as well as identification of configurational patterns. It thus enables the clinician to estimate the practical consequences of an individual's hearing impairment, but the validity of this estimate is subject to question. Since hearing is the primary communicational sense, a valid estimate of the practical consequences of hearing loss should utilize speech as the test stimulus. The desire to obtain this more valid measure led to the development of speech audiometry as a tool to supplement pure-tone techniques.

There are basically two aspects of speech audiometry which will be dealt with in this chapter. The first is the measurement of threshold sensitivity for the speech stimulus. This measure is analogous to the threshold in pure-tone audiometry and allows an estimate of the degree of hearing impairment. The second phase of speech audiometry involves the measurement of speech discrimination, that is, the ability of the listener to make fine distinctions among similar speech sounds at supra-threshold intensities. While an individual's ability to understand speech is influenced by his pure-tone threshold configuration, the former cannot always be predicted very accurately from the latter and it is this fact that makes speech audiometry an indispensable clinical tool.

II. History

The first speech audiometer (Western Electric 4-A, Fletcher, 1929) was employed as a group screening device as early as 1927. This apparatus, though historically important, does not appear to have been utilized clinically. Actually, other work of Fletcher and Steinberg (1929) and their associates at the Bell Telephone Laboratories more directly undergirds, but still predates, the clinical use of speech audiometry in the United States. These individuals were primarily concerned with the development and application of speech testing materials to be used in assessing the effectiveness of various electronic communications systems, including the telephone. From Fletcher's (1929) work emerged the concept of the articulation function which displays accuracy of speech perception (percent correct response) as a function of signal intensity. This curve allows the precise determination of the signal intensity corresponding to 50% correct response (threshold) and in addition it serves for speech audiometry a function similar to that served by the audiogram for pure tone audiometry. Thus, the development and application of the concept of the articulation function represents an important milestone in the development of speech audiometry.

Using the sentence material provided by the Bell Telephone Intelligibility Lists (Fletcher and Steinberg, 1929), Hughson and Thompson (1942) developed the monitored-live-voice technique for assessing threshold sensitivity for speech. With their technique and test materials, both of which were rather cumbersome, Hughson and Thompson described the basic relationships between threshold sensitivity for pure tone and speech stimuli. It was this work that first established the importance of threshold speech audiometry as a clinical tool.

During the early 1940s, Hudgins *et al.* (1947) at the Psycho-Acoustic Laboratory (PAL) at Harvard University developed a number of recorded speech tests, some of which employed lists of spondee words. Concurrently, at the same laboratory, Egan (1948) and others developed 50-word lists of monosyllables that, at least to a first approximation, incorporated the phonetic characteristics of American speech. During this same period the United States military services established aural rehabilitation centers, where the speech testing materials developed at the Harvard Psycho-Acoustic Laboratory were applied to a large clinical population of veterans with impaired hearing. At Deshon Hospital for example, Carhart (1946b) utilized both threshold and suprathreshold testing methods in both the initial evaluation of an individual's hearing impairment and in the subsequent selection of a hearing aid for the individual. Because the PAL PB-50 lists presumably embodied the phonetic balance of American speech, they possessed a high face validity as a clinical tool for assessing the everyday communicative efficiency of the individual and thus were a valued clinical tool in the rehabilitative centers. The methods developed in the military aural rehabilitation program were quickly adopted by clinical programs concerned with the civilian population having impaired hearing.

Thus, by the mid 1940s the basic techniques of speech audiometry had been established. On the one hand, speech audiometry employed spondee words that were very homogeneous in audibility for establishing threshold sensitivity for speech. On the other hand, monosyllabic words, highly heterogeneous in audibility but presumably embodying the appropriate phonetic balance, were used as a suprathreshold test of speech understanding. Basically, for the past 25 years, these procedures have continued to be employed clinically and the only major innovations introduced have been the refinement of testing materials for assessing speech discrimination and the application of speech audiometric procedures in the diagnosis of higher auditory pathway lesions. As will be seen, even the basic issue of the development of a standardized method for establishing the "threshold for speech" has not been addressed, although standards relating to characteristics of the speech audiometer and the testing materials for assessing threshold have been established. This chapter will concentrate on a description of current methods and materials for the measurement of threshold sensitivity and discrimination for speech as well as on the applications of these methods in the clinical setting.

III. Measurement of Threshold

A. Introduction

As just mentioned, Hughson and Thompson (1942) were the first investigators to measure the "speech reception threshold" and to define the relationships between speech and pure tone thresholds in persons with impaired hearing. They utilized the Bell Telephone Intelligibility Sentences to determine the minimum level at which a given listener could just understand the sentences. Several sentences were presented at each level. The intensity at which about two-thirds of the sentences were understood was accepted as the speech reception threshold and Hughson and Thompson found that this threshold could be established quite precisely. Furthermore, they also noted a linear relationship between the hearing loss measured for pure tones of 500, 1000, and 2000 Hz and the loss measured for the reception of speech.

Carhart (1946a) made similar comparisons and came to similar conclusions. In addition he also compared thresholds for speech as determined with Bell Telephone Intelligibility Sentences with those derived by using lists of spondees developed by the Harvard Psycho-Acoustic Laboratory. He concluded that "the words and sentences are essentially equivalent in their value as materials for measuring speech reception threshold [p. 346]." Since spondee words now represent the standard materials for the clinical measurement of speech reception threshold, the next section considers the nature of these materials in detail.

B. Materials

As mentioned earlier, Hudgins et al. (1947) developed and described a number of tests to evaluate speech intelligibility. They approached their task with the idea that familiarity, phonetic dissimilarity, normal sampling of English sounds, and homogeneity with respect to audibility were most important in the development of speech tests for diagnostic purposes. It is mainly the latter, homogeneity with respect to audibility, that is of primary importance in the selection of materials for use in measuring thresholds for speech.

Homogeneity is important for two reasons. First, it increases the probability that the articulation function relating signal intensity with the percentage of items heard correctly will rise from 0 to 100% within a narrow range of intensity levels. Assuming a constant and randomly distributed error of measurement associated with the testing procedure, it follows that the steepness of the articulation function determines the precision with which threshold for the materials can be estimated. Second, it is desirable to determine the threshold for speech with as small a number of items as possible. Thus, if the words are equally audible, the threshold measurement should not vary as a function of the particular subsample of test items used to establish it. Having established these criteria, Hudgins and his group selected words for their test from a pool of items whose audibility they had previously established.

It was on these bases that PAL Auditory Test No. 9 was developed. It consisted of 84 disyllabic equal stress words which were divided into two lists of 42 words. Each list was randomized five times and the 84 items were recorded on disks in such a way that each set of six words was reproduced at a level 4 dB lower than the previous group of six. Thus, seven sets of six words each were recorded with the last group being 24 dB weaker than the first group. This arrangement was intended to allow an articulation function to be quickly plotted as a means of estimating the threshold or 50% response level.

In their evaluation of Auditory Test No. 9 Hudgins *et al.* (1947) found a standard error of measurement of 2.4 dB with normal listeners and no significant difference in the mean scores during the administration of the six forms of the test. The standard error for listeners with impaired hearing varied from 2.1 to 2.8 dB. Thus, Hudgins and his associates concluded that with a single administration of Auditory Test No. 9, the speech reception threshold for either normal or hearing-impaired listeners would fall within 2.8 dB of the true score approximately two-thirds of the time.

Auditory Test No. 14 followed Auditory Test No. 9. The same words were used in it, but all items were recorded at the same level. Now the examiner could control the level at which the various words were presented by simply manipulating the attenuator on the audiometer. This arrangement proved to be more useful clinically.

Hirsh *et al.* (1952) reduced the total number of items from 84 to 36 in the course of developing the CID W1 and W2 versions of the spondee test. The 36 items were selected after administration of the 84 spondees to experienced and inexperienced listeners at five presentation levels in order to determine the relative audibility of the individual words. Hirsh and his group used the total number of errors for a word at all presentation levels and for all listeners to rate the test item as either "easy" or "difficult." The criterion for "easy" was one error or less for all listeners; a "difficult" word was one that was missed five or more times by all listeners. Since those words which are always identified correctly and those which are always missed can be considered as "dead weight" and of no value, Hirsh *et al.* (1952) eliminated all words in the easy and difficult categories and thus reduced the original list of 84 words to one of 36 spondees of approximately equal audibility. Six randomizations of the 36 items were generated and presented to a group of normal listeners at five intensity levels. Some words were still found to be easier, others more difficult than the average. To compensate for this difference, a new recording was made in which the "easy" words were decreased 2 dB in intensity with respect to the average while the "difficult" words were increased 2 dB in intensity. The words were then administered again at the five presentations levels.

> Analysis of the data showed that the words were now homogeneous with respect to intelligibility and variations in the thresholds of the individual words were, as adequately as could be measured by this method, chance variation [Hirsh et al., 1952, p. 325].

The articulation score for these materials rose from 0 to 100% within a range of 20 dB. An increase from 20 to 80% occurred within a range of 8 dB, yielding a slope of approximately 8% per decibel in this range. Thus, the CID W1 and W2 test materials seem well suited for the measurement of speech reception threshold.

As already implied, the CID spondee test materials were recorded in two different versions with Hirsh as talker. These disk recordings are commercially available through the Technisonic Recording Studios in St. Louis.

The first version of the test was designated as CID Auditory Test W-1. It consists of various randomizations of the words all of which are recorded at a constant level and 10 dB below the level of a 1000-Hz calibration tone recorded on the inner band of each disk. Each word is introduced by the carrier phrase "Say the word," which is recorded at the level of the calibration tone.

The second version of this test, W-2, comprises the same word orders as used in W-1 but differs from the latter test in one important way. In the production of the W-2 disks, the recording level was reduced by 3 dB after each block of three words so that the last three-word block is recorded at a level 33 dB below that of the first three-word block. In this version a carrier phrase recorded at the same level as the 1000-Hz calibration tone precedes the first nine test words. Thereafter, the carrier phrase is attenuated 3 dB with each three-word block. This particular test was designed for the rapid establishment of threshold utilizing the concept of the articulation function and the statistical concept of threshold, that is, the 50% response point. Hirsh and his co-workers suggested a specific threshold measurement technique for use in conjunction with the W-2 recordings. The essential features of the method are discussed in the following section.

C. Method

In clinical applications, the speech reception threshold is usually defined as the lowest intensity at which 50% of the test material is correctly perceived by the individual being tested. As Jerger et al. (1959)

discovered, however, there is often a good deal of variability among clinicians in specifying the meaning of the phrase "50% correct response." Such a circumstance makes for the situation wherein error may be introduced because no two individuals define threshold in exactly the same way, or because the same individual fails to employ exactly the same definition from test to test. Take, for example, the approach of Hughson and Thompson (1942). In their pioneering approach to the clinical measurement of the speech reception threshold, they defined threshold as the minimum intensity at which the individual could repeat two-thirds of the sentences correctly. They varied presentation levels so that this level was bracketed, that is, sentences were delivered both above and below this critical level. The point to be made here is that Hughson and Thompson apparently did not present the same number of sentences at each presentation level and therefore the criterion of two-thirds correct repetition was, in that sense, relative.

A more systematic approach to the definition of threshold was incorporated in the PAL Test No. 9 described earlier. Recall that this test consisted of blocks of six words recorded so that after the first block the recording level was attenuated ·by 4 dB for each succeeding block of six words. Thus, 24 dB of attenuation was provided on the recording. The method of threshold measurement suggested by Hudgins et al. (1947) required that the test be started at a presentation level high enough for the subject to repeat all of the first six words, but low enough so that within the 24-dB range of attenuation provided on the record a level would be reached at which the subject missed all six words. In short, the method suggested by the developers of PAL Test No. 9 required that for a given subject the entire range from 0 to 100% correct response be sampled.

Actually, Hudgins and his co-workers described two methods for deriving threshold with their recording. While these two techniques appeared quite different, they employed essentially the same approach and yielded equivalent results.

The first approach was a graphic method that involved the plotting of an articulation function from the subject's response data. This procedure allowed the clinician to determine the exact intensity level corresponding to 50% correct response. Recognizing that this graphic method was cumbersome and probably not clinically feasible, Hudgins and his associates proposed an alternative approach that has since been adapted by others and forms the basis of a method which the authors would recommend as a standard procedure for the clinical measurement of the speech reception threshold.

Hudgins's second method was based on the notion that since six words were presented at each 4-dB intensity interval, each word could be considered the equivalent of two-thirds of a decibel of attenuation. Thus, for each word repeated correctly by the patient, the examiner could consider that the intensity level of the words had been attenuated by two-thirds of a decibel with reference to the starting level. Operationally with this method, the examiner simply counted the number of words correctly repeated, consulted a table which listed the decibel drop across the record corresponding to a given number of correct responses and subtracted the resulting number from his starting intensity. The resultant value corresponded to the 50% response point that would have been derived via the graphic method. In order to obtain this agreement, however, Hudgins et al. (1947) assigned an attenuation value of 2 dB rather than 4 dB to the first six words. This was necessary because the test must be started at a level where the first six words are repeated correctly. Thus, in order to obtain a threshold value that corresponds to the 50% response point determined graphically, it is necessary to assume that 50% of the first block of words would have been missed had the test been started at threshold. Hence, when using this method, half the words repeated at the first intensity level are not counted.

Hirsh and his associates used a variation of this method in conjunction with CID Auditory Test W-2. As just described, this test comprised 36 spondee words recorded so that three-word blocks were separated by 3-dB steps of attenuation. Thus, the W-2 recording incorporates 33 dB of attenuation, with each word having the equivalent of 1 dB of attenuation. Operationally, the computation of threshold with this recording requires the examiner to subtract the number of words correctly repeated by the listener from the level at which the first three words were presented. It is then necessary to add 1.5 dB, the decibel equivalent of half the words presented at the first level, in order to correct the threshold value to coincide with the 50% response criterion.

A method that utilizes the essential features of that described by Hirsh et al. (1952) and that can be employed with constant level recordings will now be described. It is a procedure that has been employed successfully in clinical settings and is one which confines all clinicians to the same set of operations in the definition of threshold. Thus, we think it deserves consideration as a standard method for measurement of the spondee threshold.

As its first step, the procedure incorporates the familiarization of the patient with the test-word vocabulary. This can be accomplished simply by reading the test words in alphabetical order at a comfortable listening level and asking the patient to repeat each word. This procedure minimizes measurement error associated with test vocabulary familiarity.

Tillman and Jerger (1959) showed that this error could amount to as much as 3 or 4 dB with normal listeners. It should be noted here that some hearing-impaired patients having speech discrimination problems will be unable to repeat some of the spondee test words even at comfortable listening levels. These words should be eliminated from the test vocabulary in order to avoid measurement error, which can be quite large in some cases.

Following familiarization, the procedure is to present a single spondee word at a level 30–40 dB above the estimated threshold level. If a correct response ensues, the level is attenuated 10 dB and another word is presented. This procedure is continued until an incorrect response is obtained, whereupon a second word is presented at the same level. If this word is also missed, the intensity level of the signal is increased 10 dB and the test is then begun. If the second word is repeated, however, another 10 dB of attenuation are added and the process continues until a level is reached at which two successive words are missed. The test is then begun 10 dB above this latter intensity level.

The purpose of the exploration just described is to arrive quickly at an intensity level that is relatively close to threshold so as to avoid spending undue time in the threshold seeking process. Threshold testing is begun at the level described above by presenting two successive spondee words. The intensity level is then attenuated by 2 dB and two more words are presented. This process continues with two words being presented at each 2-dB interval until the patient misses at least five of the last six words presented. One additional constraint is imposed. The starting level selected as previously described must be sufficiently high to allow the patient to repeat at least five of the first six words correctly. If this criterion is not met, the test must be started over at a level 4–6 dB above the initial starting level. Once the patient responds correctly to at least five of the first six words, the test continues until it is terminated by at least five incorrect responses on the last six items. The clinician then merely counts the number of correct responses, decreases this total by one, and subtracts the result from the hearing level setting at which the test began. The result is the speech reception threshold that would correspond to the 50% point on the articulation function. (Decreasing the total correct responses by one in effect subtracts 50% from the first group of two words presented at the starting point.)

This method has proven to be clinically feasible in most applications and it is certainly no more time-consuming than the often unsystematic bracketing techniques. Its chief advantage is that it confines all clinicians to the same operational definition of threshold, and thus reduces variability in estimates of the speech reception threshold produced by variations in this definition.

D. Relationships between Pure-Tone Thresholds and Speech-Reception Thresholds

As early as 1929 Fletcher suggested that the average of the thresholds from 512 to 2048 Hz could be used as an estimate of the sensitivity for hearing speech. In the early 1940s Sabine (1942) and Fowler (1941 and 1942) proposed various schemes for weighting pure-tone thresholds to estimate the hearing loss for speech, and as mentioned earlier, Hughson and Thompson observed a linear relationship between the thresholds for speech measured with Bell Telephone Intelligibility Sentences and the 512–2048-Hz pure-tone thresholds of hearing-impaired persons.

Carhart (1946a) compared the accuracy of several methods for predicting speech reception thresholds from pure-tone threshold tests. After computing correlations between single pure-tone thresholds and speech-reception thresholds, between pure-tone averages and speech thresholds and deriving several regression equations and weighting systems, he found that the average of the thresholds for 512, 1024, and 2048 Hz was quite adequate for predicting a given individual's threshold sensitivity for spondees or Bell Telephone Intelligibility Sentences.

Various weighting systems for estimating threshold sensitivity for speech from pure-tone thresholds have been published during the intervening years (Fletcher, 1950; Graham, 1960; Harris et al., 1956; Kryter et al., 1962; Lightfoot et al., 1953; Quiggle et al., 1957; Siegenthaler and Strand, 1964). However, the prediction most commonly used clinically appears to be that based on the pure-tone average for the three frequencies 500, 1000, and 2000 Hz. A common variation of this procedure is to use the two-frequency average suggested by Fletcher (1950), particularly for individuals whose threshold at one of these frequencies deviates markedly from the other two. Fletcher suggested using only two of the frequencies from 500 to 2000 Hz, those two for which hearing is best.

In a recent article, Carhart (1971) examines a large number of clinical records with regard to pure-tone thresholds from 250 to 4000 Hz and speech-reception thresholds, all thresholds being expressed in decibels re the ANSI-1969 norms for pure-tone and speech audiometry. The conclusion which emerges from this work is that whenever variations in audiometric configuration are not to be taken into account, speech reception thresholds can be best estimated by subtracting 2 dB from the pure-tone average for 500 and 1000 Hz.

In a later and more extensive study Carhart and Porter (1971) examined the relationships between threshold sensitivity for pure tones and speech in a large clinical sample subdivided into various groups on the basis of the shape of the audiometric configuration. They found that only in patients with sharply falling or sharply rising configurations were the predictions of speech threshold based on hearing sensitivity at 500 and 1000 Hz substantially improved by utilizing other pure-tone thresholds in the predictive formula.

The point to be made here is that a number of relatively accurate methods exist for predicting the speech reception threshold from the pure-tone threshold. Such predictions are highly accurate for the majority of clinical patients and this has led some to conclude that the measurement of speech reception threshold is therefore largely redundant (Davis and Silverman, 1970). Others point out that whenever discrepancies between speech and pure-tone threshold sensitivity do occur they are clinically important and thus justify the time expended in measuring the speech threshold (Carhart, 1952; Carhart, 1960; Chaiklin and Ventry, 1963). Furthermore, whenever the speech threshold agrees closely with the pure-tone threshold level, it serves indirectly to establish the reliability of the pure-tone test results. Thus, while the justification for measuring the speech-reception threshold is sometimes debated, the reluctance of most clinicians to dispense with this measure attests to its value.

IV. Measurement of Auditory Discrimination

A. Introduction

Egan (1948) suggests three methods by which the degree of intelligibility of speech may be determined: (1) threshold tests, (2) subjective appraisals, and (3) articulation tests. As noted previously, threshold tests help to confirm the degree of impairment indicated by pure-tone audiometry, but they fail to provide either a complete estimate of the social adequacy of the individual's hearing or the information necessary to allow differentiation among auditory pathologies. Therefore, threshold tests fail to satisfy two of the important functions of speech hearing tests listed by Silverman and Hirsh (1955). The "subjective appraisal" approach mentioned by Egan might serve these latter purposes better than threshold testing, but such an approach is clinically less than satisfying because it seldom yields a quantitative estimate of performance. Hence, such a measure does not lend itself to the precise rank ordering of either individuals or listening conditions.

We are consequently left with Egan's third procedure, articulation testing, as our best method for obtaining diagnostic information and estimating the level of social adequacy. Egan takes the position that a quantitative estimate of speech intelligibility may be obtained by simply counting the number of individual speech elements correctly perceived by the listener during an articulation test. Granting this position, we are faced with the task of selecting a speech sample that is appropriate for use in articulation testing.

Logically, for assessing social adequacy we would choose material that is representative of everyday speech. In making this choice, we are faced with the dilemma so clearly enunciated by Silverman and Hirsh (1955) when they observed that the speech materials necessary for making diagnostic distinctions are not necessarily those that are most representative of English speech. In the discussion to follow it will become clear that individuals interested in measuring speech discrimination have chosen to emphasize the diagnostic value of the method and have been content to obtain only some relative measure of social efficiency. This choice has been reflected to a large extent in the materials developed for testing articulation.

B. Materials

1. PHONETICALLY BALANCED WORD LISTS

Carhart (1965b) has made the point that a test of speech discrimination, as contrasted with a threshold test, must comprise largely nonredundant items if the individual's inabilities to make fine distinctions between consonants and vowels are to be detected. Several types of material would satisfy this criterion, but items such as individual phonemes or nonsense syllables have not been widely used for two reasons. First, these items are quite abstract and thus prove too difficult for some individuals. Second, as Lehiste and Peterson (1959) observed, items devoid of symbolic content tend to measure "recognizability" as opposed to the "intelligibility" assessed by meaningful words. It is for these reasons that monosyllabic words have been chosen by many as the test material for assessing speech intelligibility. Furthermore, as Carhart (1965b) has pointed out, monosyllables are sufficiently unpredictable for clinical patients that the individual speech elements must be perceived if correct identification is to occur.

a. Harvard PAL PB-50 Lists. The first speech-discrimination test materials to utilize monosyllabic words and to incorporate the concept of phonetic balance were the PB-50 lists developed at the Harvard Psycho-Acoustic Laboratory (Egan, 1948). This test consists of 20 lists of 50 words each. According to Egan, the words for each list were selected so as to satisfy the following criteria: (1) monosyllabic structure, (2) equal average difficulty and equal range of difficulty, (3) words in common usage, (4) equal phonetic composition, and (5) phonetic composition representative of English speech. The last criterion was satisfied by basing the phonetic composition of each word list on the composition of a sample of 100,000 words reported by Dewey (1923). For a number of reasons detailed by Egan, the "phonetic balance" of the PB-50 word lists was less than perfect. However, the test was the first to incorporate this concept of phonetic balance and it was this concept that gave these test materials high "face validity" as a method for assessing speech intelligibility.

Two facts reported by Egan are worth repeating here. First, he noted that each of the PB-50 lists contained 50 words because attempts to meet the criteria for list formation with only 25 words failed. Second, he observed that a significant difference exists between the intelligibility of words and that of sentences. Thus, he indirectly cautions against placing too much importance on a particular word-articulation score at least in any absolute sense.

Despite the limitations of the Harvard PAL PB-50 word lists and the fact that they were never recorded in their entirety for commercial distribution, this set of materials represents a milestone in the development of speech-discrimination testing. These materials received extensive application in the audiological management of hearing-impaired veterans in the aural rehabilitation centers established by the United States military services in the late years of World War II, and the usefulness of the materials and the technique was thereby demonstrated.

Several of the 20 lists were subsequently placed on disk recordings at Central Institute for the Deaf with Rush Hughes as the talker. Because of certain unique vocal characteristics of this talker, these recordings represent a relatively difficult test of speech discrimination and they never received widespread clinical application. Nevertheless, they were used quite effectively by some clinicians in rank ordering individuals with minor speech-discrimination problems (Thurlow et al., 1949). Furthermore, the Hughes's recordings of the PAL PB-50 word lists were used by Walsh and Silverman (1946) and by Davis (1948) in the development of the Social Adequacy Index and hence retain historical importance.

b. Central Institute for the Deaf Auditory Test W-22. A threefold develop a new test of speech discrimination utilizing monosyllabic words dissatisfaction with the PAL PB-50 tests led Hirsh et al. (1952) to and the concept of phonetic balance. This dissatisfaction with the PAL PB-50 lists arose because: (1) the phonetic balance of the lists was imperfect, (2) the test vocabulary contained a substantial number of rare words, and (3) no suitably standard recording of the materials had been made commercially available. Hirsh and his associates imposed criteria that ensured formation of monosyllabic word lists that were more adequate in phonetic balance and that were composed of more familiar items than characterized the PAL PB-50 lists. Four 50-word lists were developed and recorded in six different word orders, first on magnetic tape and subsequently on unbreakable disks for commercial distribution.

Hirsh *et al.* (1952) reported data indicating that the four lists of the CID W-22 test were reasonably equivalent in difficulty, at least when used to measure speech discrimination for individuals with normal hearing. Over its linear portion, between approximately 20 and 80% correct response, the articulation function yielded for these materials by normal listeners rose at the rate of approximately 6% per decibel increase in signal intensity. This was almost twice as steep as the function for the Hughes recordings of the PAL PB-50 lists and it indicates that the CID W-22 test is a much less demanding test of speech discrimination than the Hughes recording of the PAL PB-50 lists. Those who had used the latter so successfully to differentiate among individuals with mild discrimination losses were frustrated by their attempts to employ the W-22 test for the same purpose. For example, in speaking of the responses to W-22 words by patients with otosclerosis, Walsh (1964) complained that "everybody either gets 100% or 30%." On the other hand, those who had attempted to differentiate among individuals with severe discrimination losses using the Hughes recordings and who had met with little or no success found in the CID W-22 a test which allowed them to accomplish this task. These observations are intended merely to underscore a point so well made previously by Carhart (1965b). Namely, the clinician must define the clinical criteria that a particular test of speech discrimination must satisfy and then select a specific test on this basis. No one test is likely to satisfy all criteria.

c. Lehiste-Peterson CNC Word Lists. In their approach to the study of speech intelligibility, Lehiste and Peterson (1959) observed that the individual's own linguistic background will significantly influence his judgments regarding the speech he hears. They further emphasized that the particular phonetic manifestations that characterize a given speech element will vary as a function of the element which it precedes and follows. In this context they developed the concept of "perceptual phonetics" which they defined as "phonemics" and they took the position that it is really not possible to develop lists of words that are phonetically balanced. Instead they contended that it was possible only to develop lists of words that were in certain respects phonemically balanced.

They pointed to the imperfect "phonemic balance" of the Harvard PB-50 lists as the factor which motivated their development of new test materials.

For reasons not made perfectly clear, Lehiste and Peterson limited their test materials to monosyllables of the consonant–vowel–consonant type. They referred to the vowel as the "syllable nucleus" and hence chose to call their test items CNC words. For their pool of potential test words, Lehiste and Peterson selected all monosyllables of the CNC variety listed by Thorndike and Lorge (1952) as occurring at least once per million words. This criterion yielded a group of 1263 monosyllables. Lehiste and Peterson chose to base their scheme of phonemic balance for a given list on the phonemic composition of their entire group of 1263 words rather than on some estimate of the overall phonemic composition of English speech. Nevertheless, if one disregards the fact that the Harvard PB-50 lists contained both words of consonant–vowel and vowel–consonant type, while the Lehiste–Peterson lists excluded such words, the scheme of phonemic balance for the two tests is not radically different.

From the pool of 1263 words, Lehiste and Peterson formed 10 lists of 50 words each. While each list conformed closely to their projected plan for phonemic balance, no one list fit the proposed balance perfectly. Nevertheless, the 10 lists that emerged in 1959 represented the most rigorously phonemically balanced test materials yet available. In 1962, Peterson and Lehiste published 10 revised lists of CNC materials (Peterson and Lehiste, 1962). The revision was based on criteria designed to eliminate unfamiliar words that appeared in the original version. The same scheme of phonemic balance undergirds both sets of CNC word lists.

For a specific research project Tillman et al. (1963a) and later Tillman and Carhart (1966) compiled lists of 50 CNC words, all of which conformed more perfectly to the phonemic balance advocated by Lehiste and Peterson than did the original lists. Although none of the new lists duplicated those published by Lehiste and Peterson, they were selected from the same pool of 1263 CNC monosyllables and thus were, in essence, Lehiste–Peterson lists. Two of these lists were recorded on magnetic tape by a male talker with General American dialect. This particular recording of the Lehiste–Peterson materials was designated Northwestern University Auditory Test No. 4. A second version comprising the two lists of Northwestern University Test No. 4 and two new 50-word lists was later recorded by a different male talker as well as a female talker. The dialect of the male can be described as General America, Southern Fringe (southwest Oklahoma region), while that of the female was General American. These latter recordings were designated Northwestern

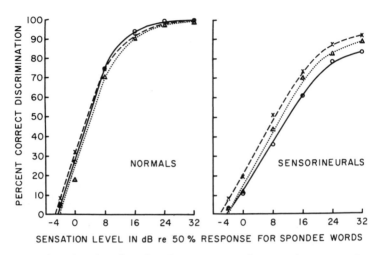

SENSATION LEVEL IN dB re 50 % RESPONSE FOR SPONDEE WORDS

FIG. 1. Ariculation functions based on average of test and retest performances of normal-hearing subjects and patients with sensorineural-type hearing impairments on three different recordings of identical speech discrimination test materials. ○—○, NU No. 4; ×--×, NU No. 6-M; △ ··· △ NU, No. 6-F.

University Auditory Test No. 6-M and No. 6-F, respectively. Figure 1 displays the articulation functions yielded by each of these three CNC discrimination tests by normal-hearing subjects and by patients with sensorineural-type hearing impairments. A given subject group listened to only one of the three tests in each of two sessions. The number of subjects per group varied from 12 to 24. The data from which the functions in the figure were drawn are listed in Table I.

The effects of talker differences on the performance of a speech discrimination test are quite apparent in these data. Cognizance of just such effects led Lehiste and Peterson to the concept of phonemic balance in the first place and later led Kreul et al. (1969) to state that only the actual recordings of given word lists as spoken by a particular individual should be considered to represent the test material, not just the word lists per se. Nevertheless, it is apparent from the data reported here that the effects of talker differences for these materials were minor and relatively constant as a function of sensation level of presentation. While it is apparent that subject type exerted significant influence on the slope of the articulation function for either of the two types of subjects, the slope of the articulation function was essentially equivalent for all three tests.

In general it is the slope of the articulation function for a given test that determines the precision with which it will separate the performance of individuals or the performance of a single individual under several different listening conditions. Lacking a standardized test, the clinician must assess the characteristics of the particular speech discrimination test he chooses to employ, for only when he knows these characteristics can he make valid comparisons between scores yielded on his test and those from other tests administered under equivalent listening conditions. From this point of view it is obvious that no standardized test is possible unless recorded tests are employed, that is, because of talker differences tests administered via monitored-live-voice defy standardization.

d. Final Comment. Although no standard test for the clinical assessment of speech discrimination has yet been adopted, monosyllabic words of the phonetically or phonemically balanced type have received by far the most widespread application. These materials have been accepted as a measure of the individual's efficiency in everyday hearing, probably because of their face validity provided by the phonetic balancing. Nevertheless, no one has conducted the experiments necessary to establish the validity of these test measures. It would appear that clinicians utilize the PB-type test because of the diagnostic, prognostic, or rehabilitative

TABLE I

AVERAGE OF TEST AND RETEST DISCRIMINATION
SCORES IN PERCENT FOR LISTS 1 AND 2 YIELDED
BY NORMAL-HEARING AND SENSORINEURAL
HEARING-IMPAIRED SUBJECTS FOR NORTHWESTERN
UNIVERSITY TESTS NO. 4, NO. 6-M, AND NO. 6-F

S.L.[a]	Test No. 4	Test No. 6-M	Test No. 6-F
Normal group			
−4	5.3	8.4	4.4
0	27.2	32.0	17.5
8	74.8	74.7	70.4
16	93.8	91.6	90.0
24	99.1	97.6	97.0
32	99.6	99.4	98.7
Hearing-impaired group			
−4	3.3	8.2	3.1
0	10.8	19.6	11.6
8	36.1	51.2	43.8
16	61.0	73.6	70.0
24	78.7	87.4	82.6
32	83.6	91.9	89.0

[a] Sensation level of presentation in decibels re intensity required for 50% response to spondee words.

information it yields, even though many of them have apparently accepted the notion that performance on this type of test provides only a very relative measure of social efficiency. This point is underscored by the number of individuals who have argued either that discrimination can be as effectively measured with 25-word PB lists as with the 50-word lists (Burke *et al.*, 1965; Campanelli, 1962; Elpern, 1961; Resnick, 1962; Shutts *et al.*, 1964) or that the concept of phonetic balance is not an important consideration (Tobias, 1964).

Many other materials and procedures have been proposed as effective approaches to the clinical measurements of speech discrimination. Some of these will be discussed in the following subsections. The point to be made here, however, is that there presently exists no test that can be accepted as a valid means for assessing the everyday listening efficiency of an individual patient.

2. MULTIPLE-CHOICE-TYPE TESTS

A multitude of multiple-choice-type speech discrimination tests have appeared in the past decade. This closed-message-set approach to articulation testing has usually been aimed at the evaluation of speech transmission systems and widespread clinical use of this approach has not yet been reported. In recent years, however, a number of studies have been completed which have compared the relative clinical effectiveness of the multiple-choice-type test with the more traditional PB-type monosyllabic word test. No attempt is made here to give exhaustive coverage to this type of test. Instead, a representative sample of such tests will be covered in the hope of conveying the principles involved and of defining the relationships between this approach and the more traditional clinical approach discussed in the previous section.

a. Fairbanks's Rhyme Test. The first of the multiple-choice tests to utilize rhyming monosyllables as the test material was proposed by Fairbanks (1958). This test consists of 50 sets of five rhyming monosyllables. For a given stimulus word, the subject is required only to add an initial consonant to a stem provided on his answer sheet. Thus, the test probes only the phonemic differentiation of the initial consonant or consonant–vowel transition in monosyllabic words. As such, this test fails to enjoy the same aura of "face validity" associated with the PB-type materials and perhaps as a result this version of the Rhyme Test never received widespread clinical use.

For two reasons Fairbanks's Rhyme Test must be considered an important development in the area of speech-discrimination testing First, it represented one of the earliest moves in the direction of the "closed message set" as a means of assessing speech discrimination. It is true that Fairbanks's test was not truly a "closed response set" since he indicates that for each test word the average adult subject had perhaps eight or nine potential responses available to him. Nevertheless, this test was much more restrictive in this regard than the PB-type test. Second, the original Rhyme Test has served as the pattern for the development of a number of subsequent tests.

b. *Modified Rhyme Test (MRT)*. Motivated by the desire for a speech-intelligibility test that could be employed in the assessment of communications systems without the need for an extensively trained listening crew, House *et al.* (1963, 1965) developed a modification of Fairbanks's Rhyme Test. The new instrument consisted of six equivalent lists of 50 words each. In developing these materials House and his associates took no strict account of either word familiarity or phonetic balance. The format of the test is such that the subject is given a response sheet containing all 300 items in the test arranged in six columns of 50 words each. For each stimulus word the subject selects a response from among the six alternatives in a given row. Thus, the Modified Rhyme Test represents a truly closed response set. Furthermore, this test assesses consonantal discrimination in both initial and final positions of the monosyllabic stimulus words.

Although no extensive clinical application of this test has been reported, House and his co-workers evaluated its performance with normal-hearing observers at varying speech-to-noise ratios. These data suggested that the various forms of the test were statistically equivalent and that continued exposures to the test failed to produce improved performance, that is, practice effects were negligible.

Kryter and Whitman (1965) compared performance on the Modified Rhyme Test with that on the 1000-item PAL PB-50 test using the same listening crew and various speech-to-noise ratios. They reported that in the performance region from 50 to 80% correct for the MRT, scores on the PB test were approximately 25% lower. They concluded that although the Modified Rhyme Test is distinctly less complicated in administration and scoring, that is, it lends itself to automation, it is not so demanding a task as that presented by the PAL PB-50 test insofar as word intelligibility in noise is concerned.

Kreul *et al.* (1968) have recently attempted to adapt the Modified Rhyme Test to make it a clinically useful tool. They felt that the format and test items were simple enough to be used with a wide range of the clinical population and that when used in conjunction with a masking noise, the test would be capable of rank ordering patients with respect to their everyday listening ability.

These investigators mixed the test items with noise before recording the composite signal on magnetic tape. On the basis of the performance of a group of normal-hearing subjects Kreul and his associates selected three signal-to-noise ratios to be stored on their tape. These ratios were chosen so as to produce target discrimination scores of 96, 83, and 75% for normals. Three different talkers were involved in the recording process.

As a test of the accuracy of the target scores suggested by Kreul *et al.* (1968) Beyer *et al.* (1969) administered this new test to 27 normal listeners. These latter investigators found no statistically significant differences among lists but did detect a significant talker effect. Furthermore, the average scores yielded by this listening crew fell some 2 to 3% below the target scores stated in the original report.

This proposed test is currently undergoing extensive clinical validation. To date, the data from this program have not been made available. However, because of its simplified format, which minimizes problems of administration and scoring as well as problems associated with practice effects, this proposed new test would appear to be a potentially useful clinical tool.

c. Phonetically Balanced Rhyme Test (PBRT). Because the two rhyme tests just discussed assess only phoneme differentiation in initial and final positions, Clarke (1965) was motivated to develop a test that would include pivotal phonemes in the medial as well as final positions in the monosyllabic word. Clarke's test was perhaps the most carefully constructed of all the rhyme-type tests. He not only took into account factors such as word familiarity and orthographic constance of the test-word stems, but he also selected test items so as to obtain lists of 50 words each that preserved the representation of the phonemes and phoneme transitions that characterized the parent population of monosyllables used in constructing the test. In this respect he adopted the approach used earlier by Lehiste and Peterson (1959).

Clarke's Phonetically Balanced Rhyme Test (PBRT) is actually three tests. The three tests of the PBRT each measure phoneme differentiation in only one position, that is, initial, medial, or final. It thus appears necessary to administer three tests, one of each type, in order to take advantage of the careful phonemic balance that this test incorporates. Each test of the PBRT consists of five equivalent forms of 50 items each. In the test administration the subject is provided with a sheet containing five columns of 50 words each, and during the administration of a particular form of a given test the subject selects his response to the stimulus word from among the five choices in a given row. In this respect, the PBRT represents a slightly more closed-response-set than the Modified Rhyme Test.

It should be stated that Clarke and his co-workers developed the PBRT as a method for assessing the efficiency of communications systems and not as a clinical tool. Hence, while Clarke reports extensive data that define the characteristics of his test and allow a comparison between it and other discrimination tests along a number of dimensions, the test apparently has not been applied clinically.

d. Multiple-Choice Discrimination Test (MCDT). Recognizing that the CID Auditory Test W-22 often yields relatively high scores even in some patients who report significant difficulty in speech discrimination, Schultz and Schubert (1969) reported a method for utilizing this test in a closed-message-set format. Their primary goals were to develop a test which would minimize word familiarity effects and systematize phoneme substitution choices.

The test format for the MCDT was quite similar to that for the Rhyme Test and Modified Rhyme Test discussed earlier. However, the MCDT differs from these two tests in that for a given stimulus word, alternative choices are available that allow confusion in either the initial or final phonemes.

Schultz and Schubert report preliminary normative data obtained in noise for the MCDT and they compare its characteristics with more traditional tests of speech discrimination. They also report an error matrix yielded by 48 hypoacousic patients tested with the MCDT. They emphasize, however, that their report is a preliminary evaluation of a prototype test whose clinical value remains to be established.

e. Final Comment. As stated earlier, there are many other speech-discrimination tests that utilize the single word stimulus–response and the closed-message format. Those discussed here represent some of the more recent and in the judgment of the authors some of the more promising tests from a clinical point of view. Most of these tests were originally conceived as methods for assessing the efficiency of speech transmitting systems rather than as clinical tools. Much research and clinical application remains to be accomplished before the relative value of the various tests can be described accurately. The obvious advantages of the multiple-choice approach in simplicity and objectivity of presentation and scoring should ensure that the needed evaluative work will be accomplished.

3. SENTENCE TESTS

A number of speech hearing tests involving the sentence as the basic test item have been developed. In most instances these materials have been intended, not for clinical use, but for assessing communications systems. Some have been utilized for measuring threshold sensitivity for speech, such as the Harvard PAL Test No. 12 (Hudgins *et al.*, 1947) and the Bell Telephone Laboratory Intelligibility Word Lists (Hughson and Thompson, 1942). With two exceptions, however, no set of sentence materials has been developed for the express purpose of assessing the individual's capacity for speech discrimination.

The first exception is represented by a group of 100 sentences developed and recorded at the Central Institute for the Deaf (Davis and Silverman, 1970; Silverman and Hirsh, 1955). On the basis of a rather rigid set of criteria these sentences were constructed to represent "everyday American speech." Responses to each set of 10 sentences are scored on the basis of 50 key words contained therein. Sentence length varies from 2 to 12 words. The recordings of these materials have not been made commercially available and no "test" per se has yet been developed from them. They were in fact conceived for use in validating other speech discrimination tests rather than as a primary test of speech discrimination.

The second exception is represented by the Synthetic Sentence Identification Test (SSI) developed by Speaks and Jerger (1965). They were interested in exploring the perception of speech as a function of changes in temporal parameters and hence were unable to utilize test materials consisting of isolated words. They chose the sentence as their basic test unit, but recognized two major problems inherent in this approach. First, in a real sentence, meaning may be conveyed by only one or two key words. Second, formation of equivalent lists of sentences is inordinately difficult due to factors such as word familiarity, word and sentence length, and syntactical structure. Speaks and Jerger felt that they could retain the advantages of the sentence as the basic test unit and yet avoid the problems just enumerated by constructing "artificial" or "synthetic" sentences. The sentences subsequently developed by these investigators are artificial in the sense that they are not "real" sentences and synthetic in the sense that the sequence of words in each sentence unit followed specifiable rules of syntax. The sentences were constructed as follows.

Words for all sentences were chosen from the 1000 most common English words as designated by Thorndike and Lorge (1944). Sentences designated as first-order approximations to real sentences were formed simply by drawing successive words randomly from this 1000-word pool. Second-order approximation sentences were constructed by choosing the initial word randomly, and then by asking one individual to select the second word after having been told the first word, a second individual to select the third word after having been informed of the second word, etc. The word selectors were constrained in their choice of words only by the requirement that the word drawn must be one that might reasonably follow the preceding word in a declarative or imperative sentence. Third-order approximations were based on what Speaks and Jerger term the "conditional probabilities" of word triplets. Although five-, seven-, and nine-word sentences were constructed, only the latter two word lengths were used for the third-order sentences. For a given test, sentence length was held constant and the syllable number per sentence was also closely controlled.

Various tests composed of 10 sentences each were developed. The test administration involves the clo.ed-message-set format in that the subject is seated before a panel containing the 10 sentences with a response button opposite each sentence. Following each presentation, his task is merely to push the button opposite the sentence that he thinks he has heard. He is informed if his response is correct and his performance is expressed as the percentage of correct responses to the 10 stimuli.

Jerger, Speaks, and their associates have subjected these sentence materials to extensive experimental and clinical analysis. Their findings can be briefly summarized as follows. First, the articulation function emerging from the presentation of the synthetic sentences in quiet is extremely steep. Incidentally, Speaks and Jerger refer to this function as the performance–intensity (PI) function and Speaks (1967b) showed it to rise at the rate of approximatly 10% per decibel increase in signal intensity over the range of 20–80% response. If anything, the steepness of this PI function increased under very restrictive filtering of either the low-pass or high-pass varieties (Speaks, 1967a). Furthermore, even when low-pass filtered at 125 Hz or high-pass filtered at 7000 Hz, performance on the synthetic sentences always reached 100% if the materials were presented at sufficiently high intensity levels. Jerger and Jerger (1967) reported a similar finding when they used the SSI task clinically with patients having lesions of the eighth cranial nerve. These results would tend to suggest that consonantal differentiation is probably not required for the correct identification of these materials presented in quiet.

Speaks et al. (1967) later found that mixing the SSI materials with white noise failed to change the slope of the PI function. However, they also determined that the slope of the function could be significantly flattened if the listener was forced to monitor the sentences in the presence of the competing speech of the same talker who had recorded the sentences. They eventually selected a message-to-competition ratio of 0 dB as a useful ratio for clinical applications and they used the symbol MCR to identify the SSI test administered in the presence of competing speech. Comparisons between the MCR test and conventional speech-discrimination tests administered in quiet revealed that those patients with flat audiometric contours tended to achieve similar scores on the two measures (Speaks *et al.*, 1970a). However, in patients whose audiometric contours sloped toward greater losses in the high frequencies, the MCR test tended to yield higher scores than the conventional PB test. This suggested to Speaks and his co-workers that the SSI–MCR test is more sensitive to low-frequency than to high-frequency threshold sensitivity. Some of Speaks's earlier work had also suggested this, in that the PI function for the sentence materials was found to resemble rather closely that known to characterize spondiac words (Speaks, 1967b).

The SSI–MCR test approach has been employed by Speaks, Jerger, and their associates in a variety of clinical–experimental situations. It may well be, as Jerger and Thelin (1968) observe, that the SSI procedure represents a reasonably valid measure of the individual's ability to understand running speech and a more realistic approach to this assessment than that provided by monosyllabic word tests. However, much remains to be learned before the validity of this statement is established.

C. Standardization: Materials and Methods

In 1960 the American Standards Association, now called the American National Standards Institute, adopted a method for measuring monosyllabic word intelligibility (ASA, 1960). This method, however was intended for the assessment of communications systems and not as a clinical approach. In the almost three decades that speech audiometry has been utilized, no standard testing methods have ever been devised. It is true that an American standard specifying the requirements that must be met by clinical speech audiometers has existed since 1953 (ASA, 1953). That document also specified the reference threshold sound pressure level for speech and outlined the procedures to be followed in expressing the sound pressure level generated by a speech signal. Only very recently these standards have been revised and updated (ANSI, 1969). This new standard specifies the reference threshold sound pressure level for intelligible speech as 19 dB above 0.0002 microbar (0.0002 μbar) based on 50% intelligibility for spondee words. It should be noted that this reference threshold sound pressure level of 19 dB is a coupler pressure that applies to the Western Electric type 705-A earphone and the National Bureau of Standards 9-A coupler. The standard suggests that for the Telephonics TDH-39 earphone, the earphone most often supplied by manufacturers of speech audiometers in the United States, the reference threshold sound pressure level should be 20 dB above 0.0002 μbar.

Thus, clinical speech audiometry in the United States is undergirded by a standard that specifies a reference threshold sound pressure level, a method for expressing the sound pressure level of speech, the electro-acoustic performance characteristics required of speech audiometers and even the type of materials to be employed in establishing the speech reception threshold. (For details see ANSI, 1969.) Curiously, the standard is silent not only with respect to a method for threshold measurement, but also in regard to the suprathreshold measurement of speech intelligibility. It is precisely this lack of standardized materials and procedures, coupled with the enormous complexities involved in the clinical measurement of speech intelligibility that has led to the proliferation of materials and procedures described in the previous section.

Obviously, the choice of both test materials and methods of presentation will differ according to the particular clinical goal. As the next section will make clear, there are several separate and distinct reasons for the clinical assessment of speech intelligibility, and it thus seems unlikely that any one standard set of materials or any single standard method for the clinical assessment of speech intelligibility will ever be adopted. Nevertheless, if speech audiometry is to continue as a viable clinical tool and if its results are to have any universal meaning, certain issues must be faced.

First, one or more sets of speech-discrimination test materials needs to be selected and then the research called for by Silverman and Hirsh (1955) must be conducted. Namely, the validity of the test or tests as measures of everyday receptive communicative efficiency must be established.

Next, the standard materials must be recorded in some fashion so that all clinicians will be able to use the same test materials. The effects produced by varying the "talker" of the test materials have already been reported and these effects must be eliminated if a meaningful standard is to be achieved.

Finally, some minimal requirements relating to test administration need to be established. The concept and usefulness of the PB–MAX are familiar to everyone. However, it is now apparent that it is fruitless to argue that this score can be derived for all clinical patients via the presentation of the test materials at any one intensity level. It is also clear that to plot an entire articulation curve for each individual or each listening condition is not clinically feasible. Under certain conditions, however, the administration of a discrimination test at two different intensity levels can yield far more than twice the information provided by either of the two alone. The point is that no clinical standard for the measurement of speech discrimination will ever provide answers to all or even the majority of clinical problems. Nevertheless, adoption of a standard set of recorded materials and specification of at least minimal procedural requirements is sorely needed to bring order out of chaos.

V. Applications of Speech Audiometry

A. Introduction

Because of the great stability of the relationship between threshold sensitivity for pure-tone and speech stimuli, some authorities, as noted earlier, have taken the position that the measurement of speech reception threshold is largely redundant (Davis and Silverman, 1970). Recognizing that good agreement can be expected between speech and pure-tone sensitivity in the majority of clinical patients, others have emphasized that exceptions to clinical expectations are often critically important. In fact, one of the more reliable indicators of pseudohypoacousis is a speech-reception threshold that is significantly lower (better) than would have been predicted on the basis of the individual's pure-tone audiogram (Carhart, 1952; Chaiklin and Ventry, 1963).

In addition to this diagnostic application, threshold speech audiometry can have other useful applications. For example, the clinician cannot easily assess the threshold shift provided for the individual by a wearable hearing aid using pure-tone audiometry and thus for this purpose speech-threshold testing is almost indispensable.

Other examples could be cited that would "justify" the need for threshold speech audiometry. However, most would agree that the diagnostic and rehabilitative applications of this clinical procedure are somewhat more limited than those of suprathreshold discrimination testing both in quiet and in competition. Therefore, in the remainder of this section, emphasis will focus almost exclusively on the clinical applications of speech-discrimination testing.

B. Diagnostic

In this section, attention is focused entirely on the diagnostic applications of routine speech discrimination testing. The diagnostic uses of the so-called sensitized speech audiometric procedures merit special consideration in another chapter of this book.

Reference has already been made to Walsh's use of the Rush Hughes recordings of the PAL PB-50 lists to differentiate between patients with conductive as opposed to sensorineural hearing loss (Thurlow et al., 1949). Shambaugh (1967) points to the fact that one can expect speech discrimination loss that is out of proportion to the severity and configuration of the pure-tone audiometric loss in patients with Meniere's disease.

He emphasizes also both the qualitative and quantitative difference between patients with Meniere's disease and those with space-occupying lesions involving the eighth cranial nerve. In these latter patients, difficulties in discriminating speech are often so severe that scores of 0% are common, even when such easy test materials as the CID Auditory Test W-22 are employed.

Jerger (1960, 1964) points to the difficulties in speech discrimination that can be produced by central nervous system lesions both at the levels of the brain stem and the temporal cortex. Lesions at these sites tend not to produce losses in threshold sensitivity. Thus, a loss in speech discrimination in a patient whose pure tone audiogram is within normal limits can have real diagnostic significance. It should be emphasized, however, that variability in these diagnostic syndromes is great and unimpaired speech discrimination scores measured via conventional procedures are probably more common.

These observations lead one to the obvious conclusion that routine speech discrimination testing holds somewhat limited diagnostic value. It is undoubtedly for this reason that so many speech discrimination testing procedures employing some form of distortion in such parameters as time and frequency have been developed in the past decade or so. Nevertheless, the value of routine discrimination testing is such that it is almost never omitted in the audiological evaluation of the patient referred for diagnostic testing.

C. Rehabilitative

1. PREDICTING LEVEL OF EVERYDAY EFFICIENCY

As is obvious from the previous discussion, a number of tests and methods are currently available for measuring an individual's threshold for speech reception and his ability to understand speech at suprathreshold levels. However, there have been few systematic attempts to relate results obtained from speech reception and speech discrimination tests to the ability of the hearing-impaired individual to hear and understand speech in everyday listening situations. One purpose of the speech reception threshold is to determine the speech intensity necessary for the individual to just hear speech, understand words, sentences, or connected discourse, that is, whether he can hear soft speech, conversational level speech or only loud speech. The speech discrimination tests are intended to provide some indication as to how well he can understand speech when it is made sufficiently intense to be heard at a comfortable listening level.

An early attempt to utilize speech test results to predict the speech handling capacity of the hearing-impaired person in common work and social situations is the Social Adequacy Index of Silverman et al. (1948). This work grew out of earlier work of Walsh and Silverman in 1946. The Social Adequacy Index was defined as the average speech discrimination score obtained at three levels corresponding to soft, average, and loud speech, using the Rush Hughes recordings of the PAL PB-50 word lists (Silverman et al., 1948). After extensive analysis of speech test data and the results of a questionnaire survey of a large number of patients who had undergone fenestration surgery, it was their observation that an average score of 94% or better (SAI = 94) was within normal limits, that difficulty in hearing and understanding speech would begin with a social adequacy index of 67, and that the "threshold of social adequacy" would be reached with an average speech discrimination score of 33% (SAI = 33).

Davis modified this procedure somewhat by assuming that hearing impairment might be expected to shift the position of the articulation function along the intensity dimension or to decrease the performance level at the plateau of the function but that the shape and slope of the functon would be unaffected by hearing loss. He pointed out that the speech reception threshold (SRT) could be used to locate the point at which the articulation function would intersect the x-axis (intensity) scale and further noted that the plateau of the funcion for a given individual could be located by administering the PAL PB-50 discrimination test at a level of 110 or 120 dB re 0.0002 microbar. He then constructed a table which allowed the clinician to determine the SAI for any combination of threshold hearing level and discrimination loss. The SAI provided a unique method for the clinical evaluation of the effects of surgical or remedial procedures on the social adequacy of an individual's hearing capacity. However, as specified earlier, the research upon which the Social Adequacy Index was based, utilized the relatively difficult Rush Hughes recordings of the PAL PB-50 word lists, and therefore, use of the table published by Davis with a less difficult test such as the CID Auditory Test W-22 would result in unduly optimistic estimates of social adequacy.

A more recent attempt to relate subjective impression of hearing difficulty to speech test results is the Hearing Handicap Scale (High et al., 1964). This scale is a questionnaire completed by the hearing-impaired individual who rates the frequency of his difficulty in hearing on a five-point scale (from almost always to almost never) in various situations. Two forms of the questionnaire are available, each having 20 questions relating to various listening situations. In their evaluation of the relationship between scores on the Hearing Handicap Scale (HHS) and measures of pure-tone threshold, speech-reception threshold, and speech discrimination, High *et al.* (1964) examined 50 hearing-impaired subjects. Correlations between the results from the various audiological measurements and the Hearing Handicap Scale were computed. Relatively high correlations (0.65 or greater) were observed between the results from the Hearing Handicap Scale and either the average pure-tone threshold from 500–2000 Hz or the speech-reception threshold. However, correlations between the speech discrimination scores and the Hearing Handicap Scale data did not reach statistical significance at the 0.05 level. Thus, scores on the HHS appeared to be more closely related to threshold sensitivity than to discriminatory capacity.

Speaks *et al.* (1970b) later confirmed and extended the findings just reported. These investigators correlated scores obtained on a variety of speech test materials with scores yielded on the Hearing Handicap Scale. The strongest relationships observed linked the HHS scores with measures of threshold sensitivity. In discussing their findings, Speaks and his associates point to the fact that the majority of the items on the form of the HHS that they utilized were oriented toward loss in hearing sensitivity.

Nelson (1968) studied a group of 18 persons with sensorineural hearing loss whose speech discrimination scores on CID Auditory Test W-22 ranged from 28 to 100% (mean circa 67%). Nelson correlated results obtained from these individuals on the questionnaire of Dirks and Carhart (1962) with the W-22 discrimination test scores as well as with scores for lists of sentences selected from the synthetic sentences of Speaks and Jerger. (Mean score on the SSI test was 30 correct responses to 33 test sentences.) All speech tests were administered in quiet in a sound field at sensation levels of 30 dB and 25 dB for the W-22 and SSI tests, respectively. The reference intensity in both instances was that corresponding to 50% response to spondee words. Nelson used 24 of the 26 items from the Dirks and Carhart questionnaire but he used a 13-point rating scale as opposed to the five-point scale originally suggested. Using this scheme Nelson obtained a correlation of −0.72 between the questionnaire results and speech discrimination scores for the CID W-22 test. (This negative correlation is in the expected direction since a high score on the questionnaire suggests poor hearing while the reverse is true for the speech test.) Correlation coefficients of only −0.07 and 0.06 were obtained when the questionnaire data were compared with those from the SSI and spondee threshold tests, respectively. Recall that the characteristics of the PI functions for SSI test materials presented in quiet are very similar to those of the articulation function for spondee words. One may conclude from Nelson's findings that results from the

Dirks and Carhart questionnaire appear not to be influenced by threshold sensitivity per se, but that some relationship between speech discrimination scores for monosyllabic word lists and subjective impression of hearing difficulty does exist. This observation points up the need for the questionnaire of Dirks and Carhart to be evaluated further in clinical settings and in systematic research efforts to investigate its applicability as an index of hearing difficulty in everyday life situations and also to provide additional information regarding its relationships to various measurements of hearing for speech.

2. HEARING AID SELECTION

As mentioned previously, the earliest development and application of speech testing materials were directed toward the assessment of the effectiveness of various electronic communications systems. Likewise, the earliest application of tests employing speech stimuli with hearing aids sought to discover the relationships between electroacoustic performance characteristics of carbon-type hearing aids and speech understanding (Hartig and Newhart, 1936). These investigators used both sentences and consonant-vowel-consonant syllables with normal hearing observers to determine the effects of various nonlinear distortion characteristics in carbon-type hearing aids on speech understanding. However, it was Carhart (1946c) who first reported a systematic approach utilizing speech audiometry to assist in the selection of hearing aids for individual patients. He described the use of speech-reception threshold tests, speech discrimination tests, and various other listening experiences for the purpose of assisting veterans in choosing a hearing aid as part of their aural rehabilitation program. The philosophy, as he discussed it in a separate publication (Carhart, 1950) was not to continue testing an individual until the "best" hearing aid had been found for him, but rather to select an acceptable instrument. A different point of view was taken by Shore et al. (1960) who, on the basis of their investigation, contended that differences in speech test results with different hearing aids were not of sufficient magnitude or stability to warrant the time and effort spent in testing hearing-impaired individuals with various hearing aids. Instead, they recommended routine pure tone and speech testing to determine the extent of hearing loss, followed by counseling of the individual relative to his hearing loss, difficulties in communication he would encounter, and in the use of a hearing aid. It was up to the individual to select a hearing aid dealer for the purchase of a hearing aid.

Resnick and Becker (1963) agreed with Shore et al. (1960), but they suggested a somewhat modified procedure. After preliminary clinical evaluation, Resnick and Becker referred all hearing-impaired individuals who were judged to be potential hearing aid users directly to a hearing aid dealer. After selection of an aid by the dealer, the individual returned to the hearing clinic where he underwent speech audiometric tests to determine the adequacy of the hearing aid. As Jeffers and Smith (1964) later pointed out, it seems somewhat contradictory to take the position that speech tests are not useful in the selection of an aid, but are of value in evaluating the adequacy of a given hearing aid for a particular individual once that aid has been selected by a dealer.

Notwithstanding the position taken by Shore et al. (1960) and by Resnick and Becker, it seems clear that at least some of the recent innovations in types of hearing aids such as CROS (Harford and Barry, 1965; Harford and Dodds, 1966; Wullstein and Wigland, 1962) and BICROS (Harford, 1966) have been developed as a result of clinical efforts to assist hearing-impaired persons in the selection of hearing aids. Such innovations might never have come about had all clinicians abandoned the use of speech audiometry in their attempts to assist hearing-impaired individuals in the hearing aid selection process. Even so, it must be recognized that many clinicians have been frustrated in their attempts to differentiate among hearing aids by using speech discrimination tests administered in quiet.

In attempts to improve hearing aid selection procedures, many investigators have employed various speech tests in a background of competition of some type (competing speech, white noise, "cafeteria noise," etc.) Most of these studies have demonstrated differences in speech intelligibility with different hearing aids (Hudgins et al., 1948; Jerger, 1967; Jerger et al., 1966; Jerger and Thelin, 1968; Olsen, 1970; Olsen and Carhart, 1967; and others). The recommendation that performance with hearing aids should be tested in difficult listening conditions, that is, against noise or speech competition of some sort, has been stated often (Berry, 1939; Bleeker and Huizing, 1953; Carhart, 1946c; Carhart and Thompson, 1947; Davis et al., 1946; Fest, 1944; Holmgren, 1939; Olsen and Tillman, 1968; and others), but literature reporting the clinical application and evaluation of such suggestions is lacking. The absence of such reports, and by inference then, the absence of extensive clinical experience in the use of speech tests in noise backgrounds to assist in the selection of hearing aids, may be one of the factors that has contributed to the controversy regarding the clinical utility of the hearing aid selection process.

It is also clear that some important facets of our understanding of the difficulties encountered by hearing-impaired persons in difficult listening situations have come from speech tests conducted in noise or competing speech backgrounds. For example, the head shadow effect which can cumulate to approximately 13 dB in noisy situations for a unilateral hearing loss case or a monaural hearing aid wearer (Carhart, 1965a, 1967a,b; Nordlund and Fritzell, 1963; Olsen and Carhart, 1967; Tillman *et al.*, 1963b; Tillman *et al.*, 1970) was explored at least in part in investigations of performance with monaural and binaural hearing aids. These data have provided practical application of earlier work on the influence of the human head in sound diffraction (Sivian and White, 1933; Wiener, 1947) and of pertinent information regarding its influence on ear level hearing aids (Kasten and Lotterman, 1967; Lybarger and Barron, 1965; Temby, 1965; Wansdronk, 1959).

It is speech testing against a background competition that has also established the validity of what is probably the most common complaint of hearing-impaired persons (with or without hearing aids), that is, they can hear and understand speech reasonably well in quiet environments, but they experience great difficulty and frustration in trying to hear and understand speech of interest to them in noisy environments. This observation has been made often (Ewertsen, 1966: Hallpike, 1934; Mueller, 1953; and others). Studies which have dealt with the speech handling capacity of hearing-impaired persons have consistently shown that speech-to-competition ratios which result in only a slight reduction in speech intelligibility for normal-hearing persons can impose severe restrictions for many persons with sensorineural hearing losses (Carhart, 1967a,b; Carhart, 1970; Olsen and Carhart, 1967; Olsen and Tillman, 1968; Tillman *et al.*, 1970). This work has indicated that a given signal-to-competition ratio may represent a listening condition which can be as much as 14 dB more difficult for individuals with sensorineural hearing loss than for normal-hearing persons. This decrement becomes even greater when the speech and competition are received via hearing aids. Furthermore, the decrease in speech intelligibility is also seen to vary with different hearing aids in these more difficult listening conditions.

From this discussion it is apparent that much work needs to be done to answer questions concerning the applicability of speech audiometry for predicting with some confidence the ability of a hearing-impaired individual to hear and understand speech in everyday life situations. Also, the controversy over the value of speech audiometry in the selection of hearing aids for hearing-impaired persons is not resolved at the present time. However, it would appear that further research directed toward testing speech reception and understanding in noise backgrounds, revival of such concepts as the social adequacy index of Davis, taking into account new and different speech tests, further evaluation of questionnaires such as the Hearing Handicap Scale, the questionnaire of Dirks and Carhart, etc., may provide much needed information to relate speech audiometry results to degrees of difficulty experienced by hearing-impaired persons in everyday life situations with or without hearing aids. Such information is vitally necessary for meaningful audiological counseling and assistance to hearing-impaired individuals.

VI. Summary and Conclusions

Clinical speech audiometry actually grew out of the basic research conducted over 40 years ago by Harvey Fletcher and many others at the Bell Telephone Laboratories. This work, though motivated by very practical considerations, led to a much more comprehensive understanding of the characteristics of the auditory system than had previously existed. This work also produced the first real speech audiometer which, although never used clinically, eventually led to the clinical measurement of the speech reception threshold.

The earliest applications of speech audiometry stressed the measurement of threshold sensitivity utilizing speech testing materials developed to assess the efficiency of communications systems. Establishment of the aural rehabilitation programs by the United States military during World War II resulted in the expansion of speech audiometry to include suprathreshold testing of speech discrimination for both diagnostic and rehabilitative purposes.

As clinical speech audiometry was applied on a wider and wider front, it became apparent that the test materials and techniques available did not always lend themselves to the particular tasks at hand. The result was a flurry of research designed to yield more acceptable methods for assessing the practical consequences of hearing loss.

In 1953 the United States adopted its first set of standards defining the minimum electroacoustic requirements for clinical speech audiometers. This same document specified the standard reference threshold sound pressure level for speech and described a method for measuring the intensity of a speech signal. Still, research was lacking that would establish the validity of existing speech discrimination tests as measures of the everyday significance of hearing impairment.

In 1969 the initial United States standard for speech audiometers was revised and extended. This new document specified the type of test materials to be employed in assessing threshold hearing level for speech, but remained silent on the second and perhaps most critical phase of speech audiometry, measurements of speech discrimination or intelligibility.

Thus, the further refinement of speech audiometry awaits two critical developments. The first is the research needed to provide something more than face validity for the speech discrimination test approach. The second is the development of at least minimal standards for both materials and methods to be employed in speech discrimination testing. Speech audiometry will continue to serve useful functions both in diagnosis and rehabilitation. However, its value in this latter area will increase significantly when the two goals listed here are reached.

References

American National Standards Institute (1970). Specifications for Audiometers. ANSI S3.6-1969. American National Standards Institute, Inc., New York.

American Standards Association (1953). American Standard Specifications for Speech Audiometers. Z24.13-1953. American Standards Association, Inc., New York.

American Standards Association (1960). American Standard Method for Measurement of Monosyllabic Word Intelligibility. ASA-53.2-1960. American Standards Association, Inc., New York.

Berry, S. (1939). The use and effectiveness of hearing aids. *Laryngoscope* **49**, 912–942.

Beyer, M. R., Webster, J. C., and Dague, D. M. (1969). Revalidation of the clinical test version of the modified rhyme words. *J. Speech Hearing Res.* **12**, 374–378.

Bleeker, G. F., and Huizing, H. C. (1953). Speech audiometry and selection of hearing aids. *Proc. 1st Int. Congr. Audiol. Leiden*, 116–120.

Burke, K. S., Shutts, R. E., and King, W. P. (1965). Range of difficulty of four Harvard phonetically balanced word lists. *Laryngoscope* **75**, 289–296.

Campanelli, P. A. (1962). A measure of intra-list stability of four PAL word lists. *J. Auditory Res.* **2**, 50–55.

Carhart, R. (1946a). Monitored live-voice as a test of auditory acuity. *J. Acoust. Soc. Amer.* **17**, 339–349.

Carhart, R. (1946b). Selection of hearing aids. *Arch. Otolaryngol.* **44**, 1–18.

Carhart, R. (1946c). Tests for selection of hearing aids. *Laryngoscope* **56**, 780–794.

Carhart, R. (1950). Hearing aid selection by university clinics. *J. Speech Hearing Dis.* **15**, 103–113.

Carhart, R. (1952). Speech audiometry in clinical evaluation. *Acta Oto-Laryngol.* **41**, 18–42.

Carhart, R. (1960). The determination of hearing loss. Veterans Administration Dept. Med. & Surg. Inform. Bull. IB 10-115. U.S. Govt. Printing Office, Washington, D.C.

Carhart, R. (1965a). Monaural and binaural discrimination against competing sentences. *Int. Audiol.* **4**, 5–10.

Carhart, R. (1965b). Problems in the measurement of speech discrimination. *Arch. Otolaryngol.* **82**, 253–260.

Carhart, R. (1967a). Discussion on the first round table international audiology conference. Mexico City 1967. *Int. Audiol.* **6**, 285–289.

Carhart, R. (1967b). The advantages and limitations of a hearing aid. *Minn. Med.* **50**, 823–826.

Carhart, R. (1970). Problems of the hearing impaired in noisy social gatherings. *In* "Oto-Rhino-Laryngology: Proceedings of the Ninth International Congress," Mexico 1969. Pp. 564–568. Excerpta Medica, Amsterdam.

Carhart, R. (1971). Observations on relations between thresholds for pure tones and for speech. *J. Speech Hearing Dis.* **36**, 476–483.

Carhart, R., and Porter, L. S. (1971). Audiometric configuration and prediction of threshold for spondees. *J. Speech Hearing Res.* 14, 486–495.

Carhart, R., and Thompson, E. A. (1947). The fitting of hearing aids. *Trans. Amer. Acad. Ophthalmol. Otolaryngol.* 51, 354–361.

Chaiklin, J. B., and Ventry, I. M. (1963). Functional hearing loss. In "Modern Developments in Audiology" (J. F. Jerger, ed.). Academic Press, New York.

Clarke, F. R. (1965). Technique for evaluation of speech systems. Final Report from Stanford Research Institute on Contract DA 28-043 AMC-00227 (E). Prepared for U.S. Army Electronics Laboratories, Ft. Monmouth, New Jersey, AD-473 995.

Davis, H. (1948). The articulation area and the social adequacy index for hearing. *Laryngoscope* 58, 761–778.

Davis, H., and Silverman, S. R. (1970). "Hearing and Deafness." Holt, New York.

Davis, H., Hudgins, C. V., Marquis, R. J., Nichols, R. H., Jr., Peterson, G. E., Ross, D. A., and Stevens, S. S. (1946). The selection of hearing aids. *Laryngoscope* 56, 85–163.

Dewey, G. (1923). "Relative Frequency of English Speech Sounds." Harvard Univ. Press, Cambridge, Massachusetts.

Dirks, D. D. and Carhart, R. (1962). A survey of reactions from users of binaural and monaural hearing aids. *J. Speech Hearing Dis.* 27, 311–322.

Egan, J. P. (1948). Articulation testing methods. *Laryngoscope* 58, 955–991.

Elpern, B. S. (1961). The relative stability of half-list speech discrimination tests. *Laryngoscope* 71, 30–36.

Ewertsen, H. (1966). The fitting of hearing aids in Danish rehabilitation centers. *Int. Audiol.* 5, 384–391.

Fairbanks, G. (1958). Test of phonemic differentiation: The Rhyme test. *J. Acoust. Soc. Amer.* 30, 596–600.

Fest, T. B. (1944). Hearing aids: Recent developments. *J. Speech Hearing Dis.* 9, 135–146.

Fletcher, H. (1929). "Speech and Hearing." Van Nostrand-Reinhold, Princeton, New Jersey.

Fletcher, H. (1950). A method of calculating hearing loss for speech from the audiogram. *Acta Oto-Laryngol. Suppl.* 90, 26–37.

Fletcher, H., and Steinberg, J. C. (1929). Articulation testing methods. *Bell Syst. Tech. J.* 7, 806–854.

Fowler, E. P. (1941). Hearing standards for acceptance, disability ratings and discharge in the military service and in industry. *Trans. Amer. Acad. Ophthalmol. Otolaryngol.* 35, 243–263.

Fowler, E. P. (1942). A simple method of measuring percentage of capacity for hearing speech. *Arch. Otolaryngol.* 36, 874–890.

Graham, J. T. (1960). Evaluation of methods for predicting speech reception threshold. *Arch. Otolaryngol.* 72, 347–350.

Hallpike, C. S. (1934). Hearing aids and hearing tests. *J. Laryngol. Otol.* 49, 240–246.

Harford, E. R. (1966). Bilateral CROS two sided listening with one hearing aid. *Arch. Otolaryngol.* 84, 426–432.

Harford, E. R., and Barry, J. (1965). A rehabilitative approach to the problem of unilateral hearing impairment. *J. Speech Hearing Dis.* 30, 121–138.

Harford, E. R., and Dodds, E. (1966). The clinical application of CROS: A hearing aid for unilateral deafness. *Arch. Otolaryngol.* 83, 455–464.

Harris, J. D., Haines, H. L., and Myers, C. K. (1956). A new formula for using the audiogram to predict speech hearing loss. *Arch. Otolaryngol.* 64, 447.

Hartig, H. E., and Newhart, H. (1936). Performance characteristics of electrical hearing aids for the deaf. *Arch. Otolaryngol.* 23, 617–632.

High, W. S., Fairbanks, G., and Glorig, A. (1964). Scale for self-assessment of hearing handicap. *J. Speech Hearing Dis.* 29, 215–230.

Hirsh, I. J., Davis, H., Silverman, S. R., Reynolds, E. G., Eldert, E., and Bensen, R. W. (1952). Development of materials for speech audiometry. *J. Speech Hearing Dis.* 17, 321–337.

Holmgren, L. (1939). Hearing tests and hearing aids. *Acta Oto-Laryngol. Suppl.* 34.

House, A. S., Williams, C. E., Hecker, M. H. L., and Kryter, K. D. (1963). Psychoacoustic speech tests: A modified rhyme test. Technical Documentary Report ESD-TDR-63-403, U.S. Air Force Systems Command, Hanscom Field, Electronic Systems Division.

House, A. S., Williams, C. E., Hecker, M. H. L., and Kryter, K. D. (1965). Articulation testing methods: Consonantal differentiation with a closed response set. *J. Acoust. Soc. Amer.* 37, 158–166.

Hudgins, C. V., Hawkins, J. E., Jr. Karlin, J. E., and Stevens, S. S. (1947). The development of recorded auditory tests for measuring hearing loss for speech. *Laryngoscope* 57, 57–89.

Hudgins, C. V., Marquis, R. J., Nichols, R. H., Jr., Peterson, G. E., and Ross, D. A. (1948). The comparative performance of an experimental hearing aid and two commercial instruments. *J. Acoust. Soc. Amer.* 20, 241–248.

Hughson, W., and Thompson, E. A. (1942). Correlation of hearing acuity for speech with discrete frequency audiograms. *Arch. Otolaryngol.* 36, 526–540.

Jeffers, J., and Smith, C. R. (1964). On hearing aid selection—in part a reply to Resnick and Becker. *Asha* 6, 504–506.

Jerger, J. (1960). Audiological manifestations of lesions in the auditory nervous system. *Laryngoscope* 70, 417–425.

Jerger, J. (1964). Auditory tests for disorders of the central auditory mechanism. *In* "Neurological Aspects of Auditory and Vestibular Disorders," (B. R. Alford and W. S. Fields, eds.). Thomas, Springfield.

Jerger, J. (1967). Behavioral correlates of hearing aid performance. *Bull. Prosthet. Res.* 10-7, 62–75.

Jerger, J., and Jerger, S. (1967). Psychoacoustic comparison of cochlear and VIIIth nerve disorders. *J. Speech Hearing Res.* 10, 659–688.

Jerger, J., and Thelin, J. (1968). Effects of electroacoustic characteristics of hearing aids on speech understanding. *Bull. Prosthet. Res.* 10–10, 159–197.

Jerger, J., Carhart, R., Tillman, T. W., and Peterson, J. L. (1959). Some relations between normal hearing for pure tones and for speech. *J. Speech Hearing Res.* 2, 126–140.

Jerger, J., Malmquist, C., and Speaks, C. (1966). Comparison of some speech intelligibility tests in the evaluation of hearing aid performance. *J. Speech Hearing Res.* 9, 253–258.

Kasten, R. N., and Lotterman, S. H. (1967). Azimuth effects with ear level hearing aids. *Bull. Prosthet. Res.* 10–7, 50–61.

Kreul, E. J., Nixon, J. C., Kryter, K. D., Bell, D. W., Lang, J. S., and Schubert, E. D. (1968). A proposed clinical test of speech discrimination. *J. Speech Hearing Res.* 11, 536–553.

Kreul, E. J., Bell, D. W., and Nixon, J. C. (1969). Factors affecting speech discrimination test difficulty. *J. Speech Hearing Res.* **12**, 281–287.

Kryter, K. D., and Whitman, E. C. (1965). Some comparisons between rhyme and PB-word intelligibility tests. *J. Acoust. Soc. Amer.* **37**, 1146.

Kryter, K. D., Williams, C. E., and Green, D. M. (1962). Auditory acuity and the perception of speech. *J. Acoust. Soc. Amer.* **34**, 1217–1223.

Lehiste, I., and Peterson, G. E. (1959). Linguistic considerations in the study of speech intelligibility. *J. Acoust. Soc. Amer.* **31**, 280–286.

Lightfoot, C., Carhart, R., and Jerger, J. (1953). Efficiency of impaired ears in noise: C. perception of speech at suprathreshold levels. Project No. 21-1203-0001, Report No. 6, USAF School of Aviation Medicine, Randolph Field, Texas.

Lybarger, S. F., and Barron, F. E. (1965). Head baffle effect for different hearing aid microphone locations. *J. Acoust. Soc. Amer.* **38**, 922 (A).

Mueller, W. (1953). The fitting of hearing aids as an office procedure. *Laryngoscope* **63**, 581–592.

Nelson, D. G. (1968). An evaluation of the synthetic syntax sentence test. Master's Thesis, Vanderbilt University.

Nordlund, B., and Fritzell, B. (1963). The influence of azimuth on speech signals. *Acta Oto-Laryngol.* **56**, 632–642.

Olsen, W. O. (1970). Presbycusis and hearing aid use. *J. Acad. Rehabil. Audiol.* **3**, 34–42.

Olsen, W. O., and Carhart, R. (1967). Development of test procedures for evaluation of binaural hearing aids. *Bull. Prosthet. Res.* **10–7**, 22–49.

Olsen, W. O., and Tillman, T. W. (1968). Hearing aids and sensorineural hearing loss. *Ann. Otol. Rhinol. Laryngol.* **77**, 717–726.

Peterson, G. E., and Lehiste, I. (1962). Revised CNC lists for auditory tests. *J. Speech Hearing Dis.* **27**, 62–70.

Quiggle, R. R., Glorig, A., Delk, J. H., and Summerfield, A. B. (1957). Predicting hearing loss for speech from pure tone audiograms. *Laryngoscope* **67**, 1–15.

Resnick, D. M., (1962). Reliability of the twenty-five word phonetically balanced lists. *J. Auditory Res.* **2**, 5–12.

Resnick, D. M., and Becker, M. (1963). Hearing aid evaluation—a new approach. *Asha* **5**, 695–699.

Sabine, P. E. (1942). On estimating the percentage of loss of useful hearing. *Trans. Amer. Acad. Ophthalmol. Otolaryngol.* **46**, 179–196.

Schultz, M. C., and Schubert, E. D. (1969). A multiple choice discrimination test (MCDT). *Laryngoscope* **79**, 382–399.

Shambaugh, G. E., Jr. (1967). "Surgery of the Ear." Saunders, Philadelphia.

Shore, I., Bilger, R. C., and Hirsh, I. J. (1960). Hearing aid evaluation: Reliability of repeat measurements. *J. Speech Hearing Dis.* **25**, 152–170.

Shutts, R. E., Burke, K. S., and Creston, J. E. (1964). Derivation of twenty-five word PB lists. *J. Speech Hearing Res.* **29**, 442–447.

Siegenthaler, B. M., and Strand, R. (1964). Audiogram average methods and SRT scores. *J. Acoust. Soc. Amer.* **36**, 589–593.

Silverman, S. R., and Hirsh, I. J. (1955). Problems related to the use of speech in clinical audiometry. *Ann. Otol. Rhinol. Laryngol.* **64**, 1234–1244.

Silverman, S. R., Thurlow, W. R., Walsh, T. E., and Davis, H. (1948). Improvement in the social adequacy index of hearing following the fenestration operation. *Laryngoscope* **58**, 607–631.

Sivian, L. J., and White, S. D. (1933). Minimum audible fields. *J. Acoust. Soc. Amer.* **4**, 288–321.

Speaks, C. (1967a). Intelligibility of filtered synthetic sentences. *J. Speech Hearing Res.* **10**, 289–298.

Speaks, C. (1967b). Performance-intensity characteristics of selected verbal materials. *J. Speech Hearing Res.* **10**, 344–347.

Speaks, C., and Jerger, J. (1965). Method for measurement of speech identification. *J. Speech Hearing Res.* **8**, 185–194.

Speaks, C., Karmen, J. L., and Benitez, L. (1967). Effect of a competing message on synthetic sentence identification. *J. Speech Hearing Res.* **10**, 390–395.

Speaks, C., Jerger, J., and Trammel, J. (1970a). Comparison of sentence identification and conventional speech discrimination scores. *J. Speech Hearing Res.* **13**, 755–767.

Speaks, C., Jerger, J., and Trammel, J. (1970b). Measurement of hearing handicap, *J. Speech Hearing Res.* **13**, 768–776.

Temby, A. C. (1965). Sound diffraction in the vicinity of the human ear. *Acustica* **15**, 219–222.

Thorndike, E. L., and Lorge, I. (1944, 1952). "The Teacher's Word Book of 30,000 Words." Columbia Univ. Press, New York.

Thurlow, W. R., Davis, H., Silverman, S. R., and Walsh, T. E. (1949). Further statistical study of auditory tests in relation to the fenestration operation. *Laryngoscope* **59**, 113–129.

Tillman, T. W., and Carhart, R. (1966). An expanded test for speech discrimination utilizing CNC monosyllabic words Northwestern University Auditory Test No. 6. Technical Report No. SAM-TR-66-55, USAF School of Aerospace Medicine, Brooks Air Force Base, Texas.

Tillman, T. W., and Jerger, J. (1959). Some factors affecting the spondee threshold in normal hearing subjects. *J. Speech Hearing Res.* **2**, 141–146.

Tillman, T. W., Carhart, R., and Wilber, L. (1963a). A Test for Speech Discrimination Composed of CNC Monosyllabic Words, Northwestern University Auditory Test No. 4. Technical Documentary Report No. SAM-TDR-62-135, USAF School of Aerospace Medicine, Brooks, Air Force Base, Texas.

Tillman, T. W., Kasten, R. N., and Horner, J. S. (1963b). Effect of head shadow on reception of speech. *Asha* **5**, 778–779. (A)

Tillman, T. W., Carhart, R., and Olsen, W. O. (1970). Hearing aid efficiency in a competing speech situation. *J. Speech Hearing Res.* **13**, 789–811.

Tobias, J. V. (1964). On phonemic analysis of speech discrimination tests. *J. Speech Hearing Res.* **7**, 98–100.

Walsh, T. E. (1964). Informal comment. *Trans. Amer. Otol. Soc.* **52**, 79.

Walsh, T. E., and Silverman, S. R. (1946). Diagnosis and evaluation of fenestration. *Laryngoscope* **56**, 536–555.

Wansdronk, C. (1959). On the influence of the diffraction of sound waves around the human head on characteristics of hearing aids. *J. Acoust. Soc. Amer.* **31**, 1609–1612.

Wiener, F. M. (1947). On the diffraction of a progressive wave by the human head. *J. Acoust. Soc. Amer.* **19**, 143–146.

Wullstein, H. L., and Wigland, M. E. (1962). A hearing aid for single ear deafness and its requirements. *Acta Oto-Laryngol.* **54**, 136–142.

Chapter 3

Diagnostic Audiometry

JAMES JERGER

Baylor College of Medicine

I. Introduction

In a sense, all audiometry is diagnostic since it contributes, in some sense, to the ultimate localization of the auditory disorder. The relationship between air-conduction and bone-conduction thresholds, for example, is one of the principal bases for differentiating conductive from sensorineural hearing loss. In this chapter, however, attention will be confined to those specialized techniques that have been advanced in relatively recent years for the express purpose of sharpening the ability to differentiate among the various sites of auditory disorder.

This chapter outlines, in general terms, some useful diagnostic test procedures, and describes the expected outcomes for different sites of lesion. In addition, it presents some illustrative case material showing how the pattern of diagnostic test results changes with site of lesion.

The list of diagnostic procedures given in this chapter is by no means exhaustive. From the several score of special auditory tests that have been proposed from time to time over the past two decades, only those techniques and procedures that seem to have some possibility of enduring value have been selected for comprehensive discussion.

A. Distinction between Peripheral and Central Disorders

It is important to distinguish at the onset between tests especially suited to the evaluation of the peripheral auditory system and tests more appropriate to the evaluation of the central auditory system. Although subsequent research may alter the boundary somewhat, it seems useful, at this point, to define a line of demarcation just at the synapse between first- and second-order neurons of the afferent auditory pathway in the dorsal and ventral cochlear nuclei. Lesions distal to this boundary may be said to affect the peripheral system. The three principal loci of disorder in the peripheral system are: (1) the middle ear, (2) the cochlea, and (3) the eighth nerve.

Lesions proximal to the boundary at the first synapse may be said to affect the central auditory system. The two principal loci of disorder in the central system are: (1) the brainstem pathway in the lateral lemniscus, and (2) the primary auditory projection area (Heschl's gyrus) on the superior convolution of the temporal lobe.

The distinction between peripheral and central loci is necessary and useful because peripheral disorders modify the system's response to auditory signals in a fundamentally different way from central disorders. Hence test procedures specifically designed to differentiate among peripheral loci are usually not appropriate for the evaluation of central disorder, and vice versa.

B. Characteristics of Peripheral and Central Disorders

Peripheral disorders share some or all of the following common characteristics: (1) sensitivity loss, (2) distortion, (3) abnormal adaptation, and (4) ipsilateral symptoms.

Central disorders, on the other hand, share the common characteristics of virtually normal sensitivity and contralateral symptoms.

A characteristic common to both categories is impairment in the ability to transmit complex signals like speech. As a result, loss in the ability to understand speech is a trait common to both peripheral and central disorders.

The peripheral characteristics of sensitivity loss, distortion, and abnormal adaptation are uniquely suited to exploration with pure-tone test signals. By taking advantage of the spectral concentration of energy in pure-tone signals we can define the pattern of sensitivity loss, the nature and extent of distortion, and the time course of adaptation. In central disorders, however, these peripheral symptoms are usually lacking. Hence, most tests based on pure-tone signals are usually performed well by the patient with central disorder and, to this date, have proven instructive largely in a negative sense (Bocca and Calearo, 1963). It is not surprising, therefore, that tests employing pure-tone signals play a more important role in the evaluation of peripheral than central disorders, whereas tests employing speech signals are important in the evaluation of both peripheral and central disorders.

II. Peripheral Test Battery

The purpose of the peripheral test battery is to differentiate among the three possible peripheral sites: the middle ear, the cochlea, and the eighth nerve. The total battery consists of three primary and three reserve tests as follows:

Primary tests
    Impedance audiometry
    Békésy audiometry
    Performance–intensity (PI) function for phonetically balanced (PB) words

Reserve tests
    Short-increment sensitivity index (SISI) test
    Alternate binaural loudness balance (ABLB) test
    Tone decay test

A. Impedance Audiometry

The examination begins with impedance audiometry (Alberti and Kristensen, 1970; Brooks, 1969; Feldman, 1964; Jerger, 1970c; Lidén, 1969; Terkildsen and Scott-Nielsen, 1960; Thomsen, 1955; Zwislocki, 1961). This powerful procedure establishes, with little ambiguity, whether the middle ear is or is not functioning normally. Impedance audiometry yields data in three categories: (1) The tympanogram (Brooks, 1968; Jerger, 1970c; Lidén et al., 1970) is a graphic portrayal of the relation between air pressure in the external canal and impedance in the plane of the eardrum. (2) The static impedance (Bicknell and Morgan, 1968; Brooks, 1971; Feldman, 1963, 1964; Zwislocki and Feldman, 1969) is a factor proportional to the mobility of the ossicular mechanism. (3) The threshold of the stapedius reflex (Jepsen, 1963; Klockhoff, 1961; Metz, 1951; Møller, 1958) in response to pure tones of varying frequency is a sensitive index of the entire stapedius reflex arc. Middle ear disorders usually affect all three measures (Jerger, 1970c; Lidén, 1969). Chronic adhesive otitis media, for example, alters the normal shape of the tympanogram drastically, lowers the maximum static compliance[1] significantly, and abolishes the stapedius reflex.

The outcome of impedance audiometry leads to the first diagnostic decision. If the tympanogram is abnormal, and the maximum static compliance is outside the normal range, then there is strong evidence of a middle ear site. If further diagnostic information is desired, one may now turn to any of the variety of special techniques especially designed for the evaluation of conductive loss (for example, the audiometric Weber test, the audiometric Bing test, the sensorineural acuity level (SAL) test, or conventional bone-conduction audiometry).

Suppose, however, that the outcome of impedance audiometry is not consistent with a middle ear site. The tympanogram is normal and maximum static compliance is within normal limits. This establishes that the loss is sensorineural. The possibility of a middle ear site can be ruled out. Now the problem is to differentiate cochlear from eighth nerve disorder.

Here, again, impedance audiometry yields a valuable clue. If the stapedius reflex is observed when sound is presented to the ear in question, and if the reflex is observed at a sensation level less than 60 dB, then loudness recruitment is present in the test ear and a cochlear site is strongly presumed (Ewertsen et al., 1958; Jerger, 1970c; Lamb et al., 1968; Metz, 1952). If, on the other hand, the stapedius reflex cannot be demonstrated on the test ear, despite only mild-to-moderate sensitivity loss, then loudness recruitment is absent and an eighth nerve site is strongly indicated. The interpretation that absent reflexes indicate

---

[1] The static impedance of the middle ear has two principal components, one due to resistance, the other due primarily to compliance (see Chapter 10). In addition, both components may be measured either at ambient atmospheric pressure in the external canal or at that canal air pressure (usually slightly negative) which produces minimum impedance. In actual clinical diagnostic use, the most useful measure of static impedance is the compliance measured at the air pressure yielding minimum impedance (maximum compliance). In subsequent sections, this measure is termed "maximum static compliance," or simply "maximum compliance."

lack of loudness recruitment is possible, of course, only if the sensitivity loss does not exceed about 70 dB (ISO-64). If the sensitivity loss exceeds 70 dB, then the lack of reflex is ambiguous. Its absence could simply be due to the fact that the auditory signal never attains a loudness sufficient to elicit the reflex whether loudness recruitment is present or not. But if the sensitivity loss is less than 70 dB, the absence of stapedius reflex should lead to the strong presumption of eighth nerve site.

In a very small proportion of eighth nerve disorders, the reflex may be observed at some frequencies; but in these cases, careful study of the time course of the reflex will usually demonstrate pathological adaptation (Anderson et al., 1969). To test for this "reflex decay," the examiner simply holds the tone on for 20–30 sec and observes whether the reflex amplitude maintains its initial level or whether it declines rapidly to the base line.

The stapedius reflex thresholds, then, provide the basis for the second diagnostic decision, whether the loss is likely to be cochlear or eighth nerve. If reflexes are present and do not decay significantly over time, then a cochlear site is probable. If, however, despite sensitivity loss less than 70 dB the reflexes are either absent, or are present but demonstrate excessive decay over time, an eighth nerve site must be suspected. Subsequent diagnostic testing should be designed to confirm or deny this initial impression.

B. Békésy Audiometry

The most useful test procedure to administer next is Békésy audiometry (Jerger, 1960c). The first step is the set of sweep-frequency tracings for interrupted and continuous tones. The overall pattern emerging from this procedure indicates frequency regions of particular interest and value for subsequent fixed or discrete-frequency tracings. The occurrence of a Type I or Type II Békésy audiogram serves to confirm the impression of cochlear site. On the other hand, the occurrence of a Type III or Type IV pattern confirms the initial impression of an eighth nerve site (Owens, 1964). In the event of ambiguity in the classification of the conventional sweep or discrete-frequency tracings, further sharpening can often be achieved by running the continuous tone tracings again, but this time with the frequency beginning at the high end (8000–10,000 Hz) and moving in the high-to-low direction (that is, backward) in contrast to the conventional low-to-high direction. Sometimes the presence of abnormal adaptation will be revealed by a significant discrepancy between the continuous-forward trace and the continuous-backward trace even though the conventional continuous–interrupted relation is not remarkable (Jerger et al., 1972; Palva et al., 1970).

C. PI–PB Function

It is profitable to follow Békésy audiometry with a detailed study of the performance versus intensity (PI) function for PB word lists (Jerger and Jerger, 1971). In the ear with cochlear disorder, the function will typically rise to its maximum, then level off and maintain a plateau as intensity is further increased. There may be a slight decline in performance at very high speech intensities, but the effect, if present, is not substantial. In the ear with eighth nerve disorder, however, the function will typically show a pronounced "rollover" or decline in performance as speech intensity is raised above the level yielding maximum performance. The rollover phenomenon in the PI–PB function in eighth nerve sites is often quite dramatic. Performance may, for example, rise to a maximum of 70–80% at, for example, 80 dB sound pressure level (SPL), then decline to as low as 0–10% as speech level is increased to 110 dB.

D. Summary of Primary Test Battery

This primary three-test battery, consisting of impedance, Békésy, and speech audiometry, is often sufficient to produce a clear-cut picture consistent with either cochlear or eighth nerve site. In the case of cochlear site, stapedius reflex will be present [if hearing threshold level (HTL) does not exceed 70 dB], the Békésy audiogram will be Type I or Type II, and the PI–PB function will show little or no rollover. In the case of eighth nerve site, the stapedius reflex will either be absent or show abnormal decay, the Békésy audiogram will be Type III or Type IV, and the PI–PB function will typically show a marked "rollover."

In many patients, however, a variety of circumstances may conspire against a clear and unambiguous result. The hearing loss may be so great that absence of the reflex is no longer diagnostic; or the reflex, if present, may decay as much in the good ear as in the bad ear, a not-uncommon problem at frequencies in the region of 4000 Hz. The severity of loss may make the distinction between a Type II and a Type III Békésy audiogram difficult; or the Békésy outcome may simply not be sufficiently valid and reliable to classify. Similarly, the loss in PB performance may be so severe that the PI–PB function never rises high enough to achieve rollover.

E. Reserve Tests

Under any or all of these circumstances it will often prove advantageous to administer a further battery of reserve tests; the SISI test (Jerger *et al.*, 1959; Owens, 1965), the tone-decay test (Carhart, 1957;

Hopkinson and Thomas, 1967; Parker and Decker, 1971), and the ABLB test (Graham, 1967; Jerger and Harford, 1960). Since these three "backup" tests are not quite so adversely affected by degree of loss as the primary tests, they can often yield valuable information when the primary tests cannot.

The SISI test result should be positive in cochlear disorders but negative in eighth nerve disorders. The tone decay test should be negative in cochlear disorders but positive in eighth nerve disorders. Finally, the ABLB test should reflect the presence of loudness recruitment in cochlear disorders but not in eighth nerve disorders.

F. Frequency Dependence of Peripheral Signs

One complicating factor in the interpretation of all tests in the peripheral battery, both primary and reserve, is the frequency dependence of test results. In cochlear disorders the symptomatology is uniquely related to test frequency. Cochlear signs are, by and large, high-frequency signs. There is usually little indication of abnormality at frequencies of 250 or 500 Hz. Cochlear signs are usually evident only at frequencies above 1000 Hz. The SISI score, for example, will usually be quite low (0–20%) at 250 and 500 Hz, questionable (40–60%) at 1000 Hz, and very high (80–100%) at 2000, 3000, and 4000 Hz. Similarly, the tone decay test in cochlear disorders ordinarily shows little decay at 250 and 500 Hz, but mild to moderate decay (10–20 dB) at 2000, 3000, and 4000 Hz. And, of course, the Type II Békésy tracing is defined by the fact that the continuous trace usually falls below the interrupted trace at frequencies above 300–1000 Hz but seldom below this range.

It is a useful point of diagnostic distinction that eighth nerve disorders typically do not exhibit this frequency dependence. The abnormalities characterizing the eighth nerve site may appear at any point on the frequency scale and may occupy only a small segment, or the bulk, of the range of test frequencies. Abnormal adaptation, for example, may appear at 4000 Hz only, or may be present at frequencies as low as 125 Hz. In the analysis of diagnostic test results, therefore, it is useful to consider the frequency range over which signs and symptoms appear. In general, eighth nerve signs appearing in the low-frequency range below 1000 Hz should be given more weight than the same symptoms when they occur only in the 4000-Hz region.

G. Qualifications

The overall strategy of the peripheral test battery is recapitulated, in simplified schematic fashion, in Figure 1. Here are summarized the expected outcomes of the various tests for each of the three possible

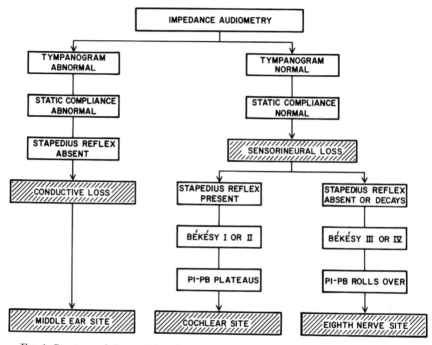

FIG. 1. Strategy of the peripheral test battery. Tympanogram and static compliance determine whether loss is conductive or sensorineural. Stapedius reflexes, Békésy audiograms, and PI–PB functions determine whether sensorineural site is cochlear or eighth nerve.

sites: middle ear, cochlea, and eighth nerve. It should be emphasized, at this point, that the schemata of Figure 1 represent only the likely or expected outcome at each site. It should not be interpreted to mean that all patients will fit this pattern precisely. Inevitably the fit between idealized expectation and reality will be less than perfect.

Furthermore, it is absolutely critical that *site* of disorder not be confused with *type* of disorder. Since acoustic tumors account for a substantial proportion of eighth nerve disorders, there is a tendency to equate such tumors with eighth nerve site (Brand and Rosenberg, 1963; Naunton, 1967), thereby blurring the distinction between site of disorder and type of disorder. One unfortunate consequence of this blurred distinction is the expectation that all patients with acoustic tumors should show only eighth nerve signs.

Let it be reemphasized, therefore, that an acoustic tumor is not necessarily synonymous with an exclusively eighth nerve site. Hood and his associates have emphasized for many years that acoustic tumors and, indeed, many other neoplasms of the cerebellopontine angle can affect the cochlea as well as the eighth nerve (Dix and Hood, 1953; Hood, 1969). It is certainly conceivable that in some patients with an acoustic tumor, cochlear signs may be quite pronounced and may effectively mask concomitant eighth nerve signs. If, therefore, a patient with a surgically confirmed acoustic tumor yields a preoperative picture consistent with a cochlear site, this does not necessarily indicate a failure of diagnostic audiometry. The auditory findings may simply be reflecting the fact of concomitant cochlear involvement. Rather, if there is a "failure" in this situation, it is the failure of nature to provide *types* of auditory disorder that always bear one-to-one correspondence with *sites* of disorder. Diagnostic audiometry is necessarily limited to *site* of disorder. It claims only that certain test outcomes are the inevitable consequence of disorders at certain sites, that the patient's behavioral response to appropriately constituted auditory tasks will be uniquely modified by the site of the auditory disorder. It can make no claim to identify the type of disorder. Thus, the presence of predominantly cochlear signs does not necessarily preclude the possibility of an acoustic tumor. Nor does the presence of predominantly eighth nerve signs necessarily preclude the possibility of a primarily cochlear disorder. In the case of multiple sites of disorder we do not yet possess techniques for assessing the relative contributions of the multiple sites to the modification of test performance. The challenge to the audiologist in this situation is twofold: first, to interpret, in proper perspective, to his medical colleagues the role and contribution of diagnostic audiometry to otologic and otoneurologic diagnosis; second, to sharpen existing tools and to develop, if necessary, new tools for increasing the sensitivity of the peripheral test battery to the relative contributions of disorders at both the cochlear and eighth nerve levels.

H. Some Revealing Statistics

The actual statistics on the outcome of diagnostic audiometry in patients with acoustic tumors are interesting. The most extensive series of patients was reported by Johnson (1968). His results indicate that if only two diagnostic tests—SISI and Békésy—are administered, 54% of patients with acoustic tumors will show eighth nerve signs on both tests, and 60–70% will show eighth nerve signs on at least one test. Only about 20% will show cochlear signs on both tests. These results are extremely encouraging, especially in view of the high probability of concomitant cochlear disorder in acoustic tumors, either because of interruption of the cochlear blood supply (Perez de Moura, 1967) or because of changes in the chemistry of the cochlear fluids (Benitez *et al.*, 1967; Perez de Moura, 1967). Johnson's data show that despite the fact that acoustic tumors may produce lesions in both the cochlea and the eighth nerve, the eighth nerve symptoms predominate.

More detailed findings are provided by Buxton (1970). This investigator surveyed the literature from 1948 to 1970 and found 73 papers reporting some diagnostic test data on patients with either medically diagnosed Meniere's disease or surgically confirmed acoustic tumor. Buxton then tabulated results according to whether the outcome of a particular test was or was not consistent with the site of disorder (cochlear in the case of Meniere's disease, and eighth nerve in the case of acoustic tumor).

The SISI test result was considered cochlear if the reported score exceeded 60%, eighth nerve if the score was less than 60%. The tone decay test (TDT) result was considered cochlear if the decay did not exceed 30 dB, and eighth nerve if decay exceeded 30 dB. Types I or II Békésy audiograms were considered cochlear, while Types III or IV were considered eighth nerve. The alternate binaural loudness balance (ABLB) test was considered cochlear if loudness recruitment was partial or complete, and eighth nerve if loudness recruitment was absent.

Table I summarizes Buxton's findings. Each entry for a particular site includes the number of studies reporting data (N_s), the number of patients for whom data were reported (N_p), and the percentage of patients whose results on that test were consistent with expectation. One of the most striking findings revealed by the data of Table I is the remarkable stability of the percentages across the various tests. With the single exception of the TDT, all percentages are between 95 and 98 for patients with Meniere's disease. In other words, with the exception of TDT, the false-positive rate (that is, false-positive for eighth

TABLE I

PERCENTAGE OF PATIENTS WITH MENIERE'S DISEASE AND ACOUSTIC TUMOR SHOWING EXPECTED OUTCOMES ON VARIOUS DIAGNOSTIC TESTS[a]

	Disorder					
	Meniere's			Acoustic tumor		
Test	N_s[b]	N_p[c]	Percentage	N_s	N_p	Percentage
SISI	5	76	95	15	272	80
TDT	9	301	73	13	90	76
Békésy	6	177	98	16	283	67
ABLB	15	504	96	17	118	67

[a] From Buxton (1970).
[b] N_s = number of studies reporting data.
[c] N_p = number of patients reported.

nerve site) in true cochlear disorders varied from 2 to 5%. In the case of TDT, however, the false-positive rate was 27%. This relatively high false-positive rate is probably related to the nature of the response required from the patient. Reporting the moment when a signal disappears from consciousness is a judgment plagued by procedural error, especially in the case of naive listeners. It is not surprising, therefore, that the TDT shows a high false-positive rate. The three other procedures do not seem to be subject to this limitation, probably because they emphasize the detection of signal onset rather than signal disappearance. This is especially true of SISI, and determines at least half of the judgments required by Békésy audiometry. The best single test for cochlear site would appear to be Békésy audiometry (98% accurate), although the differences among Békésy, SISI, and ABLB are not great.

In the case of patients with acoustic tumor, Buxton's survey shows results in remarkable agreement with Johnson's data cited earlier. The expected outcome ranges from 67 to 80%. Thus the false-negative rate (that is, false-negative for eighth nerve site) ranges from 20 to 33%. The SISI test (80%) shows the highest rate of expected outcome, but TDT is not far behind at 76%. Both Békésy and ABLB are 67% accurate. As noted earlier, the high false-negative rate in patients with acoustic tumor is undoubtedly related to the expected occurrence of cochlear as well as eighth nerve disorder in many of these patients. Interestingly, the best test of these four, from an overall point of view, is SISI. Its combined false-identification rate for both Meniere's disease and acoustic tumor is only 25%. The TDT fares least well with a combined false-identification rate of 51%.

Because diagnostic audiometry is concerned with site, not type, of auditory disorder, it is not a method for diagnosing acoustic tumors. It does, however, provide site information that may be extremely helpful in supplementing other diagnostic data. The following principles of interpretation must, however, be borne in mind:

I. Principles of Test Interpretation

1. An eighth nerve pattern on diagnostic audiometry does not necessarily mean that an acoustic tumor is present. The eighth nerve signs indicate only eighth nerve site. Acoustic tumor is only one of several types of disorder that have an eighth nerve site. Although acoustic tumors are probably the most common source of auditory disorder at the eighth nerve level, viral infection, vascular insult, trauma, and multiple sclerosis are other etiologies of hearing loss that must be considered.

2. A cochlear pattern on diagnostic audiometry does not necessarily mean that an acoustic tumor is not present. There is a definite probability (20% in Johnson's series) that the patient with acoustic tumor will

show only cochlear signs on both SISI and Békésy. It is a reasonable assumption that, in these patients, the cochlea is involved to a relatively greater extent than the eighth nerve and the cochlear signs override the eighth nerve signs. The challenge to the audiologist is to devise test procedures that will reveal the eighth nerve involvement in spite of cochlear signs.

Viewed in this context, diagnostic audiometry can assist in the otoneurologic diagnosis of acoustic tumor in the following ways:

1. Eighth nerve signs in any patient with unilateral or asymmetrical hearing loss should alert one to the possibility of an acoustic tumor, with the understanding, however, that there are other types of disorders that can cause eighth nerve hearing loss.

2. If the patient's history and other physical findings are not clear-cut but suggest the possibility of an acoustic tumor, diagnostic audiometry can supplement the overall picture by either confirming or failing to confirm that the hearing loss has an eighth nerve site, with the understanding that consistent cochlear findings, while unlikely, do not necessarily rule out the possibility of acoustic tumor.

3. If the patient's history and other physical findings are strongly suggestive of an acoustic tumor, diagnostic audiometry can supplement the overall picture by confirming that the hearing loss has an eighth nerve site; again, however, with the qualification that failure to demonstrate eighth nerve signs does not necessarily rule out the possibility of acoustic tumor.

III. Central Test Battery

A. Central System Defined

The central auditory system may be broadly defined as that portion of the total auditory system lying within the central nervous system. It includes chiefly the brainstem pathways (Jungert, 1958) and the primary auditory projection areas on the superior temporal gyri (Tunturi, 1960). The central auditory system consists of two crossed pathways. Each pathway begins at the synapse between first- and second-order neurons in the cochlear nuclei, then crosses to the opposite side of the brain either directly or via the superior olivary complex. The pathway then rises in the lateral lemniscus to the medial geniculate body in the thalamus. From this synaptic level fourth-order neurons, the "auditory radiations," project to a small area on the superior gyrus of the temporal lobe, Heschl's gyrus or the primary auditory area on the cerebral cortex.

This primary auditory area is by no means the end of the system. We know very little, however, about the subsequent pathways beyond this point. We can only speculate that further pathways ultimately link auditory cortex with language centers in the precentral and parietal areas, and with association areas linked to other sensory inputs (Penfield and Roberts, 1959).

We do know that each of the two crossed pathways is rather elaborately interconnected with the other pathways throughout the course of second- and third-order neurons (Jungert, 1958). Furthermore, fourth-order neurons are probably interconnected via the corpus callosum (Milner *et al.*, 1968).

Interestingly, we will see later that some manifestations of central auditory disorder reflect this elaborate interconnection while other manifestations seem to be unaware of its existence. Furthermore, we will see that the crossed pathway concept has demonstrable reality. Lesions of either pathway proximal to the crossover point in the brainstem will invariably produce symptoms in the ear opposite to the affected side of the brain, that is, in the ear to which the crossed pathway is, in effect, connected.

B. The Italian Pioneers

It has often been observed that science seldom proceeds with a steady, even pace. Rather, it often languishes on a given plateau of knowledge for long periods until some dramatic breakthrough, some significant new insight rapidly accelerates the ascent to new heights of understanding. In the case of central auditory disorders, a 100-year dry spell ended abruptly with the publication of the now-classic paper, "Testing 'Cortical' Hearing in Temporal Lobe Tumors," by the Italian Bocca and his colleagues (1955). These investigators showed for the first time that in patients with unilateral temporal lobe disease, a deficit in speech understanding could be demonstrated on the ear contralateral to the affected temporal lobe. This unilateral deficit was demonstrable despite virtually normal pure-tone sensitivity in both ears. They showed, further, that the unilateral deficit could be enhanced by systematically increasing the difficulty of the speech intelligibility task either through low-pass filtering, temporal interruption, or acceleration. These fundamental observations formed the basis for a renewed attack on the problem of central auditory disorder.

The next significant development was Calearo's (1957) observation that patients with central auditory disorder often demonstrated deficits in the ability to fuse binaural, coherent messages (that is, the same signal to both ears). This fundamental observation was subsequently elaborated by Matzker (1957, 1958), Linden (1964), Ohta *et al.* (1967), and Antonelli (1970a). Concurrently Kimura (1961), in Montreal, opened a Pandora's box (Berlin and Lowe, 1972; Kimura, 1963, 1967; Milner, 1962; Studdert-Kennedy and Shankweiler, 1970) with the observation that patients with temporal lobe disorders showed deficits in the ability to attend and to respond appropriately to binaural, noncoherent messages (Broadbent, 1956) (that is, different signals to the two ears). The binaural noncoherent paradigm is called "dichotic" listening.

These fundamental observations form the theoretical foundation for the clinical evaluation of central auditory problems. Test procedures are based on the following basic tenets:

1. The patient will ordinarily show no significant "hearing loss," in the sense of decreased sensitivity for pure tones, on either ear (Antonelli *et al.*, 1963; Parker *et al.*, 1968).

2. The patient will ordinarily demonstrate little or no difficulty with pure-tone tasks of the type so useful in the evaluation of peripheral disorders (Bocca and Calearo, 1963; Jerger, 1964; Lidén, 1969).

3. The primary symptom will be difficulty in understanding speech presented to the ear opposite the affected side of the brain (Antonelli, 1970b; Jerger, 1960a, Lidén, 1969).

4. Speech intelligibility tasks involving binaural, noncoherent signals (simultaneous dichotic listening) will be especially sensitive to temporal lobe disorders (Dobie and Simmons, 1971; Feldmann, 1967; Katz *et al.*, 1963; Kimura, 1961; Sparks *et al.*, 1970).

C. Problems in Central Test Construction

Within this frame of reference, the construction of a central auditory test battery is largely a strategic problem of designing test procedures that tap the patient's performance potential at precisely the proper level of difficulty and with a minimum of error variance. The problem of test difficulty cannot be overemphasized. In the case of peripheral auditory disorders, the homogeneity of patient performance is usually so good that a given level of difficulty in a listening task is suitable for the vast majority of patients. In the case of central auditory disorder, however, such homogeneity does not exist. A listening task that is vastly too difficult for one patient may be surprisingly simple for another. In order to demonstrate the presence of central disorder effectively, therefore, it is necessary to adjust the difficulty of the listening task to match the extent of the patient's disorder. This is a basic weakness of many of the scores of test procedures that have been proposed for the evaluation of central auditory disorder during the past decade. They may work well with the patients on whom they were developed, but the level of difficulty cannot be manipulated to meet the needs of all patients with central auditory disorder.

The central test battery proposed below enjoys no theoretical advantage over the many other available procedures. It is based on the same basic principles. Its salient feature, however, is that the procedures have been designed in such a way that there is substantial flexibility in the extent to which the difficulty of the listening task can be adjusted to meet the needs of virtually any patient.

The primary central test battery consists of three speech-audiometric procedures: (1) The performance–intensity function for PB words (PI–PB) (Jerger and Jerger, 1971). (2) Synthetic sentence identification (SSI) in the presence of an ipsilateral competing message (SSI–ICM) (Jerger, 1970a, 1970b; Jerger et al., 1968; Speaks and Jerger, 1965). (3) Synthetic sentence identification in the presence of a contralateral competing message (SSI–CCM) (Jerger, 1970b).

D. PI–PB Function

The PI–PB function is useful in central disorders for two reasons. First, it performs an important role as a screening technique for detecting central problems. Any patient who shows a consistent ear difference on PI–PB functions in the absence of a pure-tone sensitivity difference sufficient to account for the ear difference on a peripheral basis must be suspected of central auditory disorder. Second, the PI–PB functions help to define the extent of the central problem. The performance deficit will typically appear on the ear contralateral to the affected side of the brain. In addition, rollover of the PI–PB function may occur. The presence of rollover, in the absence of sensitivity loss, is a further confirmatory sign of a central problem. The PI–PB function works well as a screening device primarily because, for patients with central disorder, PB word repetition is usually a relatively difficult listening task. Hence an ear difference of 20–30% is often demonstrable.

There are many patients, however, for whom PI–PB does not function as a satisfactory detector. In some, the task is not sufficiently difficult. In others, there may be an ear difference but its magnitude is too small to be considered significant. For these patients the staggered spondee word test of Katz et al. (1963) is recommended as a supplementary screening technique. This test presents the listener with an extraordinarily difficult listening situation. Different spondee words are presented simultaneously to the two ears, but with a time separation such that the final syllable of one word coincides in time with the initial syllable of the other word. The listener's task is to repeat all four syllables heard. The test is based on the principle that patients with central disorders have difficulty handling simultaneous dichotic messages (in this case the time-coincident syllables of the two spondee words).

E. Synthetic Sentence Identification Tests (SSI–ICM and SSI–CCM)

If either screening technique suggests the possibility of a central lesion, the sentence identification procedures (SSI–ICM and SSI–CCM) can be used to explore the problem in greater detail.

The materials for SSI are artificial or synthetic sentences constructed as approximations to real English sentences according to rules governing the probabilities of word sequence (Speaks and Jerger, 1965). For the evaluation of central auditory disorders it is sufficient to use a single list of 10 such synthetic sentences. An example of such a list of third-order approximations is shown in Table II. Each of the 10 sentences is exactly seven words in length and contains nine syllables (±1 syllable).

The patient has this printed list or closed message set in front of him at all times. The 10 sentences are presented successively to the test earphone in random order. After the presentation of each sentence, the patient must locate the sentence in the closed set and press a response button corresponding to the sentence number. In succeeding test conditions the same 10 sentences are presented over and over, but each time in a different random order. The competing message is simply continuous discourse, preferably recorded by the same talker who records the sen-

TABLE II
EXAMPLE MESSAGE SET CONSISTING OF
10 ALTERNATIVE SYNTHETIC SENTENCES,
CONSTRUCTED AS THIRD-ORDER
APPROXIMATIONS TO REAL SENTENCES

Alternative sentences

1. Small boat with a picture has become
2. Built the government with the force almost
3. Go change your car color is red
4. Forward march said the boy had a
5. March around without a care in your
6. That neighbor who said business is better
7. Battle cry and be better than ever
8. Down by the time is real enough
9. Agree with him only to find out
10. Women view men with green paper should

tences. For the ipsilateral competing message condition (ICM) the sentences (message) and the continuous discourse (competition) are mixed and presented to the same earphone. Then, by varying the relative levels of message (M) and competition (C), a listening task of virtually any degree of difficulty can be presented to the subject. In actual testing this message-to-competition ratio (MCR) is varied to define a function extending from 100% to 10–20% correct identification.

When the message and the competition are at the same level (MCR = 0 dB), most normals perform at 100%, but at MCR = −10 dB, average normal performance is only 80%. At MCR's of −20 and −30 dB, normal performance drops to 55% and 20% respectively.

The SSI–ICM procedure appears to be particularly sensitive to brainstem lesions. A patient with an intraaxial tumor of the brainstem on the right side, for example, will typically show a large performance deficit on SSI–ICM when signals are presented to the left ear, but relatively normal results when signals are presented to the right ear. Patients with temporal lobe lesions may show an ear difference on SSI–ICM, but the effect will be relatively less severe than in the case of brainstem disorder.

For the contralateral competing message condition (CCM), the sentences and the competition are presented to opposite ears. If the sentences are presented to the right ear (test ear), then the competition is heard in the left ear. Again, as in the case of SSI–ICM, the message competition ratio (MCR) is varied over a considerable range. Now however, the normal listener will have little difficulty even at extremely unfavorable MCR's. Over the range from MCR = 0 dB to MCR = −40 dB, normal performance will hold at 100%. The CCM condition is, however, especially sensitive to disorders at the level of the temporal lobe. A patient with left temporal lobe lesion, for example, will typically perform normally when the sentence goes to the left ear and the competition to the right ear. He will show a performance deficit, however, when the sentence goes to the right ear and the competition goes to the left ear. Patients with brainstem disorder, on the other hand, ordinarily have little difficulty with the CCM condition.

The patient's relative performance on the two tasks, SSI–ICM and SSI–CCM, can, therefore, assist in the differentiation of brainstem and temporal lobe sites. A relatively greater performance deficit for ICM than for CCM suggests a brainstem site, whereas a relatively greater deficit for CCM than for ICM suggests a temporal lobe lesion. In some patients the effect may be seen in pure form. The patient with brainstem disorder shows an ear difference on ICM but no abnormality whatever on CCM. More commonly, however, central auditory disorder at any level has at least some effect on any speech audiometric measure. It is the relative configuration of results, therefore, that contributes diagnostic information. Patients with brainstem disorders typically show relatively more difficulty with a difficult monaural task than with dichotic presentation. Conversely, patients with temporal lobe disorders typically show relatively more difficulty with simultaneous dichotic message tasks than with difficult monaural tasks.

F. Other Tests of Interest

It is often interesting to carry out further exploration of central problems with certain tests borrowed from the peripheral battery. On impedance audiometry, for example, the stapedius reflex (Giacomelli and Mozzo, 1964; Greisen and Rasmussen, 1970) may be absent when signals are presented to the ear opposite the affected side of the brain. In rare cases the reflex may be absent from both ears. In still others, however, it will be present in both ears.

Abnormal adaptation seems to be distributed in similar fashion (Antonelli, 1970a; Parker et al., 1962). Many brainstems and virtually all temporal lobes show Type I Békésy audiograms and no significant tone decay on either ear. In some brainstems, however, a Type IV Békésy audiogram and abnormal tone decay may be observed on one or both ears.

Finally, the instrumentation necessary for the SISI test can be used to advantage in central auditory problems by constructing psychometric functions for intensity discrimination (that is, percentage-correct response versus increment size) (Hodgson, 1967; Jerger et al., 1969; Swisher, 1967; Zhukovich and Khortseva, 1965). Such functions often demonstrate startling deficits in intensity discrimination on the ear opposite the affected side of the brain.

IV. Illustrative Cases

The following pages show diagnostic test results in 10 patients with lesions at each of the five possible sites of auditory disorder; the middle ear, the cochlea, the eighth nerve, the brainstem, and the temporal lobe.

The findings in these 10 patients illustrate the general principle that the behavioral manifestations of disorders at different sites within the auditory system are determined by the unique function of that site in the chain of events leading ultimately to auditory perception (Jerger, 1960a). The general principle is illustrated in Figure 2. Disorders of the middle ear, for example, reflect only the effects of the altered acoustic

O NONE ⊖ QUESTIONABLE ◎ SLIGHT ◍ MODERATE ● SEVERE	SITE				
	PERIPHERAL			CENTRAL	
	MIDDLE EAR	COCHLEA	VIIIth NERVE	BRAIN-STEM	TEMPORAL LOBE
SENSITIVITY LOSS	●	◍	◎	⊖	O
DISTORTION	⊖	●	⊖	⊖	O
ABNORMAL ADAPTATION	O	◎	●	⊖	O
SPEECH PROCESSING	O	◎	◍	●	◍
EAR SYMPTOMS OBSERVED ON	IPSI	IPSI	IPSI	CONTRA	CONTRA

Fɪɢ. 2. Schematic illustration of relation between site of auditory disorder and nature of behavioral manifestations.

impedance of a mechanical vibratory system. There is a loss in sensitivity, but other important characteristics of the system are normal. Disorders of the cochlea reflect the effects of damage to the system's biological amplifier. In addition to sensitivity loss, there is considerable signal distortion. At the eighth nerve site the analog-input signal is coded into the unique digital language of the nervous system. Disorders at this site, therefore, affect the system's ability to code and transmit complex signals (for example, speech). Sensitivity loss for pure tones will still be present, but, as compared with comparable degrees of sensitivity loss due to cochlea lesion, there will be disproportionate loss in the capacity for adequately coding complex input signals. The brainstem pathway plays a similar role in the transmission of complex signals; hence, lesions at this site will reflect the same inability to convey a complex signal, like speech, through that portion of the system. Sensitivity loss will have largely disappeared at this level, however, probably because of the multiple alternate paths that simple signals can follow through the brainstem.

The extreme and apparently exclusive sensitivity of the simultaneous dichotic listening paradigm to temporal lobe damage suggests that at least one important function of this segment of the afferent auditory pathway is the creation and maintenance of "auditory space" and the assignment of spatial location to events occurring in that space.

While many of these concepts are highly speculative, there does seem to be an orderly and meaningful relationship between site of disorder and the nature of the auditory task that best demonstrates the disorder. This relationship forms the basis of diagnostic audiometry, both its historical antecedents and its modern development.

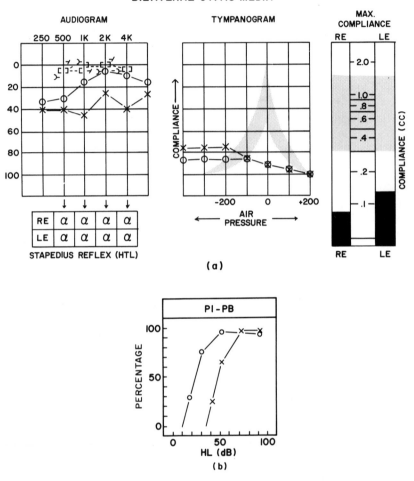

Fig. 3. A 14-year-old female with bilateral otitis media. (a) Audiogram shows a mild conductive loss, greater on the left ear. Tympanograms are type "B," indicating little change in compliance as air pressure in the external canal is varied from +200 to −400 mm H$_2$O. Shaded area is range of normal tympanograms. Maximum static compliance, expressed in cubic centimeters, is well below the normal (shaded) range of 0.3–1.6 cc in both ears. Stapedius reflexes are absent (α) at all four test frequencies in both ears. (b) PI–PB functions rise to high levels, then plateau as speech level is increased.

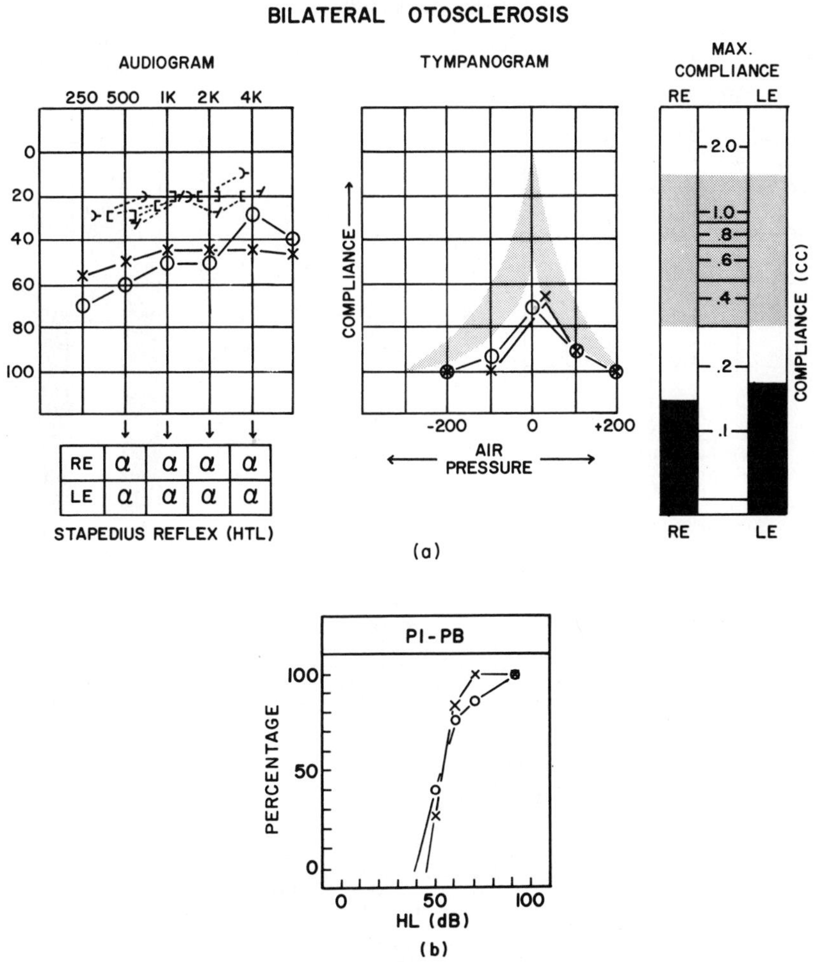

BILATERAL OTOSCLEROSIS

AUDIOGRAM

TYMPANOGRAM

MAX. COMPLIANCE

| RE | α | α | α | α |
| LE | α | α | α | α |

STAPEDIUS REFLEX (HTL)

(a)

(b)

Fig. 4. A 36-year-old female with bilateral otosclerosis. (a) Audiogram shows moderate conductive loss, slightly greater in the right ear. Tympanograms are type "A" but very shallow (A_S). Maximum static compliance is well below the normal range in both ears. Stapedius reflexes are absent bilaterally. (b) PI–PB functions rise to high levels.

JAMES JERGER

NOISE EXPOSURE

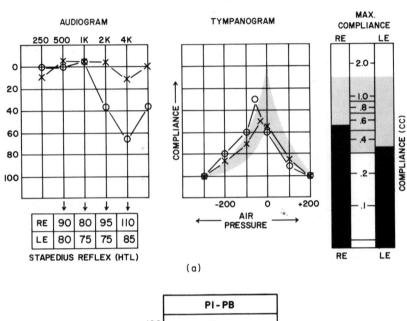

AUDIOGRAM

RE	90	80	95	110
LE	80	75	75	85

STAPEDIUS REFLEX (HTL)

TYMPANOGRAM

MAX.
COMPLIANCE

(a)

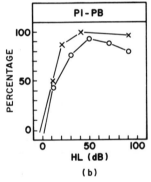

(b)

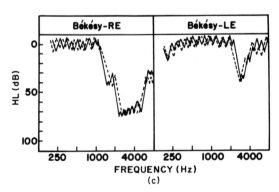

(c)

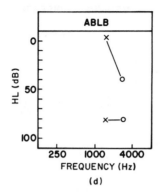

(d)

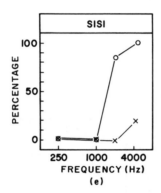

(e)

FIG. 5. A 23-year-old male with a history of excessive exposure to gunfire. (a) Audiogram shows sensorineural notch at 4000 Hz, slight in the left ear but substantial in the right ear. Tympanograms are type "A" and in the normal range except for a slight but insignificant negative pressure in the right middle ear. Maximum static compliance is within the normal range on both ears. Stapedius reflexes are present at all test frequencies. The reduced sensation levels of the reflexes at 2000 and 4000 Hz in the right ear indicate that loudness recruitment is present at these frequencies. Tympanogram and normal maximum compliance on right ear indicate that loss is sensorineural. (b) PI–PB functions rise to high levels, then plateau. There is only slight decline in performance on the right ear as speech intensity is raised to very high levels. (c) Békésy audiograms for interrupted (– – –) and continuous (——) signals are Type I in both ears. (d) Alternate binaural loudness balance test (ABLB) shows complete recruitment at 2000 Hz. (e) SISI test shows abnormally high scores at 2000 and 4000 Hz in the right ear, but normal results in the left ear.

Overall configuration of results in this patient is consistent with a cochlear site.

MENIERE'S DISEASE

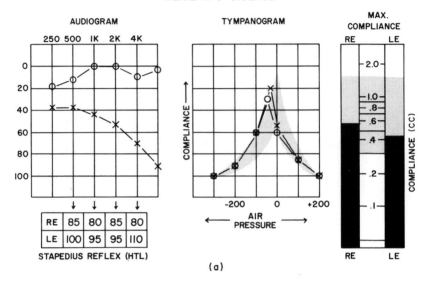

(a)

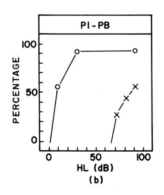

(b)

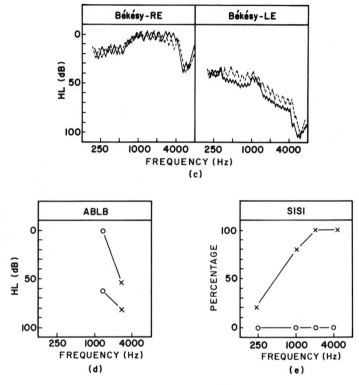

FIG. 6. A 46-year-old female with Meniere's disease on the left ear. (a) Normal tympanograms and normal maximum static compliance indicate that the moderate sensitivity loss on the left ear is sensorineural. Presence of stapedius reflexes at reduced sensation levels on the left ear indicates that loudness recruitment is present. (b) PI–PB function shows considerably reduced PB$_{max}$ on the left ear, but function continues to climb up to highest speech level tested. (c) Békésy audiogram is Type I on the right ear. Type II on the left ear. (d) ABLB shows partial recruitment at 2000 Hz. (e) SISI scores are normal on the right ear, but abnormally high at 1000, 2000, and 4000 Hz on the left ear.

Overall configuration of results is consistent with a cochlear site.

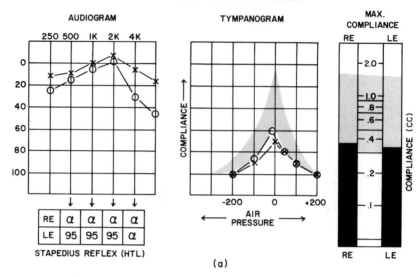

RIGHT ACOUSTIC TUMOR

(a)

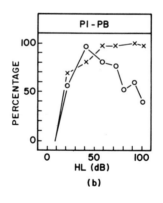

(b)

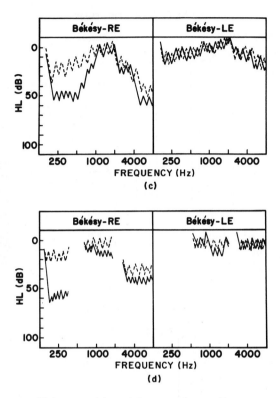

FIG. 7. A 45-year-old-female with a right acoustic neurilemmoma. (a) Audiogram shows only a very mild, high-frequency sensitivity loss on the right ear. Tympanograms are at the shallow end of the normal range. Maximum static compliance is in the normal range. Absence of stapedius reflexes when sound is presented to the right ear indicates not only that loudness recruitment is absent on this ear but that there is a substantial suprathreshold loudness "loss." Absence of stapedius reflex at 4000 Hz on left ear probably has no pathologic significance. (b) PI–PB function is normal on the left ear but shows substantial rollover on the right ear. PB_{max} scores are actually identical on the two ears, but poor performance at high speech intensity levels on the right ear is a retrocochlear sign. (c) Sweep frequency Békésy audiograms are Type I on the left ear and Type IV on the right ear. (d) Fixed frequency Békésy tracings confirm the Type IV configuration (large separation between thresholds for interrupted and continuous signals at low frequencies) on the right ear.

Overall configuration of results is consistent with an eighth nerve site.

JAMES JERGER

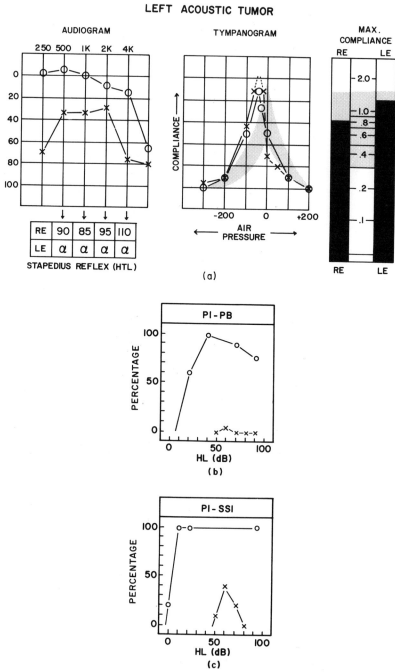

LEFT ACOUSTIC TUMOR

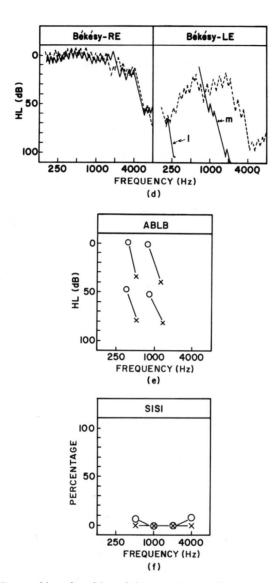

Fig. 8. A 35-year-old male with a left acoustic neurilemmoma. (a) Audiogram shows only a moderate sensitivity loss on the left ear. Tympanograms are normal except for slight negative shift. Maximum static compliance is in the normal range. Absence of stapedius reflex when sound is presented to left ear indicates that loudness recruitment is absent on left ear. (b) PI–PB functions show that PB performance is essentially unmeasurable on the left ear. (c) PI functions for synthetic sentence identification (SSI) permit some measurement of speech understanding on left ear. PI function shows rollover (decreasing performance as speech intensity is raised above maximum). (d) Békésy audiogram is Type I on right ear, but Type III on left ear, whether continuous trace is initiated at very low frequency (1) or in midfrequency region (m) trace falls rapidly to equipment limit. (e) ABLB confirms that recruitment is absent at 500 and 1000 Hz. (f) SISI scores are in the normal range on both ears.

Overall configuration of results is consistent with an eighth nerve site.

LEFT BRAINSTEM TUMOR

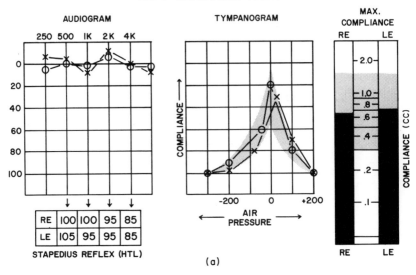

(a)

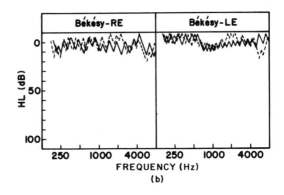

FREQUENCY (Hz)

(b)

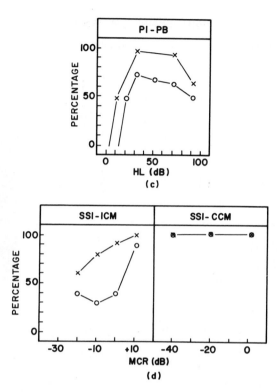

FIG. 9. A 17-year-old female with a pontine glioma eccentric to the left. (a) Audiogram, tympanograms, maximum compliance, and stapedius reflexes are all normal. (b) Békésy audiograms are Type I. (c) PI–PB functions show reduced PB_{max} on right ear and some rollover on both ears. (d) Synthetic sentence identification (SSI) scores in the presence of an ipsilateral competing message (ICM) show a marked performance deficit on the right ear as the message-to-competition ratio (MCR) is varied over the range from +10 to −30 dB. In the case of contralateral competition (CCM), however, performance is unimpaired. In all SSI conditions the sentence (message) level is held constant at 50 dB SPL.

Note that all speech intelligibility deficits appear on ear opposite to affected side of brain stem. Overall configuration of results is consistent with a disorder of the auditory pathway on the left side of the brain stem.

RIGHT BRAINSTEM TUMOR

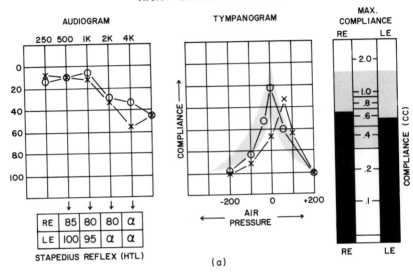

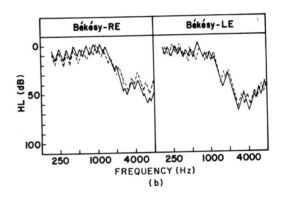

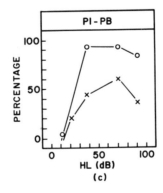

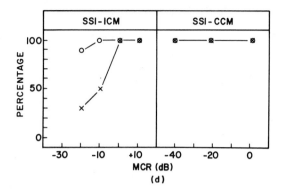

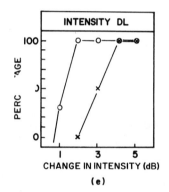

Fig. 10. A 28-year-old male with a pontine glioma eccentric to the right. (a) Audiogram shows a moderate high-frequency sensitivity loss, slightly greater at 4000 Hz in the left ear. Tympanograms are relatively normal. Slight positive displacement of left tympanogram is unusual but not pathologically significant. Absence of stapedius reflexes at 4000 Hz on both ears cannot be considered significant because of low but definite incidence of absent reflexes at this frequency in otherwise normal ears. Absence of reflex at 2000 Hz in left ear suggests aberrant suprathreshold loudness function at 2000 Hz in this ear. (b) Békésy audiograms are Type I in both ears. (c) PI–PB functions show substantial loss in PB_{max} on left ear. (d) SSI–ICM shows performance deficit on left ear at MCR's of −10 and −20 dB. SSI–CCM is performed without difficulty on either ear. (e) Psychometric functions for intensity discrimination show markedly poorer performance on left ear. $F = 1000$ Hz.

Note again that performance deficits appear on ear opposite the affected side of brain. Overall configuration of results is consistent with disorder of auditory pathway on right side of brainstem.

RIGHT TEMPORAL LOBE TUMOR

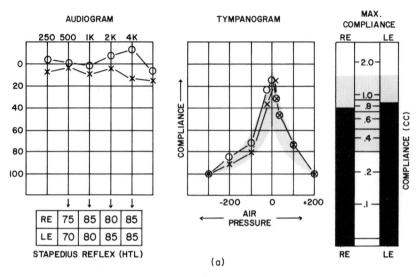

(a)

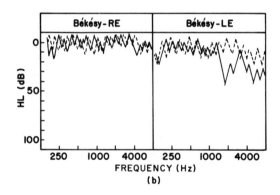

(b)

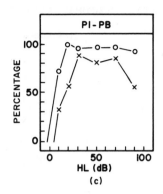

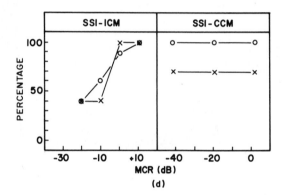

FIG. 11. A 42-year-old- female with a glioma in the right temporal lobe. (a) Audiogram, tympanograms, maximum static compliance, and stapedius reflexes are all within normal limits. (b) The Békésy audiogram is Type I on the right ear, but is slightly abnormal above 1000 Hz on the left ear. (c) PI–PB functions show slightly reduced maximum and moderate rollover on left ear. (d) SSI–ICM performance shows little ear difference, but SSI–CCM condition shows performance deficit on left ear.

Overall configuration of results is consistent with a disorder at the temporal lobe level on right side of brain.

LEFT TEMPORAL LOBE CVA

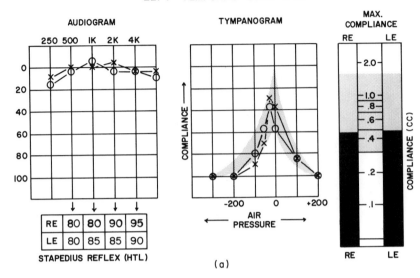

(a)

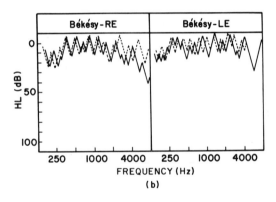

(b)

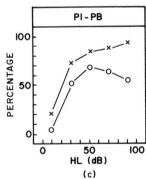

(c)

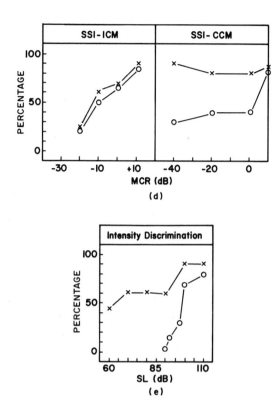

Fig. 12. A 69-year-old female who sustained left cerebrovascular insult. Although patient was aphasic she was able to perform all tests satisfactorily. (a) Audiogram, tympanograms, maximum static compliance, and stapedius reflexes are all within normal limits. (b) Békésy audiograms are Type I in both ears. (c) PI–PB function on left ear rises slowly but eventually reaches 90% level at high speech intensities. On right ear, however, PB$_{max}$ is reduced to 70% and slight rollover occurs. (d) SSI–ICM functions show little ear difference, but SSI–CCM condition shows marked performance deficit on the right ear. (e) Detection of a 1.0-dB intensity increment shows a substantial ear difference at test sensation levels from 60 to 95 dB. $F = 1000$ Hz; $\Delta I = 1$ dB.

Overall configuration of results is consistent with a disorder at the temporal lobe level on left side of brain. Note that left-sided lesion affects performance on right ear in a manner indistinguishable from the effect that a right-sided lesion has on left ear performance. The outcome on these tests of relatively elementary auditory perception is symmetric despite the fact that left hemisphere is dominant for language and may produce concomitant aphasia.

ACKNOWLEDGMENT

The preparation of this chapter was supported by PHS Research Grant number NS08542 from the National Institute of Neurological Diseases and Stroke.

References

Alberti, P., and Kristensen, R. (1970). The clinical application of impedance audiometry. A preliminary appraisal of an electroacoustic impedance bridge. *Laryngoscope* **80,** 735–746.

Anderson, H., Barr, B., and Wedenberg, E. (1969). Intra-aural reflexes in retrocochlear lesions. *In* "Nobel Symposium 10: Disorders of the Skull Base Region" (C. Hamberger and J. Wersall.), pp. 49–55. Almqvist and Wiskell, Stockholm.

Antonelli, A. (1970a). Sensitized speech tests: Results in brain-stem lesions and diffusive CNS diseases. *In* "Speech Audiometry" (C. Røjskjaer, ed.), pp. 130–139. Second Danavox Symposium, Odense, Denmark.

Antonelli, A. (1970b). Sensitized speech tests: Results in lesions of the brain. *In* "Speech Audiometry," (C. Røjskjaer, ed.), pp. 176–183. Second Danavox Symposium, Odense, Denmark.

Antonelli, A., Calearo, C., and De Mitri, T. (1963). On the auditory function in brain stem diseases. *Int. Aud.* **2,** 55–61.

Benitez, J., Lopez-Rios, G., and Novoa. V. (1967). Bilateral acoustic neuroma. A human temporal bone report. *Arch. Otolaryngol.* **86,** 51–57.

Berlin, C., and Lowe, S. (1972). Temporal and dichotic factors in central auditory testing. *In* "Handbook of Clinical Auditory Measurement" (J. Katz, ed.). Williams and Wilkins Co., Baltimore (in press).

Bicknell, M., and Morgan, N. (1968). A clinical evaluation of the Zwislocki acoustic bridge. *J. Laryngol. Otol.* **82,** 673–691.

Bocca, E., and Calearo, C. (1963). Central hearing processes. *In* "Modern Developments in Audiology" (J. Jerger, ed.), pp. 337–370. Academic Press, New York.

Bocca, E., Calearo, C., Cassinari, V., and Migliavacca, F. (1955). Testing 'cortical' hearing in temporal lobe tumors. *Acta Oto-Laryngol.* **45,** 289–304.

Brand, S., and Rosenberg, P. (1963). Problems in auditory evaluation for neurosurgical diagnosis. *J. Speech Hearing Dis.* **28,** 355–361.

Broadbent, D. E. (1956). Successive responses to simultaneous stimuli. *Quart. J. Exp. Psychol.* **8,** 145–162.

Brooks, D. (1968). An objective method of detecting fluid in the middle ear. *Int. Aud.,* **7,** 280–286.

Brooks, D. (1969). The use of the electro-acoustic impedance bridge in the assessment of middle ear function. *Int. Aud.* **8,** 563–569.

Brooks, D. (1971). Electroacoustic impedance bridge studies on normal ears of children. *J. Speech Hearing Res.* **14,** 247–253.

Buxton, Faye. (1970). Audiological tests in cochlear and retrocochlear diagnosis: A review of the literature. Unpublished, University of Houston.

Calearo, C. (1957). Binaural summation in lesions of the temporal lobe. *Acta Oto-Laryngol.* **47,** 392–395.

Carhart, R. (1957). Clinical determination of abnormal auditory adaptation. *Arch. Otolaryngol.* **65,** 32–39.

Dix, M., and Hood, J. D. (1953). Modern developments is pure tone audiometry and their application to the clinical diagnosis of end-organ deafness. *J. Laryngol. Otol.* **67,** 343–357.

Dobie, R. A., and Simmons, F. B. (1971). A dichotic threshold test-normal and brain-damaged subjects. *J. Speech Hearing Res.* **14**, 71–81.

Ewertsen, H., Filling, S., Terkildsen, K., and Thomsen, K. A. (1958). Comparative recruitment testing. *Acta Oto-Laryngol. Suppl.* **140**, 116–122.

Feldman, A. S. (1963). Impedance measurements at the eardrum as an aid to diagnosis. *J. Speech Hearing Res.* **6**, 315–327.

Feldman, A. S. (1964). Acoustic impedance measurement as a clinical procedure. *Int. Aud.* **3**, 1–11.

Feldmann, H. (1967). The diagnosis of central disturbances of hearing. *Deut. Med. Wochenschr.* **92**, 377–383.

Giacomelli, F., and Mozzo, W. (1964). An experimental and clinical study on the influence of the brain stem reticular formation on the stapedial reflex. *Int. Aud.* **3**, 42–44.

Graham, A. (1967). Alternate loudness balance techniques. *In* "Sensorineural Hearing Processes and Disorders" (A. Graham, ed.), pp. 245–257. Little, Brown, Boston, Massachusetts.

Greisen, O., and Rasmussen, P. E. (1970). Stapedius muscle reflexes and oto-neurological examinations in brain-stem tumors. *Acta Oto-Laryngol.* **70**, 366–370.

Hodgson, W. R. (1967). Audiological report of a patient with left hemispherectomy. *J. Speech Hearing Dis.* **32**, 39–45.

Hood, J. D. (1969). Basic audiological requirements in neuro-otology. *J. Laryngol. Otol.* **83**, 695–711.

Hopkinson, N. T., and Thomas, S. (1967). Two tests of tone decay: Their contribution to diagnostic decisions. *Ann. Otol. Rhinol. Laryngol.* **76**, 189–203.

Jepsen, O. (1963). Middle-ear muscle reflexes in man. *In* "Modern Developments in Audiology" (J. Jerger, ed.), pp. 193–239. Academic Press, New York.

Jerger, J. (1960a). Audiological manifestations of lesions in the auditory nervous system. *Laryngoscope* **70**, 417–425.

Jerger, J. (1960b). Observations on auditory behavior in lesions of the central auditory pathways. *Arch. Otolaryngol.* **71**, 797–806.

Jerger, J. (1960c). Békésy audiometry in the analysis of auditory disorders. *J. Speech Hearing Res.* **3**, 275–287.

Jerger, J. (1964). Auditory tests for disorders of the central auditory mechanism. *In* "Neurological Aspects of Auditory and Vestibular Disorders" (W. Fields and B. Alford, eds.), pp. 77–93. Thomas, Springfield, Illinois.

Jerger, J. (1970a). Development of synthetic sentence identification (SSI) as a tool for speech audiometry. *In* "Speech Audiometry" (C. Røjskjaer, ed.), pp. 44–65. Second Danavox Symposium, Odense, Denmark.

Jerger, J. (1970b). Diagnostic significance of SSI test procedures: retrocochlear site. *In* "Speech Audiometry" (C. Røjskjaer, ed.), pp. 163–175. Second Danavox Symposium, Odense, Denmark.

Jerger, J. (1970c). Clinical experience with impedance audiometry. *Arch. Otolaryngol.* **93**, 311–324.

Jerger, J., and Harford, E. (1960). Alternate and simultaneous binaural balancing of pure tones. *J. Speech Hearing Res.* **3**, 15–30.

Jerger, J., and Jerger, S. (1971). Diagnostic significance of PB word functions. *Arch. Otolaryngol.* **93**, 573–580.

Jerger, J., Shedd, J., and Harford, E. (1959). On the detection of extremely small changes in sound intensity. *Arch. Otolaryngol.* **69**, 200–211.

Jerger, J., Speaks, C., and Trammell, J. (1968). A new approach to speech audiometry. *J. Speech Hearing Dis.* **33**, 318–328.

Jerger, J., Weikers, N., Sharbrough, F., and Jerger, S. (1969). Bilateral lesions of the temporal lobe: a case study. *Acta Oto-Laryngol. Suppl.* **258.**

Jerger, J., Jerger, S., and Mauldin, L. (1972). The forward-backward discrepancy in Békésy audiometry. *Arch. Otolaryngol.* (in press).

Johnson, E. (1968). Auditory findings in 200 cases of acoustic neuromas. *Arch. Otolaryngol.* **88**, 598–603.

Jungert, S. (1958). Auditory pathways in the brain stem: a neurophysiological study. *Acta Oto-Laryngol. Suppl.* **138.**

Katz, J., Basil, R., and Smith, J. (1963). A staggered spondaic word test for detecting central auditory lesions. *Ann. Otol. Rhinol. Laryngol.* **72**, 908–917.

Kimura, D. (1961). Some effects of temporal-lobe damage on auditory perception. *Can. J. Psychol.* **15**, 156–165.

Kimura, D. (1963). Speech lateralization in young children as determined by an auditory test. *J. Comp. Physiol. Psychol.* **56**, 899–902.

Kimura. D. (1967). Functional asymmetry of the brain in dichotic listening. *Cortex.* **3**, 163–178.

Klockhoff, I. (1961). Middle ear muscle reflexes in man. A clinical and experimental study with special references to diagnostic problems in hearing impairment. *Acta Oto-Laryngol. Suppl.* **164.**

Lamb, L., Peterson, J. L., and Hansen, S. (1968). Application of stapedius muscle reflex measures to diagnosis of auditory problems. *Int. Aud.* **7**, 188–189.

Lidén, G. (1969). The scope and application of current audiometric tests. *J. Laryngol. Otol.* **83**, 507–520.

Lidén, G., Peterson, J.. and Björkman, G. (1970). Tympanometry. *Arch. Otolaryngol.* **92**, 248–257.

Linden, A. (1964). Distorted speech and binaural speech resynthesis tests. *Acta Oto-Laryngol.* **58**, 32–48.

Matzker, J. (1957). The binaural test in space-occupying endo-cranial processes; a new method of otological diagnosis of brain disease. *Z. Laryngol.* **36**, 177–189.

Matzker, J. (1958). "A Test of Binaural Fusion in Central Hearing Impairment." G. Thieme, Stuttgart.

Metz, O. (1951). Studies on the contraction of the tympanic muscles as indicated by changes in the impedance of the ear. *Acta Oto-Laryngol.* **39**, 397–405.

Metz, O. (1952). Threshold of reflex contractions of muscles of middle ear and recruitment of loudness. *Arch. Oto-Laryngol.* **55**, 536–543.

Milner, B. (1962). Laterality effects in audition. *In* "Interhemispheric Relations and Cerebral Dominance " (V. Mountcastle, ed.), pp. 177–195. Johns Hopkins Press, Baltimore.

Milner, B., Taylor, L., and Sperry, R. (1968). Lateralized suppression of dichotically presented digits after commissural section in man. *Science* **161**, 184–185.

Møller, A. R. (1958). Intra-aural muscle contraction in man, examined by measuring acoustic impedance of the ear. *Laryngoscope* **68**, 48–62.

Naunton, R. F. (1967). The audiologic diagnosis of eighth nerve tumors. *Int. Aud.* **6**, 201–210.

Ohta, F., Hayashi, R., and Morimoto, M. (1967). Differential diagnosis of retrocochlear deafness: binaural fusion test and binaural separation test. *Int. Aud.* **6**, 58–62.

Owens, E. (1964). Békésy tracings and site of lesion. *J. Speech Hearing Dis.* **29**, 456–468.

Owens, E. (1965). The SISI test and VIIIth nerve versus cochlear involvement. *J. Speech Hearing Dis.* **30**, 252–262.

Palva, T., Karja, J., and Palva, A. (1970). Forward vs reversed Bekesy tracings. *Arch. Otolaryngol.* **91**, 449–452.

Parker, W., and Decker, R. (1971). Detection of abnormal auditory threshold adaptation (ATA). *Arch. Otolaryngol.* **94**, 1–7.

Parker, W., Decker, R., and Gardner, W. (1962). Auditory function and intracranial lesions. *Arch. Otolaryngol.* **76**, 425–435.

Parker, W., Decker, R., and Richards, N. (1968). Auditory function and lesions of the pons. *Arch. Otolaryngol.* **87**, 228–240.

Penfield, W., and Roberts, L. (1959). "Speech and Brain-Mechanisms." Princeton Univ. Press, New Jersey.

Perez de Moura, L. (1967). Inner ear pathology in acoustic neurinoma. *Arch. Otolaryngol.* **85**, 125–133.

Sparks, R., Goodglass, H., and Nickel, B. (1970). Ipsilateral versus contralateral extinction in dichotic listening resulting from hemisphere lesions. *Cortex.* **6**, 249–260.

Speaks, C., and Jerger. J. (1965). Method for measurement of speech identification. *J. Speech Hearing Res.* **8**, 185–194.

Studdert-Kennedy, M., and Shankweiler, D. (1970). Hemispheric specialization for speech perception. *J. Acoust. Soc. Amer.* **48**, 579–594.

Swisher, L. (1967). Auditory intensity discrimination in patients with temporal-lobe damage. *Cortex.* **3**, 179–193.

Terkildsen, K., and Scott-Nielsen, S. (1960). An electroacoustic impedance measuring bridge for clinical use. *Arch. Otolaryngol.* **72**, 339–346.

Thomsen, K. A. (1955). Employment of impedance measurement in otologic and oto-neurologic diagnostics. *Acta Oto-Laryngol.* **45**, 159–167.

Tunturi, A. (1960). Anatomy and physiology of the auditory cortex. *In* "Neural Mechanisms of the Auditory and Vestibular Systems" (G. Rasmussen and W. Windle, eds.), pp. 181–200. Thomas, Springfield, Illinois.

Zhukovich, A., and Khortseva, G. (1965). The differential limen of the perception of sound intensity in patients with lesions of the CNS. *Vestn. Otorinolaringol.* **1**, 7–12.

Zwislocki, J. (1961). Acoustic measurement of the middle ear function. *Ann. Otol. Rhinol. Laryngol.* **70**, 1–8.

Zwislocki, J., and Feldman, A. S. (1969). Acoustic impedance of pathological ears. Tech. Rep. LSC-S-5. Laboratory of Sensory Communication, Syracuse University.

Chapter 4

Auditory Masking

GERALD A. STUDEBAKER

Memphis State University

I. What Is Masking?

Over the past 40 or more years masking generally has been operationally defined, often as follows: "Masking is the amount by which the threshold of audibility of a sound is raised by the presence of another (masking) sound. The unit customarily used is the decibel [Amer. Nat. Standards Inst., S1.1 (1960)]." Not everyone has been willing to accept this definition. Meyer (1959), for example, insisted that the definition should be expanded to include the reduction in loudness in a stimulus that occurs under certain circumstances upon the introduction of other signals. Scharf (1964) used the term "partial masking" to refer to this loudness reduction phenomenon.

Tanner (1958) presented evidence that at least three factors other than the simple direct masking of one sound by another may cause subject performance decrements in the masking experiment. These included signal uncertainty, subject response criterion changes, and distortion in the ear produced by the addition of the masker. On the basis of these observations Tanner concluded that a problem lies in the use of an operational definition and asks "Does masking occur merely because conditions are established leading to a change in performance [p. 921]?" The answer to this question, of course, must be "no." It does not appear reasonable to this writer to lump signal uncertainty, subject response criteria changes or distortion under the heading of masking simply because some of these factors may be introduced into the masking experiment along with the masker and produce similar effects.

However, Tanner's question led Carter and Kryter (1962) to comment that for their purposes "masking refers to the limits placed on the recognition of a sound by the presence of another sound, when the time and frequency characteristics of both are known to the observer, and when he is oriented to perceive them. The definition includes intra-aural distortion products as one of the consequences of both stimuli [p. 66]."

A recently used definition of masking was one given by Deatherage and Evans (1969) who stated that masking is "the process by which the detectability of one sound, the signal, is impaired by the presence of another sound, the masker [p. 362]." This definition was devised to be consistent with signal detection theory concepts in that it does not include the word *threshold*. However, in other regards it is fundamentally unchanged from earlier definitions.

Works on the physiological correlates of masking are few. However, important contributions have been made by Teas et al. (1962) and by Finck (1966). Finck reported that a 1935 study by Derbyshire and Davis demonstrated that the action potentials (AP) recorded from the round window were amenable to masking, but that the cochlear microphonic (CM) appeared unaffected by a "hissing sound." Teas et al. (1962) stated that their results were consistent with the conclusion that "noise eliminates part of the AP [p. 1449]." Further, they concluded that "noise acts primarily by eliminating portions of the normal response at times appropriate to the frequency characteristics and level of the noise. . . . Higher levels remove more AP, but they do not appear to change the timing of the AP that remains. The effect is purely subtractive and is not accompanied by any other interactions between noise and transient [p. 1449]." (Clicks were used as test stimuli in this study.)

In 1966, Finck reported his studies on the physiology of tonal masking and related his results to the psychoacoustic pure-tone masking studies, particularly those of Small (1959). Masking was defined in terms of the pure-tone masker level required to obliterate the gross eighth nerve response to the pure-tone test signal. Comparisons with psychoacoustical data revealed remarkable similarities in several particulars with the pure-tone masking data obtained by Small on human subjects, including a notch in the data when the frequency of the masker was about 85% of the frequency of the test tone. (This is in contrast to the 50% value reported by Wegal and Lane, 1924.) Finck stated that these results" suggest that the mechanisms involved in the masking of the neural response and the detectability of a signal in simple, pure-tone masking are comparable [p. 1062]."

II. Ipsilateral Direct Masking

A. Masking of Pure Tones by Pure Tones

Three relatively recent studies of the masking of pure tones by pure tones are those of Ehmer (1959a), Small (1959), and of Carter and Kryter (1962). Both Ehmer and Small noted that when the masking tone was weak the masking pattern produced was symmetrical around the masker frequency (see Figure 1, an example from Ehmer). At higher masker levels the masking pattern became asymmetrical, with more masking above than below the frequency of the masker until at high masker levels the asymmetry was quite marked. On these points these studies are in agreement with nearly all previous work. However, Ehmer observed that the second peak (the first peak above the frequency region

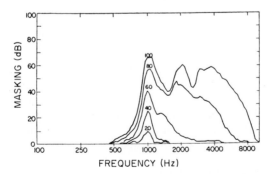

FIG. 1. Masking patterns produced by a 1000-Hz tone at various levels. Note the symmetry at low masker levels with increasing asymmetry at higher levels and the gradual emergence of a "second" peak which migrates upward in frequency as the masker level is increased. [From Ehmer (1959a).]

of the masker) did not fall at one octave above the masker frequency as observed in the Wegal and Lane (1924) results. Rather, at the lower intensity levels the peak was at about one-half octave above the frequency of the masker and then migrated upward as the masker level was increased. Only at 100 dB did the peak fall at or near the masker harmonic. Ehmer concluded that "The masking pattern of a pure tone results primarily from the activity pattern of the tone in the cochlea [p. 1120]." At low levels the activity and masking pattern are narrow. As the masker is increased "activity spreads only towards the base, while retaining a maximum at the locus of the original response. . . . Aural distortion plays a much smaller role in masking than had previously been supposed [p. 1120]." It should be noted that Carter and Kryter (1962) reported that in the frequency range below 1000 Hz the frequency of maximum masking was, at times, above the masker frequency and that it migrated upward with masker intensity increases.

Small (1959) also observed that the irregularity in the masking curve above the frequency of the masker did not fall at a one-octave separation between the masker and test tone as observed by Wegal and Lane (1924), but occurred when the masker frequency was 85% of the test tone frequency. Small concluded with Ehmer that aural harmonics were ruled out as a cause of these irregularities as had been commonly held.

In 1961, Finck reported the results of a study in which the masking patterns produced by 10-, 15-, 25-, 30-, and 150-Hz pure tones were investigated. The extent of the masking produced was relatively small but quite smooth and equal across frequency and extended well into the 2000–4000 Hz region. Furthermore, there was a notable lack of irregularities at harmonic multiples of the masker. These findings are consistent extensions of the Ehmer (1959a) study where smoother curves were found at lower masker frequencies.

Jerger et al. (1966) observed threshold shifts produced by 2-, 7- and 12-Hz maskers. Unlike Finck and Békésy, both of whom used a loudspeaker with tubes leading to the ears, Jerger et al. used a device which varied the air pressure in a small room. While few of the conditions are exactly the same, reasonable agreement is seen across the three studies although it appears that the Finck results agree somewhat better with the Békésy results than do the Jerger et al. (1966) results, particularly at the 1000-Hz test-tone frequency.

B. Masking of Pure Tones by Noise

Ehmer (1959b) demonstrated that the amount of masking produced by a narrow-band noise with the same overall level as a pure-tone masker and centered at the pure-tone masker frequency produces more masking near the center of the masker band than does the pure-tone masker. This result is thought to occur because the masker noise does not interact with the test tone as do pure-tone maskers when close to the frequency of the test tone. Above the second peak Ehmer noted that the masking produced by a tone and by a noise band of equal level and center frequency produced very nearly the same masking. Ehmer concluded that this evidence further ruled out harmonic distortion as the cause of high-frequency spread of masking because tone and noise of equal overall levels should produce substantially different harmonic distortion because of their differing spectrum levels.

A recent application of the masking of pure tones by narrow bands of noise was the effort of Carterette et al. (1969) to demonstrate Mach bands in hearing. Mach bands are visual bands of light and dark which appear under certain circumstances as visual contrast phenomena when, in fact, the objective illumination changes from place to place at a uniform rate. Mach bands in vision are thought to appear subjectively because of inhibition of retinal areas adjacent to areas receiving greater stimulation. Carterette et al. (1969) pointed out that it is difficult to explain the ability of the ear to discriminate pitch without assuming some kind of laterally inhibiting network in the cochlea. On this basis they sought evidence of edge effects using computer-generated narrow bands consisting of 56 sinusoids spaced randomly by frequency. The use of the sinusoids theoretically gave the noise an infinite attenuation rate at the cutoff frequency. (Actual attenuation rate of excitation will be less than infinite because of limitations imposed by the electronic gear and by the ear.)

Figure 2 shows some of the results obtained by Carterette et al. (1969) for four individual subjects. The many peaks and discontinuities in evidence are in contrast to earlier reports where filtered random noise was used. Carterette et al. (1969) concluded that these irregularities are consistent with laterally inhibiting networks and illustrate the equivalent of both light and dark visual bars (Mach bands). They concluded also that these data are consistent with Békésy's findings on the lateral inhibition of sensation on the skin.

Young and Wenner (1967) and Young (1969) masked white noise and high-pass and low-pass noise with pure tones of various frequency. A tone with a frequency of 800 Hz was the most effective masker of white noise, producing a 36-dB sound-pressure level (SPL) white-noise threshold when presented at 100 dB. Young concluded that the pure tones at high levels activate the entire basilar membrane and, therefore, those tones that fall at or near the mechanical resonance of the ear are the most effective maskers.

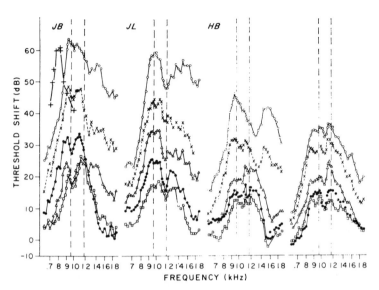

FIG. 2. Masking patterns produced by a narrow-band masker (dotted lines) with very steep skirts for four individual subjects. Note the substantial irregularities which were interpreted to represent Mach bands in hearing. □—□, 20 dB; ●—●, 30 dB; △—△, 40 dB; ×--×, 50 dB; ○—○, 60 dB. [From Carterette et al. (1969).]

C. Remote Masking

Remote masking was first identified by Bilger and Hirsh (1956). Below the low-frequency skirt of a narrow band the pure-tone threshold decreases rapidly, reaching a local minimum before increasing again with the masked threshold approximately paralleling the threshold in quiet. That portion of the curve below the minimum was called remote masking. Deatherage et al. (1957a) demonstrated that the frequency region of the remote masking could be controlled by manipulation of the envelope of the masker and concluded that remote masking is produced by an envelope detection process. This conclusion was supported by the observation of Deatherage et al. (1957b) that cochlear microphonics in the apical region of guinea pig cochleas followed the envelope of the masking noise. Contralateral remote masking will be discussed in a later section.

D. Additivity of Masking

Bilger (1959) was the first to investigate the effects of combining two types of masking. He reasoned that if two maskers summated on a simple energy basis then the amount of masking obtained when two equal masking maskers are combined should be 3 dB more than the amount of masking obtained with either masker alone. However, somewhat more masking was actually obtained. For example, when remote masking was combined with direct masking at levels where each masker alone produced equal thresholds for a 500-Hz tone, up to 3 dB of additional threshold shift (beyond the 3 dB for energy summation) was observed. Bilger concluded that the additional summation must occur within the ear or central to it.

Green (1967) used an approach similar to Bilger's but combined instead masking tones and masking noises. After being adjusted to produce equal masking of a pure tone, the white-noise and pure-tone maskers were presented together. The test tone then had to be increased by at least 6.5 dB and up to as much as 14 dB under various conditions in order to obtain threshold. Green suggested that the detection of signals in noise and the detection of a signal in the presence of a sinusoid are based on different processes. He proposed that when listening in the presence of noise the listener use a "narrow filter (critical band) in the vicinity of the signal frequencies. The width of this hypothetical filter should be as narrow as possible, because this would maximize the signal-to-noise (S/N) ratio at the output of this filter [p. 1521]." On the other hand, when a sinusoidal signal is added incoherently to a background sinusoid, a "fluctuation in the envelope of the filter output would be strong evidence that the signal had been presented. . . . This cue will become more and more effective as the width of the initial filter is increased [p. 152]." When the two types of masking are presented together, each masker type renders the system for detection in the presence of the other noise type relatively ineffective.

Henning (1969) presented a discussion and evidence which suggested that amplitude discrimination in noise, pedestal experiments and the additivity of masking are "simply different ways of exploring the same parameter space . . . [p. 430]." The Henning work demonstrates the difficulty of differentiating between certain types of masking studies and amplitude difference limen (DL) studies. He presented a model describing a three-dimensional space within which these three kinds of experiments appear very similar.

E. Critical Bands and Ratios

This area of investigation has had a long history of intensive study and has been thoroughly reviewed on a number of occasions. One of the more recent and best of these is that of Scharf (1966). For this reason discussion of this topic will be brief.

Fletcher (1940) obtained the width of the critical band on the basis of the assumption that when a pure tone is just masked by a broad-band noise, the level of the tone and the overall level of the critical band are equal. Hence, the bandwidth in decibels can be converted to a bandwidth in hertz. A band narrowing technique was also used by Fletcher in an effort to verify the calculated values, but apparently few workers believe that these results are definitive (Scharf, 1966). A series of experiments reported by Zwicker *et al.* (1957) indicated that the critical band (that is, the bandwidth of the basic analyzing system of the auditory system) is about 2.5 times as wide in hertz as obtained through the Fletcher assumption. Zwicker *et al.* (1957) suggested the term critical ratio for the Fletcher critical bands in order to distinguish them from the wider bandwidths obtained by themselves. The larger Zwicker *et al.* bandwidths now have been verified by many investigators and can be inferred from a number of other studies (Scharf, 1966).

Nevertheless, the critical ratios in decibels have proven to be very useful. It has been demonstrated repeatedly that these values provide an accurate standard for predicting and/or confirming ipsilateral noise-masked thresholds provided that the test signal frequency band is contained within the frequency bandwidth of the masker noise, and provided that the noise is at least approximately a critical band or more wide. Concerning the second proviso, Scharf (1966, p. 25) cites several studies which have shown that the threshold signal-to-noise ratio varies as the bandwidth of a very narrow band is varied. As an example of how the critical ratio values have been applied see Sanders and Rintelmann (1964).

A number of studies have demonstrated that the critical ratio is independent of masker level once above 10- to 15-dB signal level (SL). However, in two recent studies Campbell (1964) studied the masking of one noise by another noise and Campbell and Laskey (1967) studied masking of a pure tone by a pure tone and obtained somewhat different results. In each study the masker and test signals were quite similar and, in some instances, identical. They observed that the signal-to-noise ratio varied as a function of masker level, decreasing rapidly just above threshold, reaching a minimum in the 30-, 40-, or 50-dB signal-level (SL) region, then increasing to local maximum in the 60–70-dB SL region before decreasing again. The similarity of the results and of many of the signal paradigms in these studies to those of DL for intensity studies is notable except for the local maximum in the results at 60–70 dB. Campbell and Laskey (1967) pointed out that if their results were plotted on the usual test signal level by noise level graph, the deviations from a straight line would be barely visible. However, they believe that such deviations are quite real and can be detected, for example, in the Hawkins and Stevens (1950) masked speech threshold data.

Bos and deBoer (1966) carried out an experiment designed to illuminate the reasons for the differences between the critical bands of Zwicker *et al.* (1957) and those derived, in some instances, by the noise bandwidth limiting techniques of the type used by Fletcher (1940). Bos and deBoer observed that as the noise band was made very narrow, amplitude fluctuations became more prominent. These amplitude fluctuations together with the fact that the narrow-band noise becomes more and more tonelike and difficult to differentiate from the test tone causes the noise to produce more masking than it would otherwise. They concluded that the excess masking due to these causes is about 3 dB which would produce an underestimate of the critical bandwidth by a factor of about 2.

Critical ratios have been obtained for a number of animals, including at least cats, rats, chinchillas and, most recently, the bottle-nosed porpoise (Johnson, 1968). The critical ratios, and presumably the critical bands, of the chinchilla, rat, and cat are all substantially larger (wider) than man's, with the cat coming closest to man, particularly in the 250- to 1000-Hz frequency region (Scharf, 1966). The porpoise, on the other hand, produced critical ratios about equal to man's in those frequency regions where measurements have been made on both species (5000–10,000 Hz) (Johnson, 1968).

F. Ipsilateral Direct Masking of Speech

A great deal of work has been done in past years on the direct ipsilateral masking of speech and the results have been used extensively in the development of the articulation index (AI) and other procedures for the evaluation of communications systems. For an example of this application see Kryter (1962). Recent developments in the area of the ipsilateral direct masking of speech principally include studies on the effects of interrupted and modulated maskers, and the masking of speech with speech and the masking of speech using speech combined with noise maskers.

Carhart *et al.* (1966) reviewed thoroughly the earlier literature on the effects of noise modulation and noise interruption on speech reception. In their own work they observed that a 7-dB modulation of a white-noise masker yielded intelligibility functions comparable to those for continuous noise at the same average level. However, 14- and 21-dB modulations and complete interruption of the noise produced substantial improvements in intelligibility, particularly with interruption rates of one or four times per second. Under this condition, intelligibility remained at over 80% with signal-to-noise ratios as poor as —21 dB.

Wilson and Carhart (1969) studied masked spondee thresholds in the presence of various noise conditions in the same ear. The noises were interrupted or were modulated 14 dB at rates of 1, 10, and 100 times per second (50% duty cycle). No reduction in masking relative to a continuous masker occurred at low masker levels when the pulse rate was 100 times per second. Masking reduction under other conditions ranged from a fraction of a decibel to 39.3 dB for normal-hearing subjects, with the greater masking reduction at the two slower rates. Wilson and Carhart (1969) also studied a group of patients diagnosed as having cochlear otosclerosis. They observed that the "reduction in masking was less for subjects with cochlear otosclerosis . . . but otherwise the trends . . . were relatively parallel [p. 1010]."

In an associated study Dirks et al. (1969) studied the effects of pulsed masking on spondaic words, monosyllables, and synthetic sentences. The same noise conditions used by Wilson and Carhart (1969) were used. The masking of monosyllables was least with 10 interruptions per second under relatively favorable signal-to-noise conditions and least at one interruption per second at the poorest signal-to-noise ratios. The spondees were least masked at one interruption per second. The synthetic sentence results were more like the results for spondaic words than for monosyllables at the slower pulse rates.

In a study of monaurally masked speech reception, Carhart et al. (1968) noted that when a speech sound masker was added to a noise masker that produced the same amount of masking when presented alone, the additional threshold shift was considerably in excess of the 3-dB increase which would be expected on the basis of a simple power summation. Spondee thresholds were increased by 7.8 dB and monosyllable intelligibility curves were shifted by 10.5 dB. Carhart and his co-workers referred to the excess masking (the amount over 3 dB) as perceptual masking.

Carhart et al. (1969) reported further on this phenomenon. In a study of spondee thresholds they observed that the addition of a speech masker to an equal masking noise resulted in about 3.2 dB of excess masking and that the combination of two equal masking speech maskers produced 6.6 dB of excess masking. They concluded that this was not a manifestation of the excess additivity described by Bilger (1959) and by Green (1967). They did, however, see a parallel to the extent that excess masking "can be the product of cumulative interference involving two or more independent mechanisms [p. 701]." However, Carhart et al. (1969) stated that "in this case, the mechanisms depend on linguistic functions, rather than relatively simple sensory processing of the type Green describes [p. 701]." They noted further that perceptual masking was apparently independent of whether the stimuli were presented monaurally or binaurally and also that it was independent of the phase relationships or the interaural time disparities at the two ears.

III. Temporal Effects in Masking

A. Changes in Masking as a Function of Time

Under most circumstances, direct masking is stable over time (Burgeat and Hirsh, 1961; Egan, 1955) at least up to 25 min or so and probably much longer. Burgeat and Hirsh concluded that remote masking, on the other hand, does decrease over an exposure period of 5 min. Using a 2000–4000-Hz octave-band masker and a 700- or a 500-Hz test tone, they demonstrated threshold improvements as a function of exposure time for both ipsilateral and contralateral remote masking. In a parallel procedure they observed that the threshold at 3000 Hz in the presence of the same noise did not shift with time. Burgeat and Hirsh concluded that the threshold shift effect is not peripheral because it occurred in both contralateral and ipsilateral conditions.

Bilger and Melnick (1968) believed that the findings of Burgeat and Hirsh might have resulted from the change in the frequency of the test tone. Zwislocki et al. (1958) had observed that practice and motivation influenced thresholds most at low frequencies. On this basis Bilger and Melnick reasoned that the noise rather than the test-tone frequency should be changed when comparing remote and direct masking. Bilger and Melnick's results for a 500-Hz tone masked by a 2000–4000-Hz noise (remote) and a 200–4000-Hz noise (direct) showed that both the directly masked thresholds and the remotely masked thresholds improved over time. While the remotely masked thresholds shifted more, Bilger and Melnick reasoned that the changes in both instances were "akin to warmup." These results are not necessarily at variance with those of Egan (1955) because Egan noted threshold within brief test-tone presentation intervals (15 sec). Only the noise was on continuously. Bilger and Melnick, on the other hand, used interrupted tone Békésy tracings and, therefore, threshold shifts could be observed as a function of test tone on-time as well as noise on-time. The shifts under these conditions are analogous to the shifts in quiet thresholds over time (see Zwislocki et al., 1958) and are not necessarily peculiar to the masked threshold.

Most studies that showed no change in the masked threshold over time were not devised so that the changes which occur within a few milliseconds after the onset of the masker could be observed. These changes are referred to as "overshoot" because the masking is greater in the first milliseconds than later in the steady-state condition.

The basic procedure in studies of overshoot is to use a very brief [5–20 milliseconds (5–20 msec)] test-signal burst which is introduced at various times with reference to the onset or offset of a longer masker burst. Elliott (1965) and Zwicker (1965) presented detailed studies of masking overshoot in 1965. Figure 3, from Elliott (1965), is for a single listener. A test tone of 1000 Hz was presented for 5 msec at the various delays noted on the abcissa. The numbers in the figure refer to the duration of the masker. The various curves were displaced vertically for clarity. Overshoot is apparent just after the onset of the noise and just *prior* to the offset. Zwicker (1965) observed that overshoot was prominent when masker and maskee bands were different in width while little overshoot was noted when masker and test stimulus bands were similar in width. Elliott concluded that the overshoot is independent of masker duration provided that the masker exceeds 30 msec. Minimum masking occurred at 200–300 msec after masker onset.

Zwicker (1965) hypothesized that the relative bandwidths of masker and test signal is the variable directly related to the magnitude of the overshoot. Elliott (1965), however, noted that when a narrow-band noise was used, little overshoot was noted when the test-tone frequency was within the band but substantial overshoot was noted for frequencies just outside the band. This result is inconsistent with Zwicker's hypothesis, as are the results of Lankford and Stokinger (1969) who demonstrated overshoot for tones masked by tones in the ipsilateral condition

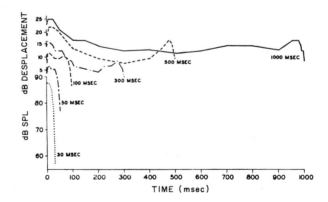

Fig. 3. Simultaneous wide-band masking of a 1000-Hz tone of 5-msec duration delayed relative to onset of masker by Δ+, which is indicated on the abcissa. The results for different masking durations are displaced vertically. [From Elliott (1965, p. 739).]

both at the onset and offset of the masker tone. They (Stokinger and Lankford, 1969) also observed overshoot for tones masked by tones in the contralateral condition both at onset and offset.

Green (1969) reported a series of experiments with which he attempted to define "the necessary and sufficient conditions needed to obtain overshoot [p. 940]." He noted that when test signal and masker were near each other in frequency, little overshoot was observed. When test tone and masker differed in frequency as much as 30–40 dB of overshoot was seen when masker and test tone are turned on and off together. (These values are substantially larger than those reported by previous investigators.) After stating that the differences among his observers in this experiment were greater than for any other psychological experiment he had ever carried out, an observation which is apparently consistent with that of other researchers, Green presents three hypotheses to explain overshoot. The first is based on equilibration of the neural system. The second is based on a time-varying critical band which takes a brief but finite time to organize (that is, to become narrow in bandwidth). The third proposal is one called "energy spatter." This hypothesis is based on the well-known physical fact that short-duration stimuli have a relatively broad spectra, becoming wider as the signal duration is decreased.

B. Backward and Forward Masking

Backward and forward masking refer to those threshold shifts which occur when the test stimulus is presented before the masker onset (backward) or after the masker offset (forward). Figure 4, taken from Elliott (1962b), illustrates the general nature and magnitude of these effects when masker and test tone are presented to the same ear. When masker and test tone are presented to opposite ears, backward masking is still

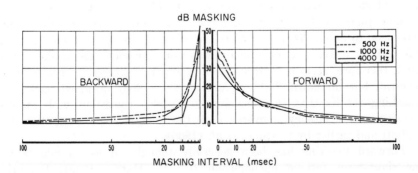

FIG. 4. Monotic forward and backward masking produced at three frequencies by a broad-band masker. [From Elliott (1962b).]

evident though much reduced. Some very small forward masking may also be in evidence (Elliott, 1962b).

Pickett (1959) observed that backward and forward masked threshold shifts were larger for shorter test-tone durations. The largest shifts occurred with a 5-msec test signal duration. He also noted that greater shifts occurred at higher masker levels, but he concluded that the interstimulus interval is the single most important determinant of the amount of backward masking, with very little masking apparent with an interval of greater than 25 msec.

Raab (1961) studied both forward and backward masking of clicks by clicks. He concluded that forward masking is consistent with earlier measures of recovery of electrophysiologic function of the eighth nerve but that backward masking is not and, therefore, must be related "to some more central mechanism."

Elliott (1962a, 1962b) demonstrated both monotic and dichotic backward masking. Figure 4 illustrates her results with a 90-dB broad-band masker. Note at very brief interstimulus intervals that backward masking was greater than forward. There was some frequency effect at less than 15 msec in the forward condition and over a longer interval in the backward condition. Elliott tentatively put forth the theory that backward masking occurs when the subsequent stronger masker produces more rapid synaptic transmissions with the result that the neural signal produced by the strong masker may arrive at the higher neural centers at or before the arrival time of the neural activity due to the prior but weaker test signal.

Wright (1964a,b) theorized that backward masking consists of three phases. The first phase is that closest to the masker (out to about 25 msec) where he observed that the amount of masking was dependent on the masker level. This phase may be accounted for by the neurophysiologic explanation given by Elliott. The other two phases were a long phase and a transition phase. The long phase extended from about 50 to about 200 msec before the masker with a transition between 25 and 50 msec. The long phase was not dependent on masker level and, therefore, seemed to result from a separate process, perhaps more central, but unknown. Babkoff and Sutton (1968) obtained backward masking results that they concluded are also consistent with an intensity–neural latency conversion of the general type suggestion by Elliott and earlier by Guttman et al. (1960).

Forward masking has been generally thought of as an adaptation or short-term fatigue phenomenon (C. M. Harris, 1959). Recently Deatherage and Evans (1969) concluded that some forward masking is not a result of fatigue or adaptation of the peripheral mechanism.

Their conclusion was based on the observation that some forward masking is noted in the dichotic situation (Elliott, 1965) and on their own results which also showed forward masking in several "crossed" (binaural) conditions. This led them to the tentative statement that their observation "suggests that peripheral adaptation is not an adequate explanation for this type of masking but instead, or perhaps additionally, is a phenomenon attributable in part to more centrally located neural structures [p. 370]."

Residual masking is a term which is also used to refer to the threshold shifts observed in a short interval after the cessation of a masker. When this term is used it usually indicates that the purpose of the study was to investigate the masking effect of one pure tone on another pure tone of differing frequency. In order to escape the beats and other interference phenomena associated with the simultaneous presentations of pure tones, the test tone is presented just after (up to about 200 msec) the masker tone is turned off (Ehmer and Ehmer, 1969; C. M. Harris, 1959).

In 1964 Pollack presented the results of an experiment involving the additivity of forward and backward masking. As in the earlier reviewed experiments on additivity and multiple maskers, the question was posed as to whether two equally effective maskers would produce a 3-dB masking increase when combined. Pollack observed between 7 and 22 dB of additional masking with combined forward and backward masking under various conditions!

IV. Binaural Masking Effects

A. Contralateral Effects

In this section are discussed those experiments wherein a test signal was presented to one ear while the masker was presented to the other. The topics include central masking and contralateral remote masking.

Contralateral remote masking (CRM) is that elevation in threshold observed at relatively low frequencies in one ear when a high-pass filtered noise is presented to the opposite ear. Ward (1961), in an extensive investigation, concluded that CRM is largely the result of the acoustic reflex which is activated by the unilateral high-frequency noise. Bilger (1966) took issue with this conclusion. Bilger compared normal control subjects with subjects who had cut stapedius muscles and demonstrated no differences in either ipsilateral or contralateral remote masking between the two groups. Hence, the acoustic reflex could not account for remote masking of either type.

In 1967 Ward again reviewed the subject and agreed that the stapedial reflex does not account for contralateral remote masking. Ward concluded that "CRM represents primarily central masking arising at one or more centers receiving afferent innervation from both right and left ears and that the change in time of CRM can be ascribed to adaptation processes [p. 593]."

Also in 1967, Gjaevenes and Vigran concluded that the CRM is "most probably caused by the middle-ear muscle reflex [p. 580]." However, they felt they could not decide whether other mechanisms were involved. Then, in a follow-up work Gjaevenes *et al.* (1969) calculated the expected threshold shift due to the acoustic reflex on the basis of eardrum impedance measurements made with and without the contralateral noise. These calculations indicated that the observed CRM was substantially bigger than could be accounted for by eardrum impedance changes. Therefore, they concluded with Bilger (1966) and Ward (1967) that central factors are predominant.

Recently, Keith and Anderson (1969) reported the results of a remote masking study using subjects with high-frequency hearing losses. They observed that when the noise was located in the frequency region of the hearing loss, less remote masking resulted. This, together with other evidence, was taken to indicate that the acoustic reflex is a significant factor in remote masking. They felt "a dual mechanism of acoustic reflex plus cochlear activity" must be invoked to explain all the available evidence.

Definitions of central masking normally include the concept that any direct masking effect on the test ear through physical crossover of sound energy to the test ear is excluded. Also, acoustic reflex effects are generally excluded. However, CRM may be considered by some to be a form of central masking.

Ingham (1959) observed that central masking was greatest at test-tone frequencies within about 30 Hz of a masker-tone frequency which was presented to the opposite ear. Sherrick and Mangabeira-Albernaz (1961) noted that central masking was greater for high frequencies and concluded, therefore, that it could not be produced by the aural reflex. They also demonstrated that the effect was much greater when masker and test signal were pulsed on and off together than when the masker was steady and test signal only was pulsed. Furthermore, when the masker was a pure tone, central masking was greater as the test-signal frequency approached the masker frequency and that gradually the task was one of localization.

Dirks and Malmquist (1965) used five combinations of pulsed and continuous masker noises and test tones in a central masking experiment.

The greatest threshold shifts appeared when signal and masker were both on continuously or when they were pulsed on and off together. When the test signal was pulsed and the masker was continuous very little central masking was seen (about 1 dB).

Dirks and Norris (1966) studied the effect of masker level on the central masking effect. Sherrick and Mangabeira-Albernaz (1961) had observed a 1-dB threshold increase for each 10-dB masker level increase. Dirks and Norris observed a 2-dB threshold increase for each 15-dB masker level increase. However, Dirks and Norris noted that their results were not systematic. Furthermore, it was noted in both studies that there was little or no change in central masking as a function of masker level in the test-signal-pulsed/noise-signal-continuous condition.

Zwislocki and his co-workers (Zwislocki *et al.*, 1967; Zwislocki *et al.*, 1968) in a series of experiments obtained several major findings of which Figures 5 and 6 are illustrative. Figure 5 shows the difference between the results obtained with a steady-state central masker (continuous masker tone) and transient central masker (test tone and masker tone pulsed on together). The masker was a 1000-Hz tone. Central masking was found to be highly frequency dependent and possibly related to the Zwicker *et al.* (1957) critical bands the width of which at 1000 Hz is noted in Figure 5. Figure 6 illustrates the effect of delaying the onset of the test signal relative to that of the masker onset. Threshold shifts as great as 11 dB were noted for this subject for simultaneous onset of masker and test tone, with the shift decreasing to about 2–3 dB at 160 msec. Zwislocki and his co-workers felt that this result may

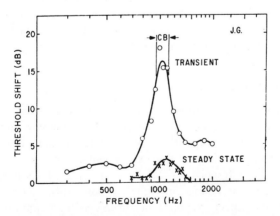

Fig. 5. Frequency distributions of the central masking produced by a contralateral 1000-Hz tone. The "transient" curve is produced when test tone and masker tone are turned on together and "steady-state" is produced when the masker is on 160 msec or more before the test tone. [From Zwislocki *et al.* (1968).]

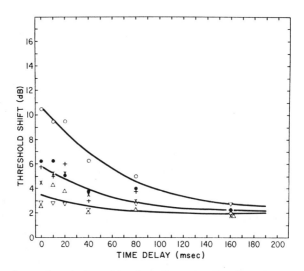

FIG. 6. The decay of central masking from "transient" to "steady-state" conditions for a single observer. ○, 950 Hz; ●, 500; ✕, 600; +, 1100; △, 300; ▽, 2000 Hz. [From Zwislocki *et al.* (1968).]

account for the pulsed versus continuous masker and test signal results obtained by earlier investigators. The parallels between these results and those of studies of overshoot are notable and suggest that ipsilateral overshoot may be, at least in part, a central phenomenon. This conclusion is also suggested by the results of Stokinger and Lankford (1969).

Zwislocki *et al.* (1967, 1968) observed that the central masking effect noted with simultaneous onset was masker level dependent, producing about a 1-dB increase for every 2-dB increase in masker level. The "steady state" masking was independent of masker level, a result which is consistent with the studies noted earlier.

B. Masking Level Differences

The articles on this subject during the past 10 years alone are so extensive in number and type that an entire chapter could be easily devoted to this topic alone. The review which follows must necessarily exclude even mention of many fine experiments.

Masking level difference, or MLD, is a term which may be defined operationally as that change in signal-to-noise ratio necessary to maintain equivalent subject response performance to monaurally or binaurally presented test signals when a binaural masker is presented in place of a monaural masker or when, principally, the phase, interaural correlation or interaural time of arrival relation of a binaural masker or test signal is (are) modified. The early work in this area was summarized and analyzed by Jeffress *et al.* (1956).

The earliest work with MLD's was carried out by manipulating the phase of the masker and test signals at the two ears. For example, the signals at the two ears were made homophasic (in phase) or antiphasic (180° out of phase). A typical experiment was to present tone and noise to one ear (Nm — Sm, to use the symbolization of Jeffress *et al.*, 1956 and subsequently)[1] and vary the signal-to-noise ratio until the desired performance level was obtained from the subject. Then the noise was added to the opposite ear as well and it was observed that in order to maintain the same subject performance the signal-to-noise ratio had to be reduced. The change in the ratio required is the MLD. (Of course, other measures can be used, such as changes in subject performance or *d'*.) In another experiment noise and tone were presented to both ears both in phase (N0–S0) as the reference condition and then the phase of one of the signals was reversed, for example, to N0–Sπ. A substantial improvement in masked threshold resulted (Jeffress *et. al.*, 1956).

Diercks and Jeffress (1962), on the basis of their own work and earlier studies, presented a hierarchy of MLD conditions in the order of increasing signal detectability. The three conditions that produce the poorest detection are Nπ–Sπ, N0–S0, and Nm–Sm (Diercks and Jeffress, 1962). These were reported to produce about equal masked thresholds and are used as the reference conditions in most MLD studies. The following conditions produce increasingly large MLD's, Nu–Sπ, Nu–S0, Nπ–Sm, N0–Sm. The best detection is obtained in the antiphasic conditions Nπ–S0 and N0–Sπ (Diercks and Jeffress, 1962).

Noise correlation is a concept which needs explanation. When a noise from a single source is split and led to earphones on the two ears, the noise at the two ears is in perfect positive correlation (+1.0) if in phase, and in perfect negative correlation (−1.0) if out of phase. The noise at the two ears is completely uncorrelated (0.0) if a separate noise source supplies the noise for each ear. When a combination of uncorrelated and perfectly correlated noise is desired, three noise generators can be used, one going to both ears and one of each of the others going to one ear. The extent of the noise correlation is determined

---

[1] The symbolization used by Jeffress *et al.* (1956) as recently modified will be used throughout this chapter. It includes, principally, S and N as signal and noise and several modifiers. The modifiers "m" means a monaural presentation, "0" means in phase at the two ears, "π" means out of phase at the two ears, and "u" means the noise at the two ears is uncorrelated.

by the relative levels of the correlated and uncorrelated noise signals. Another method is to send one source to both ears and a second noise source to one ear. The formulas needed to calculate the correlation for each of these cases and their derivation were given by Jeffress and Robinson in 1962.

Figure 7 reproduces a figure first presented by Durlach (1960) which summarized several studies on antiphasic MLD's along with a prediction based on Durlach's equalization–cancellation (EC) model which will be discussed later. The general size of the antiphasic MLD is about 15 dB at low frequencies, decreasing in size through the midfrequency range.

Figure 8 shows the effects of noise correlation on the MLD for signal in phase and for signal out of phase. These data are from Robinson and Jeffress (1963). In order to facilitate the comparison, Robinson and Jeffress reversed the abcissa for the S0 condition so that the two curves approximately parallel each other in the figure, rather than crossing. The MLD extended from 0 dB with $S\pi$ and noise at -1.0 correlation (which is equivalent to $N\pi$) to about 12–15 dB with the noise at $+1.0$ correlation (or N0). With S0 the same results were obtained but in reverse with respect to the noise correlation. Note that there was only about a 3-dB difference between $S\pi$–Nu and $S\pi$–Nπ. Also note that the MLD decreased very quickly as the noise correlation was reduced from 1.0 or -1.0.

Langford and Jeffress (1964) studied the effect of "cross-correlated" noise on the masked threshold. Noise cross correlation was accomplished by time delaying the noise going to one ear relative to the noise from

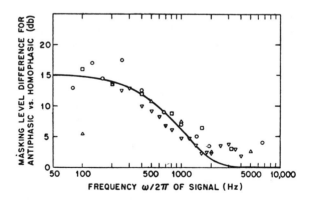

FIG. 7. Antiphasic MLD's as a function of frequency of the test tone as obtained by various investigators and a prediction from the EC model. △, Hirsh; ▽, Hirsh and Burgeat; ○, Webster; ☐, Durlach;—theory. [From Durlach (1960).]

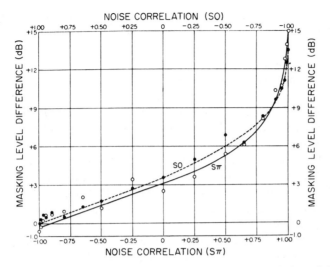

FIG. 8. MLD's as a function of interaural noise correlation with $S0$ and $S\pi$ signals. The top abcissa is for $S0$ and the bottom for $S\pi$. [From Robinson and Jeffress (1963).]

the same source (correlated) going to the other ear. Figure 9 reproduces a Langford and Jeffress figure showing the MLD for in-phase and out-of-phase signals as a function of the noise interaural delay. The alteration of the two curves is very evident. The data were interpreted to mean that the binaural system is able to effect a correlation between the events at the two ears even though the time of arrival differs somewhat, at least up to about 9 msec. At 0 msec delay the MLD for the

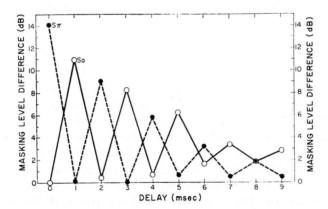

FIG. 9. MLD's for $S0$ and $S\pi$ as a function of the interaural time delay of correlated noise. [From Langford and Jeffress (1964).]

S0 condition was 0 dB and for the S_π condition the MLD was about 14 dB because the noise was perfectly correlated, which is equivalent to N0. It was hypothesized that only the components in the noise around the frequency of the test tone (500 Hz) are influential and that this narrow band influences the auditory system as would a pure tone located at the center of the band. When delayed, the components in the 500-Hz centered narrow band are put out of phase with respect to each other at the two ears. Assuming the narrow band behaved like a pure tone, a half-period time delay would put the signals at the two ears 180° out of phase. Hence, the MLD with an S0 signal will be maximum and the MLD with a S_π signal will be minimum with a half-period delay. Because the half period of 500 Hz is 1 msec, the results for this frequency should reverse in 1-msec intervals as was the case as illustrated in Figure 9.

In a study of interaural time delays Zerlin (1966) concluded that the MLD increases with interaural delay time in a manner similar to that for analogous interaural phase differences. Rilling and Jeffress (1965) in a comparison of interaural phase and time delays using tones and narrow bands as test signals observed that when the signal noise had an independent source that tones and narrow-band noise showed the same MLD's as a result of temporal delays and concluded that "there is essentially no difference in detectability between a given phase shift for the central frequency of a narrow band of noise and a corresponding time delay [p. 206]."

The MLD is generally assumed to be produced by a narrow band within the broad-band masking noise immediately surrounding the frequency of the test tone. Langford and Jeffress (1964) estimated the band to be about 100 Hz wide at 500 Hz. Sondhi and Guttman (1966) cite some unpublished works in which the bandwidths were found to be 133 Hz at 500 Hz and 90 Hz at 500 Hz. Sondhi and Guttman (1966) obtained effective bandwidths of 200 Hz at 500 Hz and 125 Hz at 250 Hz which are considerably wider than the earlier estimates.

Mulligan et al. (1967) reported a study which demonstrated that only a narrow band around the frequency of the test tone is effective in producing the MLD. Masking level differences were obtained with a medium band noise (3100 Hz wide), a narrow band noise (1600 Hz wide), and a medium band noise with a hole in it about a critical bandwidth wide and centered at the test-tone frequency. When set at equal spectral levels, the first two noises produced equal MLD's in spite of the different overall levels. The third noise produced much smaller MLD's. Mulligan et al. (1967) concluded that the MLD depends upon the relative levels, phase, and correlation of the paired critical bands of the two ears.

Two theories or models devised to encompass and explain MLD's have received extensive consideration. These are the Webster–Jeffress model (Jeffress et al., 1956) and the EC (equalization–cancellation) model of Durlach (1960). More recently Schenkel (1967) proposed what he calls the accumulation theory.

According to the Webster–Jeffress model (also called the Jeffress model, the delay-line model, or the interaural-difference model), the outputs of the corresponding filter sections (critical bands) from the two ears are compared through use of delay nets which compensate for the delay in the signal delivered to one ear and thereby provide the system with the information necessary for localization. The Webster hypothesis is then added. The Webster hypothesis is that with a noise presentation, the ear's filter delivers to the subsequent detector a signal which for short intervals can "be considered a tone to which the signal-tone is added in random phase. . . . When the interaural conditions are homophasic, the phase change [produced by the addition of the test signal] at each ear will be in the same direction and no interaural phase shift will result [Jeffress et al. (1956, p. 420)]." However, if the phase of either test tone or noise is reversed in phase at the two ears relative to the other, the phase change produced by the addition of the tone will produce a phase advance in one ear and a delay in the other. The resulting time difference "can be detected by some central mechanism [p. 420]"; presumably by the localization mechanism mentioned above.

In 1960 Durlach presented the EC (equalization–cancellation) model. The first step occurs when "the auditory system attempts to eliminate the masking components by transforming the total signal in one ear relative to the total signal in the other ear until the masking components are exactly the same in both ears (the E process), and then subtracting the total signal in one ear from the total signal in the other ear (the C process) [Durlach (1963, p. 1207)]." If the test signal has the same phase relationship at the two ears as the noise, it will be canceled with the noise. If the test signal has a phase relationship at the two ears which is different from that of the noise, the EC process will cancel the noise but not the tone. This model leads to the conclusion that the noise should not mask the tone at all in the antiphasic condition. Because this clearly is not the case, Durlach (1963) proposed that the "processing is assumed to be corrupted by various types of errors [p. 1206]." These include, principally, jitter in the E mechanism which may result in slightly different signals being delivered to the C mechanism from the two sides. A set of critical-band filters is assumed for each ear and, as for all theories of MLD, it is assumed that processing takes place in critical band pairs from the two ears.

The Schenkel (1967) "accumulation" model was explained using a theoretical circuit. Schenkel proposed that the signal-plus-noise inputs from the two ears are fed to each of three devices which compare the instantaneous amplitudes of the two inputs by adding them and by subtracting each from the other (that is, A + B, A − B, and B − A). The results of this processing are then sent on to a discriminator section where they are added to the unprocessed inputs from each ear in six identical but separate discriminator mechanisms. "Accumulation" of the signal has resulted in producing an algebraic threefold increase in signal relative to noise as compared to the monaural condition in two of the discriminators. Schenkel went on to state that detection will result if the signal-to-noise value is great enough in any one or more of the discriminators.

Diercks and Jeffress (1962) presented evidence to support the hypothesis that absolute threshold is really a masked threshold with the noise supplied internally. Their experiment concerned the 3-dB improvement in threshold which is seen commonly with binaural signal presentations relative to monaural presentations. They observed a 2.8-dB improvement when the tones at the two ears were presented homophasically, but with antiphasic tones the improvement was 3.7 dB or 0.9 dB greater than with S0. These results suggested to Diercks and Jeffress that the absolute threshold is a masked threshold and also that "the 'self' noise is made up of three components, one unique to one ear, one to the other, and one common to both. The last creates a small positive correlation [p. 984]." (Recall the three-noise-source arrangement described earlier.) On this basis Diercks and Jeffress concluded that the 3-dB binaural summation phenomenon may be a binaural masking phenomenon rather than a result of neurophysiological energy summation.

McFaddin (1968) presented evidence that he felt supported the work of Diercks and Jeffress (1962) and then went on to estimate the extent of the correlations of the internal noise. His estimate was arrived at indirectly by using the apparent 4.5-dB release from masking that he inferred for the "unmasked" condition. Using the results from the earlier work by Robinson and Jeffress (1963), the internaural correlation necessary to produce this MLD was noted. The answer was +0.35.

G. G. Harris (1968), on the basis of various assumptions, calculated the level of the Brownian motion of the cochlear partition. Various conceivable assumptions resulted in answers ranging from +22 to −33 dB signal-to-noise ratios at normal threshold and, therefore, Harris felt that it was not as yet possible to determine whether cochlear partition Brownian noise is the noise which establishes normal threshold.

C. MLD's for Speech

During the past 4 or 5 years a substantial amount of work has appeared on MLD's for speech signals. In 1963 Feldman demonstrated that monaurally masked speech discrimination scores were improved when the noise was added also to the opposite ear. He further noted that MLD's can be produced by an interaural time delay of either speech or noise signals. He concluded that the MLD's for speech test signals are dependent on the frequencies below 1200 Hz.

In 1966 Carhart and his associates published the first of a series of extensive works on MLD's using speech test signals. In this first study they observed a 4.5-dB release from masking for monosyllable word intelligibility when a continuous noise was made antiphasic (Carhart et al., 1966).

Levitt and Rabiner (1967a,b) investigated changes in the detectability and intelligibility of speech as a function of interaural phase. For the N0 — Sπ case they observed an MLD for the *detection* of single words of 13 dB and concluded that the result was determined principally by the frequencies below 500 Hz. This MLD value is quite close to the MLD obtained for the detection of pure-tone test signals in this frequency region. The MLD for intelligibility of single words was 6 dB and was not so dependent on low frequencies. On the basis of their work and that of others, Levitt and Rabiner (1967b) proposed that the binaural gain in intelligibility resulting from binaural listening can be calculated by correcting the articulation index (AI) by the frequency-dependent release from masking for pure tones produced by the binaural conditions in question.

Carhart et al. (1967) investigated the effects of interaural time delays on the release from masking. The MLD's became greater as the time delays were increased from 0.1 to 0.8 msec, but they observed that the MLD's for time delays were never as great as for the antiphasic condition and often fell far short. It was also found that antiphasic intelligibility MLD's were 7 dB for spondees and 4 dB for monosyllables.

Carhart et al. (1968) observed that the ability to attribute a specific location to a sound "is distinct from the capacity to achieve intelligibility for speech under various interaural conditions [p. 1230]." In several instances the greatest binaural release was obtained under conditions wherein the subject had the most difficulty in assigning a location to the signal or the noise. This finding is in agreement with the results of Flanagan and Watson (1966) who used pulse trains as the test stimuli, but is in apparent disagreement with some early explanations of MLD's based on apparent locations (azimuths) of noise and test signals.

Carhart *et al.* (1969) observed that the perceptual masking which results when maskers are combined and when at least one is a speech masker is essentially equivalent in homophasic, antiphasic, and time-delayed conditions supporting the Carhart *et al.* contention that masking involves at least two essentially independent stages. The first stage is that one which is the subject of the theoretical MLD models discussed in the previous section. The second stage is that one revealed when the system is called upon to perform two sorting operations as when a speech masker is combined with other masking signals.

V. Clinical Applications

The application of masking noises for clinical purposes can be divided into two general areas. In one the noise and test signals are presented to the same ear or ears for the purpose of detecting abnormal masking patterns, reducing the intelligibility of speech, detecting nonorganic hearing loss, and so on. The second category is one in which the purpose is to keep one ear masked while the other is being tested. Rainville-based procedures are included in this latter category.

A. Masking the Same Ear(s)

Noise audiometry is a procedure that is over 40 years old and it continues to be promoted by European writers (Langenbeck, 1965). As presently used, noise audiometry is a procedure in which pure-tone thresholds are obtained in the presence of a broad-band noise. Differential diagnosis is based on the "ease" with which pure tones are masked (Langenbeck, 1965). For example, Langenbeck states that in "acoustic nerve lesions the tones in the region of the lesion can be masked with abnormal ease; the intensity of tones . . . must be much greater than the noise, to become audible [p. 133]."

A number of papers, however, have refuted the claims of the noise audiometry proponents; particularly Jerger *et al.* (1960), Jerger and Waller (1962), and Palva *et al.* (1953). Jerger *et al.* (1960), for example, observed no differences in the signal-to-noise ratios among patients with otosclerosis, otitis media, sensorineural hearing loss, or presbycusis. Palva *et al.* (1953) earlier had reached the same conclusion. Finally, Jerger and Waller (1962) carefully tested a patient who was confirmed to have had a retrocochlear lesion and found that signal-to-noise ratios at masked threshold were equal to those found in normal ears and observed that the signal-to-noise ratio at threshold did not change over a period of several minutes' exposure.

Harbert and Young (1965) reported that in their experience eighth nerve hearing-loss patients produce masked threshold at test-signal levels at or above the white-noise level rather than 15–20 dB below the noise level as in other persons. They showed two examples of eighth nerve lesions where the masked threshold level for pure tones at the center of a critical-band noise was 5–10 dB above the noise-band level, in contrast to their own results and those of others for all other types of sensorineural hearing losses. These results are, of course, in agreement with Langenbeck.

A possible source of the differing opinions concerning noise audiometry may lie in what Langenbeck called the "clear tone" threshold. He acknowledged that it is above the best detection threshold but insisted that it is this threshold that must be used in noise audiometry. Harbert and Young (1965), used Békésy audiometry and they also have recommended using the "tonal" threshold (Harbert and Young, 1964).

The use of narrow band maskers to measure high- and low-frequency spread of masking has found some application as a means of differentiating between various auditory system pathologies. Harbert and Young (1965), Jerger et al. (1960), and Rittmanic (1962). demonstrated that ears which exhibited sensorineural hearing loss were subject to more high- and low frequency spread of masking than were normal and conductively impaired ears. Martin and Pickett (1970) observed a high degree of intersubject variability in the high-frequency spread of masking for both normal hearing and sensorineural hearing loss groups. They observed that the amount of upward spread was not strongly related to the degree of hearing loss and that persons with similar audiograms produced markedly different masking spread pictures. Martin and Pickett did not relate their results to factors other than the degree of hearing loss.

No retrocochlear pathology cases were evaluated by Jerger et al. (1960), Martin and Pickett (1970), or Rittmanic (1962). Harbert and Young (1965), however, did report masking-spread data on the two eighth nerve lesion cases mentioned earlier. These eighth nerve lesion patients were said to be representative of a larger number of cases. Each of the two cases reported showed very extensive high- and low-frequency masking spread which was substantially in excess of that seen with any other pathology type. It would seem that masking and masking spread in cases of eighth nerve pathology may not as yet be entirely resolved.

Katz (1969) presented what he called the continuous tone masking test (CTM). In this procedure the patient is called upon to trace his threshold (Békésy audiometry) for a pulsed tone in presence of an ipsilateral continuous tone masker of the same frequency presented at various levels. Those with cochlear hearing losses are reported to produce thresholds at the smallest signal-to-noise ratios, with normal hearers at slightly larger signal-to-noise ratios and those with retrocochlear pathology at much larger signal-to-noise ratios. Only one example of each type is reported. The relationship between this procedure and DL for intensity procedures requires clarification.

Bess and Clack (1969) studied tone on tone masking in subjects with sensorineural losses. They observed highly divergent patterns from patient to patient but noted generally much greater masking than normal at test tone frequencies above that of the pure-tone masker. Occasionally a tone at the first harmonic was masked more than were test tones near the frequency of the masker. In spite of the large intersubject variability, Bess and Clack noted a high degree of relationship between the amount of high-frequency masking spread and poor speech discrimination ability.

Young and Wenner (1968) studied the influence of a masking noise in the same ear on SISI test results. They observed, in agreement with earlier studies, that the signal-to-noise ratio was the only significant variable in determining DLI when the test tone was at least 60 dB above normal threshold. They also noted that the masked SISI scores with a given increment size went from 0 to 100% over a very small signal-to-noise ratio range, often as little as 5 dB.

Olsen and Carhart (1967) observed that a noise masker produced 5 dB greater masking of monosyllabic speech signals in the case of young adult persons with sensorineural hearing loss than observed in those with normal hearing. In the case of those with presbycusis the difference between those with hearing loss and those with normal hearing increasd to 8 dB. When sentences were used as the masker, the normal–abnormal performance disparity increased another 6 dB. Groen (1969) used a noise masker shaped to approximately equal the spectrum of cocktail party noise and observed that the signal-to-noise ratio had to be increased by 8 dB in order that presbycusics could understand monosyllables as well as normal listeners.

B. Masking the Contralateral Ear

It is well known that when a test signal is delivered by earphone to one ear of a patient, the signal also arrives at the opposite ear at an attenuated level, usually about 50–60 dB lower. With bone-conduction vibrator presentations, the signal level at the opposite ear is probably only about 0–10 dB less than at the presentation ear. The difference between the presentation level and the level at the opposite ear is referred to as the interaural attenuation (IA). Whenever the presentation level minus the IA is greater than the threshold of the nontest ear, then the nontest ear may have a significant influence on the test result. When this is not desired, noise is usually applied to the nontest ear at a level sufficient to prevent it.

The sensorineural acuity level (SAL) is briefly discussed in this section. While this procedure does present the masking noise to both ears, nevertheless, the purpose is to test one ear at a time. The SAL was first described by Jerger and Tillman in 1960. A more recent description of how it is applied was presented by Jerger and Jerger (1965). The main advantages of the procedure are that it can be standardized in an environment that does not need to be very quiet and that it substitutes the IA of air conduction for that of bone conduction (Jerger and Jerger, 1965).

After its initial introduction, the procedure soon met with a number of criticisms. Principal among these were (1) limited intensity level range with low frequency test tones (a fault it shares with standard bone-conduction tests), (2) difficulties associated with occluding the ears with earphones, and (3) excessive high-frequency spread of masking in the case of those with sesorineural hearing losses (Tillman, 1963).

Jerger and Jerger (1965) summarized previous work on the test and took issue with some of the conclusions reached by others. Only those aspects related to masking will be discussed here. Jerger and Jerger (1965) noted that there was no noise duration effect for at least 56-min exposures and they concluded that there is a one-to-one relation between the noise level and the SAL result. They observed that the correlation of the noise in the two ears did produce an MLD, but that it was the same in those persons with various hearing losses as in normal listeners and thereby should not affect the SAL test results. They pointed out, however, that retrocochlear pathologies may produce quite different results as a result of noise correlation because "timing relations may be quite aberrant [p. 113]." Finally, Jerger and Jerger reported that they did not observe the large disagreement between SAL and conventional bone-conduction audiometry in the high frequencies noted by Tillman (1963). They presented evidence which they believed suggested that the Tillman results may have been artifactual.

Whatever one's position is concerning the SAL as a substitute or adjunct to conventional bone-conduction testing, a familiarity with unilateral masking procedures is also necessary. In 1967 I (Studebaker,

1967) summarized the conclusions reached by many previous investigators and drew some conclusions based on this review. Among these were that narrow-band noises centered at the test-tone frequency are the preferred maskers of pure tones. Narrow bands need be less intense and each narrow-band noise can be calibrated independently so that the masking level dial on the audiometer always indicates the noise effective level.

Each clinician should have at his disposal some means of calibrating his masking noises. This may be done by obtaining the thresholds of normal-hearing persons for the test signals desired in the presence of the available noise (see Studebaker, 1967 or Coles and Priede, 1970) or by measuring the level of the noise in the frequency region of the test signal, calculating the noise spectrum level and then, through the use of the critical ratios, obtaining the noise effective levels.

In 1967 I also reviewed various masking procedures and concluded that the most successful procedures are those based, in one way or another, on the threshold shift phenomenon. The procedure proposed by Hood (1957) appears to be the most popular (however, I suspect that the "I guess that's about right" approach is still the most popular of all) in this country and elsewhere (Coles and Priede, 1970). This approach consists of applying the masking noise to the nontest ear at an effective level of 10-dB SL. If the apparent threshold of the test ear changes, then the noise level is increased further. This is repeated until noise level increases in one ear do not produce further changes in the apparent threshold of the other ear. This procedure is popular, probably because it is simple to carry out and it is easy to understand. There are some disadvantages associated with using the low effective levels and the safety of the procedure is increased if at least two effective levels, say 10- and 20-dB SL, are used routinely in order to avoid the possibility of undermasking with particular patients.

A second procedure is one presented in detail by Konig (1963). With this procedure a specially built audiometer is required. For routine cases the procedure is nearly totally automatic, but in problem cases, additional manual steps need to be taken. (See Konig, 1963 for a complete description.)

In 1964 and 1967 I described a method in which the noise is presented at a relatively high effective level. The purpose was to produce a large threshold shift, if one were to occur, in order to reduce the number of sometimes equivocable threshold shifts that are produced by low effective level noise presentations. The procedure can be used with automatic equipment of the type described by Konig (1963) and the noise presentation level is always a known number of decibels below the over-masking level. A major disadvantage is that the basis for the procedure is somewhat difficult to grasp (Studebaker, 1967).

C. The Influence of Masking the Nontest Ear on Clinical Test Results

The effect of a contralateral noise on pure-tone air-conduction thresholds was reviewed in the section on central masking. In these studies the elevations in the thresholds for interrupted tones of greater than moderate duration in the presence of continuous contralateral noise (the usual clinical conditions) were shown to be about 1–3 dB (Dirks and Malmquist, 1965; Zwislocki et al., 1967; Zwislocki et al., 1968).

In the case of bone-conduction tests the influence of a unilateral masker on threshold is somewhat larger, particularly if the bone-conduction vibrator is placed at the forehead (Studebaker, 1962; Dirks and Malmquist, 1964). The threshold shift was observed in these studies to be around 4 or 5 dB with mastoid vibrator placement and around 7 or 8 dB with forehead vibrator placement. The larger threshold shifts observed in bone-conduction testing were thought to occur because unmasked bone-conduction thresholds are really binaural thresholds, particularly with the vibrator placed at the forehead. The introduction of a masking noise to one ear removes the participation of this ear and, therefore, the masked thresholds are monaural thresholds which of course, are somewhat poorer than binaural. These threshold shifts presumably summate with those produced as a central masking effect (Studebaker, 1962; Dirks and Malmquist, 1964).

With exception of several works by Blegvad, remarkably little published work is to be found on the influence of contralateral noise on typical clinical auditory tests. In 1967 Blegvad and Terkildsen (1967) applied contralateral noise at 0, 50, 70, and 90 dB while obtaining intensive DL's in the opposite ear with a modified SISI procedure. With normal listeners the contralateral noise increased the size of the DLI at 250 Hz possibly due to the acoustic reflex which probably reduces the input to the cochlea at this frequency. A decrease in DLI was noted at 1000 Hz and 4000 Hz of about 0.5 dB with the 70 and 90 dB contralateral noise levels. A 0.5 dB DLI change should have a substantial influence on the outcome of a SISI test. However, it must be noted that only infrequently do circumstances dictate the need for contralateral masking with SISI test.

Blegvad (1967) evaluated the effect of contralateral noise on Békésy tracings produced by normal listeners and in 1968 he (Blegvad, 1968) also reported a similar study in which he used persons with unilateral sensorineural hearing loss. He noted that the separation between continuous and interrupted tone tracings was increased by the contralateral noise, particularly in the hearing loss group. The continuous versus interrupted tracing separation increased as much as 25 dB and 10 or 15 dB increases were not unusual among those with sensorineural hearing losses. A shortening of excursion size was also noted and was more noticeable in the hearing loss group. Blegvad noted that seven Type I tracings were changed to Type II's; seven Type II's were changed to Type IV's and three Type I's were changed to Type IV's. However, none were changed to Type III.

Grimes and Feldman (1969) compared Békésy tracings with broadband and narrow-band noises in the opposite ear. They observed that when the noise bands were narrow enough to approach the critical bandwidth, some subject confusion resulted. This confusion produced substantial elevations in the continuous tone thresholds (as much as 40 dB in the presence of a high-frequency hearing loss). For this reason Grimes and Feldman strongly recommended against using narrow-band masking noises which approach the critical bandwidth at any test signal frequency in continuous-tone Békésy audiometry.

There is extremely little information published which bears directly on the point of the effect of contralateral noise on clinical speech hearing test results. The data from two studies, one by Martin et al. (1965) and one by Martin (1966) suggest that the shift in SRT is about 2 or 3 dB and that discrimination scores are virtually unaffected except in those cases where some crossover to the better ear might be expected in the unmasked condition.

VI. Comment

Several areas seem to this writer to be in great need of study. One is that area discussed in the paragraphs just above. Very little is known about the effects of the routinely used contralateral noises upon clinical auditory tests other than pure tone absolute threshold. Blegvad's results suggest that very significant effects may exist.

Other areas calling for study are the application of the extensive literature on MLD's to the clinical situation and to the investigation of the nature of impaired auditory system. Carhart and his associates have made great strides in the area of speech signal MLD's. These ultimately may be of great usefulness in arriving at a better understanding of binaural hearing in the speech communication process and, thereby, at a better understanding of communication with a defective auditory system.

It seems that many questions concerning spread of masking, critical-band masking and the role of instructions to the patient, particularly patients with eighth nerve lesions, are not answered satisfactorily as yet. Other nearly untapped areas include additivity of masking and forward and backward masking in the defective auditory system. Overall, the impression gained in the preparation of this chapter is that the vast literature on the psychophysics of masking has found only very limited application in the development of research tools for the study of defective hearing or of clinical tools outside of the contralateral masking problem. A greater number of research efforts on the psychophysics of masking were published between 1960 and 1970 than in all of previous history combined. Perhaps the next 10 years will see a comparable increase in the efforts to apply this knowledge.

References

American National Standards Inst. (1960). Acoustical terminology. S1.1-1960, New York.

Babkoff, H., and Sutton, S. (1968). Monaural temporal masking of transients. *J. Acoust. Soc. Amer.* **44**, 1373–1378.

Bess, F. H., and Clack, T. D. (1969). Monaural masking patterns in normal and abnormal listeners. Paper presented at the 78th meeting of the Acoust. Soc. Amer., San Diego, Calif.

Bilger, R. C. (1959). Additivity of different types of masking. *J. Acoust. Soc. Amer.* **31**, 1107–1109.

Bilger, R. C. (1966). Remote masking in the absence of intra-aural muscles. *J. Acoust. Soc. Amer.* **39**, 103–108.

Bilger, R. C., and Hirsh, I. J. (1956). Masking of tones by bands of noise. *J. Acoust. Soc. Amer.* **28**, 623–630.

Bilger, R. C., and Melnick, W. (1968). Shifts in masking with time. *J. Acoust. Soc. Amer.* **44**, 941–944.

Blegvad, B. (1967). Contralateral masking and Bekesy audiometry in normal listeners. *Acta Oto-Laryngol.* **64**, 157–165.

Blegvad, B. (1968). Bekesy audiometry and clinical masking. *Acta Oto-Laryngol.* **66**, 229–240.

Blegvad, B., and Terkildsen, K. (1967). Contralateral masking and the SISI-test in normal listeners. *Acta Oto-Laryngol.* **63**, 556–563.

Bos, C. E., and deBoer, E. (1966). Masking and discrimination. *J. Acoust. Soc. Amer.* **39**, 708–715.

Burgeat, M., and Hirsh, I. J. (1961). Changes in masking with time. *J. Acoust. Soc. Amer.* **33**, 963–965.

Campbell, R. A. (1964). Masker level and noise-signal detection. *J. Acoust. Soc. Amer.* **36**, 570–575.

Campbell, R. A., and Lasky, E. Z. (1967). Masker level and sinusoidal-signal detection. *J. Acoust. Soc. Amer.* **42**, 972–976.

Carhart, R., Tillman, T. W., and Johnson, K. R. (1966). Binaural masking of speech by periodically modulated noise. *J. Acoust. Soc. Amer.* **39**, 1037–1050.

Carhart, R., Tillman, T. W., and Johnson, K. R. (1967). Release of masking for speech through interaural time delay. *J. Acoust. Soc. Amer.*, **42**, 124–138.

Carhart, R., Tillman, T. W., and Johnson, K. R. (1968). Effects of interaural

150   GERALD A. STUDEBAKER

time delays on masking by two competing signals. *J. Acoust. Soc. Amer.* **43**, 1223–1230.

Carhart, R., Tillman, T. W., and Gretis, E. S. (1969). Perceptual masking in multiple sound background. *J. Acoust. Soc. Amer.* **45**, 694–703.

Carter, N. L., and Kryter, K. D. (1962). Masking of pure tones and speech. *J. Auditory Res.* **2**, 66–98.

Carterette, E. C., Friedman, M P., and Lovell, J. D. (1969). Mach bands in hearing *J. Acoust. Soc. Amer.* **45**, 986–998.

Coles, R. R. A., and Priede, V. M. (1970). On the misdiagnosis resulting from incorrect use of masking. *J. Laryngol. Otol.* **84**, 41–63.

Deatherage, B. H., and Evans, T. R. (1969). Binaural masking: Backward, forward, and simultaneous effects. *J. Acoust. Soc. Amer.* **46**, 362–371.

Deatherage, B. H., Bilger, R. C., and Eldredge, D. H. (1957a). Remote masking in selected frequency regions. *J. Acoust. Soc. Amer.* **29**, 512–514.

Deatherage, B. H., Davis, H., and Eldredge, D. H. (1957b). Physiological evidence for the masking of low frequencies by high. *J. Acoust. Soc. Amer.* **29**, 132–137.

Diercks, K. J., and Jeffress, L. A. (1962). Interaural phase and the absolute thresholds for tone. *J. Acoust. Soc. Amer.* **34**, 981–984.

Dirks, D. D., and Malmquist, C. (1964). Changes in bone-conduction thresholds produced by masking in the non-test ear. *J. Speech Hearing Res.* **7**, 271–287.

Dirks, D. D., and Norris, J. C. (1966). Shifts in auditory thresholds produced by pulsed and continuous contralateral masking. *J. Acoust. Soc. Amer.* **37**, 631–637.

Dirks, D. D., and Norris, J. C. (1966). Shifts in auditory thresholds produced by ipsilateral and contralateral maskers at low-intensity levels. *J. Acoust. Soc. Amer.* **40**, 12–19.

Dirks, D. D., Wilson, R. H., and Bower, D. R. (1969). Effect of pulsed masking on selected speech materials. *J. Acoust. Soc. Amer.* **46**, 898–906.

Durlach, N. I. (1960). Note on the equalization and cancellation theory of binaural masking level differences. *J. Acoust. Soc. Amer.* **32**, 1075–1076.

Durlach, N. I. (1963). Equalization and cancellation theory of binaural masking-level differences. *J. Acoust. Soc. Amer.* **35**, 1206–1218.

Egan, J. P. (1955). Independence of the masking audiogram from the perstimulatory fatigue of an auditory stimulus. *J. Acoust. Soc. Amer.* **27**, 737–740.

Ehmer, R. H. (1959a). Masking patterns of tones. *J. Acoust. Soc. Amer.* **31**, 1115–1120.

Ehmer, R. H. (1959b). Masking by tones vs. noise bands. *J. Acoust. Soc. Amer.* **31**, 1253–1256.

Ehmer, R. H., and Ehmer, B. J. (1969). Frequency pattern of residual masking by pure tones measured on the Békésy audiometer. *J. Acoust. Soc. Amer.* **46**, 1445–1448.

Elliott, L. L. (1962a). Backward masking: Monotic and dichotic conditions. *J. Acoust. Soc. Amer.* **34**, 1108–1115.

Elliott, L. L. (1962b). Backward and forward masking of probe tones of different frequencies. *J. Acoust. Soc. Amer.* **34**, 1116–1118.

Elliott, L. L. (1965). Changes in the simultaneous masked threshold of brief tones. *J. Acoust. Soc. Amer.* **38**, 738–746.

Feldman, H. (1963). Experiments on binaural hearing in noise. *Trans. Beltone Inst.* **18**, 1–41.

Finck, A. (1961). Low-frequency pure tone masking. *J. Acoust. Soc. Amer.* **33**, 1140–1141.

Finck, A. (1966). Physiological correlate of tonal masking. *J. Acoust. Soc. Amer.* **39**, 1056–1062.

Flanagan, J. L., and Watson, B. J. (1966). Binaural unmasking of complex signals. *J. Acoust. Soc. Amer.* **40**, 456–468.

Fletcher, H. (1940). Auditory patterns. *Rev. Mod. Phys.* **12**, 47–65.

Gjaevenes, K., and Vigran, E. (1967). Contralateral masking: An attempt to determine the role of the aural reflex. *J. Acoust. Soc. Amer.* **42**, 580–585.

Gjaevenes, K., Gran, S., and Rollag, O. (1969). Contralateral remote masking and the aural reflex. *J. Acoust. Soc. Amer.* **46**, 918–923.

Green, D. M. (1967). Additivity of masking. *J. Acoust. Soc. Amer.* **41**, 1517–1525.

Green, D. M. (1969). Masking with continuous and pulsed sinusoids. *J. Acoust. Soc. Amer.* **46**, 939–946.

Grimes, C. T., and Feldman, A. S. (1969). Comparative Békésy typing with broad and modulated narrow-band noise. *J. Speech Hearing Res.* **12**, 840–846.

Groen, J. J. (1969). Social hearing handicap; its measurement by speech audiometry in noise. *Int. Audiol.* **8**, 182–183.

Guttman, N., van Bergeijk, W. A., and David, E. E., Jr. (1960). Monaural temporal masking investigated by binaural interaction. *J. Acoust. Soc. Amer.* **32**, 1329–1336.

Harbert, F., and Young, I. M. (1964). Threshold auditory adaptation measured by tone decay test and Bekesy audiometry. *Ann. Otol. Rhinol. Laryngol.* **73**, 48–60.

Harbert, F., and Young, I. M. (1965). Spread of masking in ears showing abnormal adaptation and conduction deafness. *Acta Oto-Laryngol.* **60**, 49–58.

Harris, C. M. (1959). Residual masking at low frequencies. *J. Acoust. Soc. Amer.* **31**, 1110–1115.

Harris, G. G. (1968). Brownean motion in the cochlear partition. *J. Acoust. Soc. Amer.* **44**, 176–186.

Hawkins, J. E., Jr., and Stevens, S. S. (1950). The masking of pure tones and of speech by white noise. *J. Acoust. Soc. Amer.* **22**, 6–13.

Henning, G. B. (1969). Amplitude discrimination in noise, pedestal experiments, and additivity of masking. *J. Acoust. Soc. Amer.* **45**, 426–435.

Hood, J. D. (1957). The principles and practice of bone conduction audiometry. A review of the present position. *Proc. Roy. Soc. Med.* **50**, 689–697, and (1960), *Laryngoscope* **70**, 1211–1228.

Ingham, J. G. (1959). Variations in cross-masking with frequency. *J. Exp. Psychol.* **58**, 199–205.

Jeffress, L. A., and Robinson, D. E. (1962). Formulas for the coefficient of interaural correlation for noise. *J. Acoust Soc. Amer.* **34**, 1658–1659.

Jeffress, L. A., Blodgett, H. C., Sandel, T. T., and Wood, C. L., III. (1956). Masking of tonal signals. *J. Acoust. Soc. Amer.* **28**, 416–426.

Jerger, J., and Jerger, S. (1965). Critical evaluation of SAL audiometry. *J. Speech Hearing Res.* **8**, 103–127.

Jerger, J., and Tillman, T. W. (1960). A new method for the clinical determination of sensorineural acuity level (SAL). *Arch Otolaryngol.* **71**, 948–955.

Jerger, J., and Waller, J. (1962). Some observations on masking and on the progression of auditory signs in acoustic neurinoma. *J. Speech Hearing Dis.* **27**, 140–143.

Jerger, J. F., Tillman, T. W., and Peterson, J. L. (1960). Masking by octave bands of noise in normal and impaired ears. *J. Acoust. Soc. Amer.* **32**, 385–390.

Jerger, J., Alford, B., Coats, A., and French, B. (1966). Effects of very low frequency tones on auditory thresholds. *J. Speech Hearing Res.* **9**, 150–160.

Johnson, C. S. (1968). Masked tonal threshold in the bottlenosed porpoise. *J. Acoust. Soc. Amer.* **44**, 965–967.

Katz, J. (1969). The continuous tone masking (CTM) test for identifying site of lesion. *J. Auditory Res.* **9**, 76–80.

Keith, R. W., and Anderson, C. V. (1969). Remote masking for listeners with cochlear impairment. *J. Acoust. Soc. Amer.* **46**, 393–398.

Konig, E. (1963). The use of masking noise and its limitations in clinical audiometry. *Acta Oto-Laryngol. Suppl.* **180**.

Kryter, K. D. (1962). Methods for the calculation and use of the articulation index. *J. Acoust. Soc. Amer.* **34**, 1689–1697.

Langenbeck, B. (1965). "Textbook of Practical Audiometry." Williams and Wilkins, Baltimore.

Langford, T. L., and Jeffress, L. A. (1964). Effect of noise crosscorrelation on binaural signal detection. *J. Acoust. Soc. Amer.* **36**, 1455–1458.

Lankford, J. E., and Stokinger, T. E. (1969). Temporal relations in pure-tone ipsilateral masking. Paper presented at the 78th meeting of the Acoust. Soc Amer., San Diego, Calif.

Levitt, H., and Rabiner, L. R. (1967a). Binaural release from masking for speech and gain in intelligibility. *J. Acoust. Soc. Amer.* **42**, 601–608.

Levitt, H., and Rabiner, L. R. (1967b). Predicting binaural gain in intelligibility and release from masking for speech. *J. Acoust Soc. Amer.* **42**, 820–829.

Martin, E. S., and Pickett, J. M. (1970). Sensorineural hearing loss and upward spread of masking. *J. Speech Hearing Res.* **13**, 426–437.

Martin, F. N. (1966). Speech audiometry and clinical masking. *J. Auditory Res.* **6**, 199–203.

Martin, F. N., Bailey, H. A. T., and Pappas, J. J. (1965). The effect of central masking on threshold for speech. *J. Auditory Res.* **5**, 293–296.

McFadden, D. (1968). Masking-level differences determined with and without interaural disparities in masker intensity. *J. Acoust. Soc. Amer.* **44**, 212–223.

Meyer, M. F. (1959). Masking: Why restrict it to the threshold level? *J. Acoust. Soc. Amer.* **31**, 243.

Mulligan, B. E., Mulligan, M. J., and Stonecypher, J. E. (1967). Critical band in binaural detection. *J. Acoust. Soc. Amer.* **41**, 7–12.

Olsen, W. O., and Carhart, R. (1967). Development of test procedures for evaluation of binaural hearing aids. *Bull. Prosthetic Res.* **10**, 22–49.

Palva, T., Goodman, A., and Hirsh, I. J. (1953). Critical evaluation of noise audiometry. *Laryngoscope* **63**, 842–860.

Pickett, J. M. (1959). Backward masking. *J. Acoust. Soc. Amer.* **31**, 1613–1615.

Pollack, I. (1964). Interaction of forward and backward masking. *J. Auditory Res.* **4**, 63–67.

Raab, D. H. (1961). Forward and backward masking between acoustic clicks. *J. Acoust. Soc. Amer.* **33**, 137–139.

Rilling, M. E., and Jeffress, L. A. (1965). Narrow-band noise and tones as signals in binaural detection. *J. Acoust. Soc. Amer.* **38**, 202–206.

Rittmanic, P. A. (1962). Pure tone masking by narrow noise bands in normal and impaired ears. *J. Auditory Res.* **2**, 287–304.

Robinson, D. E., and Jeffress, L. A. (1963). Effect of varying the interaural noise correlation of the detection of tonal signals. *J. Acoust. Soc. Amer.* **35**, 1947–1952.

Sanders, J. W., and Rintelmann, W. F. (1964). Masking in audiometry. *Arch. Otolaryngol.* **80**, 541–556.

Scharf, B. (1964). Partial masking. *Acustica.* **14,** 16–23.

Scharf, B. (1966). Critical bands. Special Report LSC-S-3. Lab. Sensory Comm., Syracuse Univ.

Schenkel, K. D. (1967). Accumulation theory of binaural masked thresholds. *J. Acoust. Soc. Amer.* **41,** 20–31.

Sherrick, C. E., and Mangabeira-Albernaz, P. L. (1961). Auditory threshold shifts produced by simultaneously pulsed contralateral stimuli. *J. Acoust. Soc. Amer.* **33,** 1381–1385.

Small, A. M., Jr. (1959). Pure-tone masking. *J. Acoust. Soc. Amer.* **31,** 1619–1625.

Sondhi, M. M., and Guttman, N. (1966). Width of the spectrum effective in the binaural release of masking. *J. Acoust. Soc. Amer.* **40,** 600–606.

Stokinger, T. E., and Lankford, J. E. (1969). Temporal relations in pure tone contralateral masking. Paper presented at the 78th meeting of the Acoust. Soc. Amer., San Diego, Calif.

Studebaker, G. A. (1962). On masking in bone-conduction testing. *J. Speech Hearing Res.* **5,** 215–227.

Studebaker, G. A. (1964). Clinical masking of air- and bone-conduction stimuli. *J. Speech Hearing Dis.* **29,** 23–35.

Studebaker, G. A. (1967). Clinical masking of the non-test ear. *J. Speech Hearing Dis.* **32,** 360–371.

Tanner, W. P., Jr. (1958). What is masking? *J. Acoust. Soc. Amer.* **30,** 919–921.

Teas, D. C., Eldredge, D. H., and Davis, H. (1962). Cochlear responses to acoustic transients: an interpretation of whole nerve action potentials. *J. Acoust. Soc. Amer.* **34,** Pt. 2, 1438–1459.

Tillman, T. W. (1963). Clinical applicability of the SAL test. *Arch. Otolaryngol.* **78,** 20–32.

Ward, W. D. (1961). Studies on the aural reflex. I. contralateral remote masking as an indicator of reflex activity. *J. Acoust. Soc. Amer.* **33,** 1034–1044.

Ward, W. D. (1967). Further observations on contralateral remote masking and related phenomena. *J. Acoust. Soc. Amer.* **42,** 593–600.

Wegal, R. L., and Lane, C. E. (1924). The auditory masking of one pure tone by another and its probable relations to the dynamics of the inner ear. *Phys. Rev.* **23,** 266–285.

Wilson, R. H., and Carhart, R. (1969). Influence of pulsed masking on the threshold for spondees. *J. Acoust. Soc. Amer.* **46,** 998–1010.

Wright, H. N. (1964a). Temporal summation and backward masking. *J. Acoust. Soc. Amer.* **36,** 927–932.

Wright, H. N. (1964b). Backward masking for tones in narrow-band noise. *J. Acoust. Soc. Amer.* **36,** 2217–2221.

Young, I. M. (1969). Effects of pure-tone masking on low-pass and high-pass-filtered noise. *J. Acoust. Soc. Amer.* **45,** 1206–1209.

Young, I. M., and Wenner, C. H. (1967). Masking of white noise by pure tone, frequency-modulated tone, and narrow-band noise. *J. Acoust. Soc. Amer.* **41,** 700–706.

Young, I. M., and Wenner, C. H. (1968). Effects of masking noise on the SISI test. *J. Auditory Res.* **8,** 331–337.

Zerlin, S. (1966). Interaural time and intensity difference and the MLD. *J. Acoust. Soc. Amer.* **39,** 134–137.

Zwicker, E. (1965). Temporal effects in simultaneous masking by white-noise bursts. *J. Acoust. Soc. Amer.* **37,** 653–663.

Zwicker, E., Flottorp, G., and Stevens, S. S. (1957). Critical band width in loudness summation. *J. Acoust. Soc. Amer.* **29**, 548–557.

Zwislocki, J., Maire, F., Feldman, A. S., and Rubin, H. (1958). On the effect of practice and motivation on the threshold of audibility. *J. Acoust. Soc. Amer.* **30**, 254–262.

Zwislocki, J., Damianopoulous, E. N., Buining, E., and Glantz, J. (1967). Central masking: Some steady-state and transient effects. *Perception Psychophys.* **2**, 59–64.

Zwislocki, J., Buining, E., and Glantz, J. (1968). Frequency distribution of central masking. *J. Acoust. Soc. Amer.* **43**, 1267–1271.

Chapter 5

Measurement of Hearing in Children

ROBERT FRISINA

National Technical Institute for the Deaf

I. Introduction

The past 25 years have been marked by great interest and accomplishment in the measurement of hearing in man. This activity was accelerated in part by electronic breakthroughs during and after World War II. Measurement devices became readily available, and at the same time the need for such instrumentation was great. The aural rehabilitation programs born out of World War II provided the initial thrust and focus for new technology and widespread research efforts in measurement and understanding of the human auditory system.

Viewed in this perspective it is interesting to note that since the advent of electronic measurement devices in the 1940s, measurement of hearing in man has moved steadily downward along the age scale. Prior to World

War II, auditory research was conducted mainly with lower animals. During the latter 1940s, following the advent of precision instrumentation, adults were the primary population seen clinically as well as in research. During the early 1950s adults dominated the audiologic scene as clinical patients but the awareness that children could be tested began to unfold, albeit slowly. The mid-1950s ushered in an era of greater interest in the measurement of hearing in children that included both behavioral and electrophysiologic methods. The late 1950s and early 1960s were marked by increased activity in school age and preschool age children and an evolving interest in infant testing. By the mid and late 1960s infant testing and in fact prenatal testing became a reality.

This movement from adults to infants very probably represents only 180° in the cycle that is likely to occur. It could well be that the movement from adulthood to infancy will proceed systematically back to adulthood.

The reasons leading to this conjecture for the 1970s are first, measurement techniques developed for a variety of reasons for evaluation of adults were simply adapted downward—few if any reasons for auditory measurement and their associated methodologies originated with populations of children; second, longitudinal studies of hearing in children are likely to provide the young science of audiology an opportunity to continue its growth as a science; and third, the field of education of hearing-impaired children continues to need such audiologic information if it is to substantially enhance its educational outcomes.

This chapter makes some observations about the measurement of hearing in children, with particular emphasis on behavioral audiometry. Electrophysiologic approaches with children are treated elsewhere in this book. In the process of presenting this material, some of the unfinished business in this area of special interest becomes apparent. Introductory definitions include those of children, measurement, and hearing.

A. Children Defined

In educational circles school-age children are those ranging from 5 through 17 years. Preschool-age children are generally considered to be those below 6 years. Kindergarten-age children are the 5-year-olds. Often, ages 3 and 4 are classed as nursery-age children. The young child generally includes those from 2 to 5 years. The term *infant* is generally reserved for those children 24 months and younger. The neonatal period extends from birth to 2 months.

The question of when children differ from adults in the audiologic sense has been determined only in part. If discrete pure-tone measurements comprise the variable under consideration and the adult standardization procedure and normative data serve as the references, children as young as 3 years of age have been shown to perform in a valid manner (Eagles and Wishik, 1961). Almost all standardized audiometric procedures originated with adults serving as subjects. As a result, the average age level of children able to perform in a like manner will vary from one test to another. This variation in cutoff age is likely to relate to the complexity of demands placed on the subject. On the basis of his performance on one test, a child might not differ from an adult, whereas on another he might classify as a child.

The uniqueness of children, and hence the special considerations needed in conducting auditory measurements with them, have been related to stimulus materials, response modes, instructional modes, and levels of ability to cooperate. It has been learned that no single audiologic definition for children exists. Whether a procedure is appropriate for a given individual depends upon that individual and the manner in which the test procedure is standardized. In general, the ability of the research subject or clinical patient to participate in a specified manner is more critical than whether he is an adult or child with respect to chronological or mental age.

B. Measurement Defined

The requirement to participate in a specified manner brings us directly to the concept of measurement. Briefly stated, measurement is the assignment of numerals in a specified manner. Hence, measurement of hearing requires specification of procedure, quantification of the stimulus dimensions, and quantification of response. Many studies dealing with children have indeed satisfied these criteria. On the contrary, however, many tests (systematic observations without assignment of numerals in a specified manner to the stimulus and/or the response) have been performed under the rubric of measurement. In this context examples of tests as contrasted to measurement might include the auropalpebral reflex, the stapedial reflex, the Moro reflex, and the responses to sound field signal sources of which the dimensions have not been specified.

C. Hearing Defined

The third definition in this brief preliminary discussion concerns hearing. As circular as it may appear, there are as many definitions of hearing as there are ways of measuring responses to specified auditory stimuli. Absolute thresholds for frequency and intensity, speech reception threshold, speech discrimination, and many others define what hearing is. Since there is no direct measurement of one's perception of sound, the stimulus–response relationships in a given set of measurements determine one's definition of hearing.

The preponderance of studies related to the measurement of hearing in children have been concerned with measures of absolute threshold. This is not so unexpected in view of the language problems frequently present in children with hearing disorders. This reduces the validity of oral instructions and often precludes utilization of verbal responses. These two constraints limit the applicability of the more complex measurements which traditionally have utilized complex signals, verbal instructions, and verbal responses. The maturation, set, and sustained attention required in the more complex tasks complicate further the pursuit of more sophisticated measurements with children. Attempts to circumvent these limitations, in large part, have consisted of modifications in the methods of instruction and in the response modes.

II. Identification Tests

The subject of detection of hearing problems in children, very much with us today, is organized around three headings: studies with neonates, studies with infants other than neonates, and studies with young children.

It is interesting to note that on its way to full circle, auditory research at the 180° point suggests the following conclusions:

(1) The cochlea seems functional by about the 20th week of intrauterine life.

(2) Basic mechanisms for coding intensity and frequency appear to be operating by the 28th to 30th week of gestation.

(3) Mechanisms governing attentive behavior may not be functional until some weeks later.

(4) Functionally differentiated channels for processing acoustic information according to the frequency and organization of a stimulus envelope probably are present at birth (Eisenberg, 1970).

Behavioral audiometric threshold techniques have not been of demonstrated usefulness in the neonate but electrophysiologic measurements suggest strongly that the threshold of hearing in newborns does not differ from that of adults.

A. Studies with Neonates (Birth to 2 Months)

The auditory characteristics of neonates have been systematically observed in the past by such investigators as Buhler (1930), Ewing and Ewing (1947), and Gesell and Armatruda (1948). These early studies indicate that during the first 2 months of age the neonate's auditory behavior is somewhat circumscribed. Responses during this period are essentially all-or-none. The overt readily observable responses include startle reflex (Moro), crying responses, assumption of listening attitude to sound of human voice (near end of second month), and diminished activity in presence of bell sounds. During the neonatal period, rather intense sounds are required in order to elicit responses, and generally most children respond.

Wedenberg (1956), Hardy et al. (1959), and Froding (1960) followed these pioneering investigations with more direct concern for auditory sensitivity threshold. Wedenberg used pure-tone signals whereas the others used noisemakers as auditory stimuli. Each was seeking a means for detecting those neonates who deviate from the auditory norms of adults. Their work confirms the findings of earlier investigators in that responses to sound depend largely upon the behavioral set of the infant; and that repeatability of response varies with the extent to which the neonate is or is not engrossed in activities such as crying, deep sleep, sucking behavior, and the like. They assumed but did not prove that the threshold of hearing in neonates is near that of the adult.

More recently, a series of independent studies has been conducted in which, for the most part, electronically generated narrow- and broad-band noises have been used as the stimuli. These efforts have been aimed at detecting those who deviate from the auditory norm (Downs and Sterritt, 1964, 1967) and are concerned with learning something about the auditory characteristics of newborns (Eisenberg et al., 1964). They include attempts at detecting hearing loss in neonates and attempts to classify behavioral responses according to their natural anatomic division of the motor outputs of midbrain, medulla, cervical–thoracic cord, and the diffuse system presumably involving the reticular formation of the brain stem (Field et al., 1967); and attempts to demonstrate in newborns adaptation for pitch discrimination and localization (Leventhal and Lipsitt, 1964).

Neonatal screening efforts have increased substantially during the past several years. These efforts have led to early detection of hearing impairment in children and early educational programming. Widespread application of neonatal screening is still questioned by some on the bases of cost and effort involved in locating a relatively small number of hearing-impaired infants. Other attempts to measure auditory thresholds in neonates have in recent years included audiometers interfaced with computers and electroencephalograph machines; these efforts are reflected in the chapter related to electrophysiologic audiometry.

B. Studies with Infants (2 Months to 24 Months)

During this age span particular attention has been paid to behavioral changes in response to different types of sounds. Gesell and Armatruda (1948) called attention to auditory behavioral changes which occurred beyond the age at which startle reflexes (APR and Moro) are evident. They determined that the infant of 8 weeks ceases in large measure to be disturbed by loud sounds. He accepts them and attempts to listen or is at least interrupted by some sounds at that age. Conditioned orienting responses by 2-month-old infants were demonstrated by Koch (1967). At 3 months of age infants begin to search for sound by using their eyes (Kendall, 1964) and the auditory oculogyric reflex (AOR) appears consistently in infants above 4 months of age (Chun et al., 1960). Certain types of sounds are more readily responded to at ages 3, 4, and 5 months (Miller and DeSchweinitz, 1962) and the frequency of response appears to grow very quickly during this same period (Miller et al., 1963) and continues subsequent to this (Mendel, 1968).

At 16 weeks of age the average infant responds to a bell with varying facial expressions. The ability to turn the head toward a sound source emerges at 21–24 weeks and by the age of 28 weeks the infant is adept at localization (Chun et al., 1960; DiCarlo and Bradley, 1961). Attempt at imitation of sounds evolves at approximately 36 weeks of age and sounds begin to be associated with people, things, or actions at about 40 weeks. At 1 year of age a child comprehends "give it to me" and at 18 months is capable of carrying out more elaborate instructions given orally.

Clinical application of identification audiometry has been on the increase in recent years and is expected to continue into the 1970s. These screening techniques are gross measures and can be administered by those who have limited technical knowledge and training. If one wishes to screen on a mass basis, it is probably most practical to do so by incorporating the assistance of paraprofessionals. Under such circumstances one can expect that this approach might lead to reduced reliability and validity of the measurements; unfortunately, to date no viable alternative for mass screening of newborns and infants has appeared on the scene.

C. Studies with Young Children (24 Months to 5 Years)

Identification audiometry above 2 years of age is handled in ways similar to those used for older subjects. Threshold or diagnostic audiometric testing with this age group will be discussed later in this chapter under the section on behavioral audiometric measures. Many state and local departments of public health as well as other governmental units in education conduct ongoing auditory screening programs. The method of choice during the past several years (Geyer and Yankauer, 1956; Farrant, 1960; Ewerstein, 1966) has been the individually administered audiometric sweep check, usually with frequencies 500 through 4000 Hz included in the sweep check. More recently, a verbal auditory screening test for preschool children has been suggested (Griffing et al., 1967). In contrast to pure-tone sounds, this procedure utilizes recorded spondee words that are presented at decreasing sound intensity levels along with pictures to which the subjects respond.

Special considerations are necessary in sweep check and other forms of audiometry used with preschool-age children. The efficiency of mass screening techniques is determined from consideration of three primary variables; average time required to screen a child; percent of "false detections," that is, overreferrals in cases where no actual hearing loss exists; and the percentage of actual hearing losses detected.

III. Behavioral Audiometric Measurements

Behavioral audiometric measurements include those that require volitional responses on the part of the subject. The primary focus in this chapter is on those audiometric procedures conducted with children that satisfy this criterion. The traditional response in standard pure-tone audiometry is a voluntary behavioral response requiring the raising of a finger, the raising of a hand, or the pressing of a button. Important to this discussion is the realization that the instructions given in the standard manner (to elicit a "conditioned" response) are presented orally. Commercially available audiometers are calibrated to normative data derived from adult subjects in that manner. In the event a clinical or research subject cannot understand verbal (oral) instructions, some modification, generally in the form of demonstration or nonverbal conditioning, is employed. The former is commonly referred to as standard pure-tone audiometry. The latter modification employs some form of "play" activity in establishing a conditioned response. In the literature such procedures often are referred to as play audiometry. The conditioned (voluntary) response may be: pressing a button and being rewarded with a puppet show; placing a block in a basket and being rewarded with a smile; stacking rings on a peg and receiving applause as a reward. Animated toys have been used as rewards in audiometry with children. This type of audiometric procedure has been successful in children as young as approximately 22 months. Certain aspects of behavioral audiometry related to children are presented next in this section.

A. Standard Pure-Tone Threshold Measurement

The question of whether or not the threshold of hearing in children differs from that in adults has in large part been determined. The approach that took precedence over others was the application of adult measurement techniques over a broad range of decreasing age levels. The landmark study by Eagles and Wishik (1961) carried out under laboratory conditions with large numbers of children shows that children as young as 3 years of age can participate successfully in standard audiometry. This has been substantiated clinically many times over.

Practice effect was controlled (not allowed to occur) in their study and yet the thresholds determined were lower than the then-existing American standards. The implication is that not only can young children participate successfully in standard audiometry, but that the thresholds derived are of statistical equivalence to those in adults.

B. Modified Pure-Tone Measurement Procedures

The question of how young a subject may be for standard pure-tone audiometric procedures to remain valid is effectively answered in the Eagles and Wishik (1961) study. The fact still remains, however, that many linguistically handicapped children cannot be measured precisely by the standard procedure. The primary procedural alteration necessary is the deviation from the verbal instructions that constitute a fundamental part of the standard audiometric procedure. Verbal instructions are critical in this instance, because it is in this way that standard audiometric threshold values are determined.

Added to the limitations imposed by the linguistically involved, there is the often-expressed question of "meaningfulness" of a pure tone to a child and its possible influence on threshold sensitivity. Further complicating the task is the recognition that children, unlike adults, have very little vested in the measurement process. They commonly display anxiety toward the audiologic environment, a condition which must be overcome in order to measure hearing. Additional factors requiring consideration in the measurement of hearing with behavioral response techniques include: getting the child to accept earphones so that each ear can be measured independently; using a conditioning procedure which allows the child to associate a stimulus with a specific response that is within, or can be added to, his response repertoire; and helping the child to develop and maintain a set for the performance of the stimulus–response task.

A slight alteration in the standard procedure has been seen to enable measurement of threshold sensitivity to be lowered to 2-year-olds. The procedure (Lowell et al., 1956) involved the establishment of a conditioned response (CR) to a drumbeat, transfer of CR to pure-tone stimuli, and measurement of threshold for pure-tone stimuli utilizing the psychophysical method of serial exploration. The audiometer calibrations and test environments were controlled in a manner similar to those in the Eagles and Wishik (1961) study. The principal difference was in the "method of instruction" given the subjects prior to the determination of threshold. In spite of the procedural difference and the limited number of subjects used in the Lowell *et al.* study (1956), as compared with the large number in the Eagles and Wishik (1961) study, the threshold means are statistically equivalent. This suggests that play techniques, so called, can be used to secure threshold measures that are equivalent to standard audiometric procedures. Also, these studies question the validity of the often-expressed concern that a pure-tone stimulus is meaningless to a child of preschool age and therefore precludes his responding at intensity levels comparable to older, school-age children and adults. In a variety of ways since the conduct of these studies, the measured sensitivity thresholds in young children have been shown to be remarkably resistant to modifications in the instructional component of the measurement enterprise.

A relatively successful clinical procedure for determining pure-tone air and bone thresholds in linguistically handicapped children has been used for many years by this writer (Frisina, 1962). Briefly, the nonverbal intructional mode consists of using the bone conduction oscillator (standard equipment on the usual commercially available audiometer) to produce a tactile stimulus that can be felt when hand-held by the examiner to the hand, face, forehead, or mastoid process of the child. The tactile conditioned stimulus (CS) is paired to the response, which is the placing of a ring on a peg (CR). Once conditioned to respond to the CS, the child generalizes without intervening instructions to an auditory stimulus. Pure-tone thresholds can thus be determined by beginning with the 500-Hz tone. The child's attention to the task can be maintained by the examiner's showing a decided interest in the child's behavior. Reward in the form of a smile, applause, a nod, etc., should be provided only when a correct response has been made. It is imperative that the child know when his response is correct. It is critical, too, that incorrect responses not be reinforced. It has been found useful to determine the intensity level that consistently elicits the CR. It is recommended that 10–15-dB intervals be used in the Carhart and Jerger (1959) threshold procedure and that positive stimuli (intensity level where consistent responses occur) be interspersed frequently so as to reduce the number of false responses that a child often makes in attempting to please the examiner. It is common to find that the threshold (50% response level) is 5 dB above the zero response level and 5 dB less intense than the 100% response level. More specifically, the dB range between the consistent response level and the no-response level rarely exceeds

10 dB when the factors discussed are made part of the procedure. This technique has been of routine usefulness in children 22 months of age and older. In reality this procedure is a modified form of operant conditioning using social reward as the reinforcer and one that incorporates an intuitively based reinforcement schedule. Outside validating criteria for air-conduction pure-tone thresholds derived in this manner have been bone-conduction pure-tone thresholds, speech awareness thresholds, and speech reception thresholds. This conditioning procedure has since been tested and quantified more objectively by Frisina and Johnson (1966).

Statistically equivalent pure-tone thresholds have been derived in other types of cross-test comparisons. For example, Barr (1955) reported the results of a comparative study utilizing play audiometry and electrodermal audiometry in children ranging in age from under 2 to 6 years. The level of consistency between the two measures was on the order of that found in the study by Lowell et al. (1956) in which deaf 3- to 6-year-olds were used to compare a conditioning procedure different from that employed by Barr (1955) and that employed by Frisina and Johnson (1966).

Several modifications to the standard behavioral audiometric procedure have been used successfully for a number of years in response to the need to test young children and others for whom verbal instructions are inappropriate (Dix and Hallpike, 1947; Guilford and Haug, 1952; Knox, 1960; Myklebust, 1954; Neiman, 1957; O'Neill et al., 1961; Statten and Wishart, 1956; Wishart, 1952). More recent approaches are presented in Lloyd and Frisina (1965) as these relate to linguistically handicapped children who are difficult to test. These techniques adapt the more formal operant conditioning principles to audiometry and will be discussed next.

C. Operant Conditioning Audiometry

Clinical audiologic management of human subjects carries the responsibility for avoiding experiences that may be damaging to the individual. Operant conditioning techniques utilizing aversive stimuli have been very effective in shaping the behavior of animals. Thus, at times the temptation to employ avoidance of punishment procedures may be great in children and adults who do not, for one reason or another, participate in behavioral audiologic procedures as standardized. This frequently arises in cases of very young children and in mental retardates. For the most part, however, positive reinforcement techniques have been employed.

Operant conditioning procedures, in fact, have been introduced to the general field of audiology in response to the need to test the young child (Dix and Hallpike, 1947) and the need to obtain audiologic information in retarded subjects whose limited verbal skills and/or general functioning levels preclude success in standard audiometric procedures (Meyerson and Michael, 1960). The former procedure uses an operant discrimination paradigm for testing hearing with the tone as the positive (discriminative) stimulus and the tone-off condition as the negative (delta) stimulus. The reinforcer for the tone-on condition is appearance of a picture, or as they termed it, a peep show. The latter (Meyerson and Michael, 1960) adapted operant techniques in which tangible reinforcers such as candy and trinkets were used. Threshold was determined most effectively with a two-button arrangement by reinforcing both the tone-on and the tone-off conditions. A special bonus reward was given for a quick and accurate response from the tone-on to the tone-off state. A single-button procedure has been described more recently by Spradlin and Lloyd (1965) in which they too use tangible reinforcers.

Lloyd (1966) discusses further this approach to auditory measurement with retardates and in doing so clarifies and emphasizes reinforcement principles that are fundamental in operant conditioning audiometry. More recently Lloyd et al. (1968) elaborated on tangible reinforcement operant conditioning audiometry (TROCA) as a procedure of demonstrated usefulness in difficult-to-test patients. It is evident that the TROCA procedure offers a promising approach to those whose linguistic competencies and/or general functioning levels preclude successful application of either standard or play audiometric procedures.

D. Békésy Audiometry

The clinical and research usefulness of Békésy audiometry with adult subjects is well established. Thus, adapting children to Békésy audiometry or Békésy audiometry to children was placed high on the list of priorities by those measuring the hearing of linguistically handicapped children. An accurate assessment of hearing at an early age in such children is required for early and appropriate educational management. Békésy audiometry has the potential for contributing to more precise longitudinal studies of hearing handicapped children when test-retest data are gathered over a period of months or years. This is particularly true since precise stimulus control is possible and the nature of the response is such that examiner influence on measured performance is practically eliminated.

With these concerns in mind, Frisina and Johnson (1966) conducted a series of experiments that led to the standardization of a behavioral response technique for measurement of hearing in nonverbal children. It consists of a modified psychophysical method of adjustment and a nonverbal vibrotactile conditioning procedure for use in the administration of conventional Békésy audiometry with children who have auditory impairment, or who are suspected of having hearing problems. Over 200 subjects were used in a series of eight experiments. Hearing and deaf adults were used to obtain baseline data concerning the apparatus and procedures. Deaf children ranging in age from $12\frac{1}{2}$ years to $2\frac{1}{2}$ years were used to ascertain the efficacy of this auditory test with young children.

The basic equipment used was the GS E-800 Békésy audiometer. It was used to generate a vibrotactile stimulus, to obtain routine fixed-frequency auditory thresholds, to obtain vibrotactile thresholds via routine Békésy procedures, to obtain Modified Ascending Békésy (MAB) thresholds with both fixed frequency and variable frequencing programming, and to function as a conventional diagnostic audiometer by inserting a step attenuator calibrated in 1-dB increments.

The age level at which the standardized routine Békésy procedures no longer resulted in 50% or more success rate turned out to be the $4\frac{1}{2}$ to $5\frac{1}{2}$ age interval in which instance a 40% success rate was obtained. From the age of $5\frac{1}{2}$ years through $12\frac{1}{2}$ years and in adulthood it was found that age was not a factor in learning the vibrotactile threshold tracing task, in tracing absolute vibrotactile and auditory thresholds, in generalizing from one sense modality (tactile) to another (auditory), and in the precision with which children could track auditory threshold as revealed in the absolute threshold itself and the size of the envelope.

A modification to the E-800 audiometer was developed that would allow a single press of the response switch by the subject to measure one's ascending threshold. This procedure referred to as MAB (modified ascending Békésy) was found to be effective with children as young as $2\frac{1}{2}$ to $3\frac{1}{2}$ years of age.

Prior to, and following this study, conventional Békésy has been found to be useful with school-age children having normal and impaired hearing (Price and Falk, 1963; Hartley and Siegenthaler, 1964; Swisher and Stephens, 1968).

E. Speech Audiometry

The problems inherent in speech materials for use in audiometric measures are presented in detail by Hirsh (1952). Further complexities are introduced when one attempts to utilize such stimulus materials with children. The influence of language experience in general and the limitations imposed on the validity of speech stimuli in the linguistically handicapped compound the problems.

Young children without linguistic handicaps are capable of responding to speech stimuli in a manner comparable to adults provided vocabulary level is controlled (Siegenthaler et al., 1954). Siegenthaler and Haspiel (1966) more recently have standardized test materials for children ranging in age from 3 to 8 years. The two measures possible are the threshold by identification of pictures test (speech reception threshold), and the discrimination by identification of pictures test. These studies demonstrate further the validity of speech audiometry with young children. In addition, the relationship between the speech reception threshold and the pure-tone average (500–2000 Hz) in children has been found to be similar to that found in adults (Siegenthaler et al., 1954).

Auditory discrimination tests in addition to those standardized by Siegenthaler and Haspiel (1966) have been developed (Myatt and Landes, 1963) and modified by others (Lerman et al., 1965). It seems reasonable to assume that suprathreshold speech measures will continue to be advanced in the future. Such evaluation techniques are important in the assessment and reevaluation of hearing-impaired children undergoing various communication and educational treatments.

Speech audiometry is useful in large numbers of hearing-impaired subjects, specifically as an outside criterion with which to verify pure tone results. Data obtained from severely deaf children and adults indicate a close relationship between threshold of awareness for speech (spondaic words) and the 500-Hz threshold (Frisina, 1962). This relationship obtains in cases where the audiometric contour is flat, gradually falling, or markedly falling. However, if the curve is the rising type, the high point on the audiogram, rather than the 500-Hz threshold, is likely to be within ±5 dB of the speech awareness threshold. This relationship between pure tones and speech awareness threshold is especially useful in children void of verbal language. It provides one of the few outside criteria with which to evaluate the validity of pure-tone threshold measurements in a given patient or subject.

Speech discrimination testing that utilizes "live" voice without a speech audiometer is used widely in clinical work with speech-impaired children. The results of this type of test indicate that the ability to discriminate between pairs of speech sounds imbedded in words increases with age up to at least $4\frac{1}{2}$ to 5 years and perhaps up to 7 years. It remains evident that difficulties in assessing auditory discrimination by this means or by the utilization of speech audiometry result principally from the effects of different linguistic experiences (language styles and vocabulary) of children and the response mode (which requires selection of pictures on the part of the test constructor). Continued advancement of speech audiometric measures in children appears to be as dependent upon emergence of more evidence related to speech materials in general as on the specific relationship between speech testing and children.

IV. Summary

The past 25 years have witnessed a gradual and consistent growing interest in the measurement of hearing in children. Audiology as a young post-World War II science focused primarily upon adults during its formative years. Awareness of and interest in children has been on the increase during the past 15 years; so much so that most of the techniques developed for use with adults have in some way been applied to children.

Audiologic measures standardized specifically with children have emerged slowly. Movement from primary interest in adults to more than token interest in children is seen as an aid to the young science of audiology in becoming of age. Longitudinal studies of children with auditory handicaps are still not well developed, but need to become so. Audiology as a science has much to offer such endeavors.

It has been seen that, in the main, audiometric procedures originated with adults. As a result, the average age of children able to perform in a like manner varies considerably from one test to another. The significance of verbal language and the complexity of the demands made on the subject determine whether or not a difference exists between adults and children in the audiologic sense. In general, the ability of an individual to participate in a specified manner is more critical than whether he is an adult or child with regard to his chronological or his mental age.

When one speaks of measurement of hearing in children, the test procedures used can be differentiated on the basis of the precision of the data derived therefrom. Some tests are screening devices, essentially "go—no-go" operations. Others follow careful specification of procedure, stimulus dimensions, and quantification of responses according to predetermined rules. Gross discrete sound stimuli generally are used for screening purposes whereas continuously variable stimuli are likely to be used in measuring more specific aspects of auditory behavior.

Hearing is seen as a highly developed sensory system in man and can be specified only in terms of the way in which it is measured. As circular as it may seem, there are as many definitions of hearing as there are ways of measuring responses to specified auditory stimuli. As audiologists, however, we need be concerned with only two sets of variables; the first is the specification of the stimulus and the way in which it is presented; second is the identification and measurement of the response. The technology for producing a well-defined stimulus is available but at this time generating and maintaining comparably precise human responses leaves something to be desired. Attempts have been made, however, and these are alluded to throughout this chapter.

The status of the end organ of hearing at birth appears to be fundamentally similar in its performance characteristics to that of adults. The transducer and transmitter characteristics of the peripheral auditory nervous system appear to be functioning adult-like at birth and with time and experience allow the individual to develop a more complete mastery of his auditory system as a whole.

In recent years, much energy has been focused on identification of hearing problems in infants and very young children. The terms *screening* or *detection* in case-finding audiometry have been subsumed under the general term *identification audiometry*. During the early neonatal period, responses to sound are essentially all-or-none. Overt responses include the startle reflex (Moro) which is sometimes referred to as the acoustic muscle reflex (AMR), the auropalpebral reflex (APR), and the auditory oculogyric reflex (AOR). As a group these responses are elicited from sudden relatively intense stimuli which have a broad frequency band. Pure tones have been used to some extent, however. Increased activity in neonatal screening has been evident during the past several years throughout the United States. These efforts have led to early detection of hearing impairment in children and initiation of early educational programming for parents and their children. Other attempts to measure auditory thresholds during the neonatal period have seen the audiometer successfully interfaced with the computer and with electroencephalographic technology. With this possible exception, identification audiometry may be described most accurately as a screening test of hearing rather than the measurement of hearing. Infant screening programs beyond the neonatal period also reflect an increase in attention and activity. Careful inquiries have been made regarding the nature of responses elicited during the first 2 years of life.

Behavioral audiometric measurements include those that require volitional responses on the part of the subject. Standard or conventional audiometry as standardized on adult subjects is of demonstrated validity in linguistically normal children as young as 3 years of age. Modified methods employing play audiometry have been shown to be successful with 2-year-olds. Comparative audiometric studies have demonstrated equivalency between thresholds derived by standard and play audiometric techniques in linguistically handicapped children. The same has been found to be true in comparing electrodermal responses with play techniques. Data related to thresholds in children resulting from laboratory-controlled test procedures, stimuli, responses, and environment have suggested pure-tone threshold levels in children equivalent to the new international audiometric standards.

Formal operant conditioning procedures recently have been introduced to the field of audiology. This has occurred in response to the need to test very young children and the need to obtain audiologic information in linguistically handicapped and mentally retarded children. Frequently, retarded children have limited verbal skills and/or general levels of functioning that do not allow use of standard audiometric procedures. Positive reinforcement techniques using tangible reinforcers have been employed for the most part with considerable success in these special clinical groups.

Standard Békésy audiometry has been used with varying degrees of success in linguistically normal children and in hearing-impaired groups of children. Békésy audiometry has been adapted for use with severely hearing-impaired children as young as $4\frac{1}{2}$–$5\frac{1}{2}$ years. Ascending threshold measures using a modified Békésy audiometer have been of demonstrated usefulness in deaf children as young as $2\frac{1}{2}$–$3\frac{1}{2}$ years of age. These various approaches to Békésy audiometry with linguistically handicapped children lend themselves well to longitudinal studies of children undergoing various forms of audiologic and educational treatment. These relatively objective measures that eliminate examiner judgment of responses must be exploited further if the science of audiology and the education of deaf children are to be coupled.

Some limited progress has been made in speech audiometry with non-handicapped children. Many problems still exist in the utilization of speech materials as the stimulus for the measurment of hearing. Differential language experience in normal and linguistically handicapped children poses additional limitations. Studies with children as young as $2\frac{1}{2}$ to 3 years have indicated high reliability. Comparisons of speech reception threshold with pure-tone average (500–2000 Hz) have indicated a high degree of face validity for these materials, but absolute thresholds on large numbers of unselected children have not been measured. In a great percentage of clinical cases with speech and hearing deficits, the usefulness of suprathreshold speech audiometry is seriously curtailed. On the other hand, speech awareness threshold, as contrasted with speech reception threshold, in children with speech and hearing problems can be used as an outside criterion for testing the validity of pure-tone results. The relationship between the pure-tone threshold at 500 Hz is expected to be within ±5 dB of the speech awareness threshold. This holds for groups of audiograms which illustrate decreasing sensitivity as frequency (in hertz) increases. In the rising type of audiogram the speech awareness threshold is likely to be within ±5 dB of the high point on the audiogram. Finally, many clinical cases can identify pictures of spondaic words by pointing. As a rule the extent of success in such a procedure is directly related to the degree of hearing impairment. The presence of hearing impairment in early life results in speech and language deviations. Standard or modified forms of speech audiometry to date have not been shown to be good predictors of academic and/or speech and language success. Usefulness to date in hearing-impaired children has been principally one of threshold measurement.

Studies in infants and children concerning localization almost exclusively have been of the extracranial type. The localization phenomenon has been exploited in identification audiometric procedures. The limited cooperation possible in infants and children under 2 years of age has been the chief deterrent to earphone measurements (intracranial localization). The ability to localize in a sound field appears to be well developed by the age of 26 weeks. Failure to respond correctly when environmental conditions are carefully controlled has resulted in subjects who were later found to have had either hearing impairment or central nervous system involvements. Infants and children with moderate or greater hearing losses are not likely to localize correctly. It is possible that those with mild to moderate degrees of hearing loss predominantly in tones above 1000 Hz can perform adequately. Failure to localize, however, has been determined by subsequent testing to have occurred in a number of children with normal hearing but with central nervous system problems such as mental retardation. When stimulus and intensity are controlled audiometrically and the child is adequately managed within the test environment, failure to localize at levels above 20 dB (re audiometric zero) greatly increases the probability of hearing impairment being present. Under the same conditions mentally retarded children have been shown to localize correctly down to 20 dB.

Intracranial localization has not been studied systematically in children. Factors other than auditory probably account for preference for adults in such studies. The difficulties involved in holding the control variables constant in children has undoubtedly limited the measurements in frequency discrimination, loudness discrimination, distorted speech measurements, and other special clinical and research procedures.

Audiology has much to contribute to the basic understanding of human development. Audition plays a basic role in the growth and development of children. It is through audition that an infant develops an elaborate verbal symbol system. It is through hearing that a most expeditious means of communication is developed in a seemingly effortless manner. When one studies children with auditory deficits in the hope of understanding deviations, the complexity of the central nervous system and behavioral concomitants comes to the fore. It is time for audiology to study in depth the developing organism. The next decade, hopefully, should provide us with a few more basic advances in our understanding of audition. It is expected that innovations in audiologic measurement, tools, and techniques mentioned in this chapter, and those to be developed, will enable us to handle more adequately the linguistic and behavioral limitations presented by children about whom we want specific audiologic information.

References

Barr, B. (1955). Pure tone audiology for pre-school children. *Acta Oto-Laryngol. Suppl.* **121**.

Buhler, C. (1930). "The First Year of Life." Day, New York.

Carhart, R., and Jerger, J. (1959). Preferred method for clinical determination of pure-tone thresholds. *J. Speech Hearing Dis.* **24**, 330–345.

Chun, R., Pawsat, R., and Forster, F. (1960). Sound localization in infancy. *J. Nerv. Ment. Dis.* **130**, 472–476.

DiCarlo, L. M., and Bradley, W. (1961). A simplified auditory test for infants and young children. *Laryngoscope* **71**, 628–646.

Dix, M., and Hallpike, C. S. (1947). The peep-show: A new technique for pure tone audiometry in young children *Brit. Med. J.* **II**, 719–723.

Downs, M., and Sterritt, G. (1964). Identification audiometry for neonates: A preliminary report. *J. Auditory Res.* **4**, 69–80.

Downs, M., and Sterritt, G. (1967). A guide to newborn and infant hearing screening programs. *A.M.A. Arch. Otolaryngol.* **85**, 15–22.

Eagles, E., and Wishik, S. (1961). A study of hearing in children. *Trans. Amer. Acad. Ophthalmol. Otolaryngol.* **65**, 261–282.

Eisenberg, R. (1970). The development of hearing in man: An assessment of current status. *ASHA*, **12**, 119–123.

Eisenberg, R., Griffin, E., Coursin, D., and Hunter, M. (1964). Auditory behavior in the human neonate: A preliminary report. *J. Speech Hearing Res.* **7**, 247–269.

Ewerstein, H. (1966). Teddy-bear screening audiometry for babies. *Acta Otolaryngol.* **61**, 279–280.

Ewing, I., and Ewing, A. (1947). "Opportunity and the Deaf Child." Univ. of London Press, London.

Farrant, R. H. (1960). The audiometric testing of children in schools and kindergartens. *J. Auditory Res.* **1**, 1–24.

Field, H., Copack, P., Derbyshire, A. J. Driessen, G., and Marcus, R. (1967). Responses of newborns to auditory stimulation. *J. Auditory Res.* **7**, 271–285.

Frisina, D. (1962). Audiometric evaluation and its relation to habilitation and rehabilitation of the deaf. *Amer. Ann. Deaf* **107**, 478–481.

Frisina, D., and Johnson, D. (1966). A nonverbal hearing test for children with deafness. USOE Research Report No. 5-0962-4-11-3.

Froding, C. (1960). Acoustic investigation of newborn infants. *Acta Oto-Laryngol.* **52**, 31–40.

Gesell, A., and Armatruda, C. (1948). "Developmental diagnosis." Harper, New York.

Geyer, M., and Yankauer, A. (1956). Teacher judgment of hearing loss in children. *J. Speech Hearing Dis.* **21**, 482–486.

Griffing, T., Simonton, K., Hedgecock, L. (1967). Verbal auditory screening for preschool children. *Trans. Amer. Acad. Ophthalmol. Otolaryngol.* **71**, 105–110.

Guilford, F., and Haug, O. (1952). Diagnosis of deafness in the very young children. *A.M.A. Arch. Otolaryngol.* **55**, 101–106.

Hardy, J., Dougherty, A., and Hardy, W. (1959). Hearing responses and audiologic screening in infants. *J. Pediat.* **55**, 382–390.

Hartley, G., and Siegenthaler, B. (1964). Relationships between Békésy fixed frequency and conventional audiometry with children. *J. Auditory Res.* **4**, 15–22.

Hirsh, I. J. (1952). "The Measurement of Hearing." McGraw-Hill, New York.

Kendall, D. (1964). The audiologic examination of young children. *Volta Rev.* **66**, 734–740.

Knox, E. (1960). A method of obtaining pure-tone audiograms in young children. *J. Laryngol. Otol.* **74**, 475–479.

Koch, J. (1967). Conditional orienting reactions in two-months-old infants. *Brit. J. Psychol.* **58**, 105–110.

Lerman, J., Ross, M., and McLauchlin, R. (1965). A picture identification test for hearing-impaired children. *J. Auditory Res.* **5**, 273–278.

Leventhal, A., and Lipsitt, L., (1964). Adaptation, pitch discrimination, and sound localization in the neonate. *Child Development* **35**, 759–767.

Lloyd, L. (1966). Behavior audiometry viewed as an operant procedure. *J. Speech Hearing Dis.* **31**, 128–135.

Llyod L., and Frisina, D. (eds.) (1965). "The Audiologic Assessment of the Mentally Retarded; Proceedings of a National Conference." Univ. of Kansas Bureau of Child Research.

Lloyd, L., Spradlin, J., and Reid, M. (1968). An operant audiometric procedure for difficult-to-test patients. *J. Speech Hearing Dis.* **33**, 236–245.

Lowell, E. L., Rushford, G., Hoverston, G., and Stoner, M. (1956). Evaluation of pure tone audiometry with preschool age children. *J. Speech Hearing Dis.* **21**, 292–303.

Mendel, M. (1968). Infant responses to recorded sound. *J. Speech Hearing Res.* **11**, 811–816.

Meyerson, L., and Michael J. (1960). The measurement of sensory thresholds in exceptional children. USOE Coop. Res. Proj. No. 418, U. Houston, Houston, Texas.

Miller, J. D., and DeSchweinitz, L. (1962). Identification audiometry in young children. *Proc. 34th Mtng. Conf. Exec. Amer. Schools for Deaf*, Austin, Texas, pp. 27–30.

Miller, J., DeSchweinitz, L., and Goetzinger, C. (1963). How infants three, four, and five months of age respond to sound. *Except. Child* **30**, 149–154.

Myatt, B., and Landes, B. (1963). Assessing discrimination loss in children. *Arch. Otolaryngol.* **77**, 359–362.

Myklebust, H. (1954). "Auditory Disorders in Children." Grune and Stratton, New York.

Neiman, L. (1957). Objective examination of the auditory sensitivity in deaf-mute and hard of hearing children of pre-school age. *Deafness, Speech, Hearing Abstr.* **1** (1960), 17.

O'Neill, J., Oyer, H. J., and Hillis, J. (1961). Audiometric Procedures Used with Children. *J. Speech Hearing Dis.* **26**, 61–66.

Price, L., and Falk, V., (1963). Békésy audiometry with chidlren. *J. Speech Hearing Res.* **6**, 129–133.

Siegenthaler, B., and Haspiel, G., (1966). "Development of Two Standardized Measures of Hearing for Speech by Children." Penn State Univ. Press, Univ. Park, Pennsylvania. P. 131.

Siegenthaler, B., Pearson, J., and Lezak, R. (1954). A speech reception threshold test for children. *J. Speech Hearing Dis.* **19**, 360–366.

Spradlin, J., and Lloyd, L. (1965). Operant conditioning audiometry (OCA) with two retardates: A preliminary report. *In* "The Audiologic Assessment of the Mentally Retarded: Proceedings of a National Conference" (L. Lloyd, and D. Frisina, eds. Univ. of Kansas Bureau of Child Research). Pp. 44–58.

Statten, P., and Wishart, D. (1956). Pure tone audiometry in young children: Psycho-galvanic-skin-resistance and peep-show. *Ann. Otol. Rhinol. Laryngol.* **65**, 511–534.

Swisher, L., and Stephens, M. (1968). Békésy sweep-frequency and conventional audiometry with hearing-impaired children. *J. Auditory Res.* **8**, 26–27.

Wedenberg, E. (1956). Auditory tests on newborn infants. *Acta Oto-Laryngol.* **46**, 446–461.

Wishart, D. (1952). A critique of present day methods of hearing testing. *Laryngoscope* **62**, 1045–1068.

Chapter 6

Functional Hearing Loss

NORMA T. HOPKINSON

University of Pittsburgh

I. Introduction

A. Definition

A functional defect has been defined as one in "which structural alteration can be neither demonstrated nor inferred." In the same context, "functional" is contrasted with organic, where an organic defect is one in which "structural alteration is an important contributing cause [Wood, 1957]." In medicine, functional disease means that an organ is not functioning effectively while the tissues of that organ show no evidence of pathology.

175

Functional hearing loss has been defined operationally by Ventry and Chaiklin (1962). They describe the loss as functional when the following circumstances apply: (1) discrepancies among intertest and intratest audiological examinations cannot be explained on the basis of an organic condition, and (2) medical examinations rule out apparent organic conditions.

1. TERMS

Several other terms have been used to describe the hearing problems characterized by disparity between function and the presence of ear pathology. The most commonly used among these terms are nonorganic, psychogenic, pseudohypoacusis, and malingering.

The term *nonorganic* gained popularity as a result of the Veterans Administration program following World War II. Audiology clinics were under contract by the Veterans Administration to test the hearing of veterans applying for compensation benefits. A strictly specified series of tests was used in the Assessment of Social Efficiency Examination to determine "the organic level of hearing" or "the organic potential of the hearing mechanism." As the testing for social efficiency became more refined, nonorganic became somewhat more acceptable than functional as a more definitive description of the opposite of organic. Functional remains a more medically oriented term.

Many proponents of the term nonorganic believe it qualifies as an operational term since the inference is made only to the organs of hearing. On the other hand, proponents of the word functional contend that a significant assumption is implicit in the term nonorganic. In the strictest sense, the latter term does not allow for the fact that some unknown, unresolved organic condition could remain responsible for the problem, even though such a condition has not been identified through the audiologic test battery or the medical examinations. Neither of the terms, functional or nonorganic, implies a judgment of conscious or unconscious motivation in the listener.

The word *psychogenic* connotes unconscious motivation. The popularity of psychogenic causes has appeared to decrease among audiologists unless psychiatric diagnoses such as conversion hysteria or depression deafness in schizophrenia have been made (Davis and Fowler, 1960). Although the clinical audiologist retains an interest in whether the motives of a patient are conscious or unconscious, he is aware that the results of the audiologic tests do not provide him with that kind of information. He will seek specialized professional help for decisions regarding a patient's motivation.

Pseudohypoacusis (Carhart, 1961) is interpreted in a general way to mean simulated hearing loss or resembling hearing loss. It can be interpreted more specifically as a value judgment of pretense and imitation. The prefix "pseudo" may imply any of these words. The term avoids the same questions as its predecessors, and does not resolve problems in the terminology.

Malingering is a specific term that indicates conscious intent to deceive. Because audiologic tests are not validated for appraising motivation, in order to use the term the audiologist either must have made a value judgment or he must have received a verbal admission of feigning from the patient. Goldstein (1966) presented the thesis that all of the terms described really represent a condition of malingering. The concept of unconscious ends in psychogenic hearing loss is called invalid. The concept of an unresolved, unidentified organic cause for the inconsistencies in audiologic test results is challenged. The alternative view is that unless a patient admits feigning, the audiologist is not qualified to judge the cause of his behavior (Hopkinson, 1967). Remote, concealed physiological causes may be responsible (Chaiklin and Ventry, 1963; Cohen *et al.*, 1963; Davis and Fowler, 1960; Hopkinson, 1967; Ventry and Chaiklin, 1962; Zwislocki, 1963), although they have not been determined as yet. These causes might be like the genetic, physiochemical causes that have been found to explain some forms of schizophrenic behavior (Heston, 1970; Meltzer, 1968; Pauling, 1968; Rosenthal and Kety, 1968).

In all of these terms, the descriptions do not account for the complexity of the problem. Rarely is the hearing condition exclusively organic or functional. Usually anatomical, physiological, and psychological factors are all pertinent (Davis and Fowler, 1960).

B. Brief History

Before the 1940s the historical literature on functional hearing loss (see O'Neill and Oyer, 1966) was directed mainly toward descriptions of cases and tuning fork techniques. During and following World War II, functional hearing loss received greater attention because of higher prevalence.

Two authors recognized that malingering and psychogenic disorders represented two different causes for functional hearing loss. Atkinson (1937) coupled psychogenic disorder with hysterical causes. Hurst (1940) attributed hysterical deafness to a neurological resistance at synapses.

The Lombard and the Stenger tests, early tests for functional loss, are still used regularly. Both can be administered using pure tone and speech audiometric equipment that is calibrated to a standard reference. These tests will be described later (Section II,C,1; Section III,B,1).

C. Prevalence

Prevalence of functional hearing loss is somewhat difficult to evaluate because the functional component is often superimposed (that is, overlaid) on some degree of organic loss. The degree of overlay varies considerably, and all patients who show a mild component are not necessarily counted as functional. Functional loss may be superimposed on normal hearing as well. Other criteria used for diagnoses vary. Also, the count will differ depending on the following: (1) patient population studied, (2) age group studied, and (3) test methods used to investigate the problem.

If one attempts to evaluate malingering separately from "unconscious" motivations, the problem becomes even more difficult because the two are not separated so easily. In addition, a larger number of investigators are suggesting that these are not separable, except at the outset, and that they become related on a time continuum (Barr, 1963; Berger, 1965; Hopkinson, 1967; Zwislocki, 1963). From the point in time at which it becomes "profitable" for the child or adult to behave as though he has a hearing loss, to the point at which the problem has not become resolved, the patient may go through progressive stages of believing in the loss himself.

1. Adults

In adults, functional loss has been most prevalent in the military and in referrals from the Veterans Administration. Estimates over a period of years range from 8 to 45% in the military (Martin, 1946; Johnson et al., 1956; Zwislocki, 1963). Estimates in a Veteran's Administration sample are 15–20% (Zwislocki, 1963). In 1962 van Dishoeck summarized the responses of several specialists to a question about prevalence. The sources that combined estimates for military and insurance referrals indicated 35–50%. One of the sources reported that 100% of all patients referred for compensation purposes showed some degree of functional hearing problem (van Dishoeck, 1962).

In England referrals from industry and adult civilian life have been assigned a prevalence of less than 1% (Beagley and Knight, 1968). A survey of 30 audiology centers in the United States made in 1951 showed that the percentage of civilians with functional hearing problems was 0 in 16 of the centers, less than 5 in 11 of the centers, and 5 or more in only 3 of the centers (Zwislocki, 1963).

2. Children

Data on children who show functional loss are difficult to interpret. Some reports present percentages of functional patients without reference to a total number of patients or to a period of time. One clinic reported that 41 children or 7% of the total case load in a 12-month period were identified as functional. The age range was 6–17 years, mean age 10.9 years (Campanelli, 1963).

Maran (1966) reported in a general study of causes of hearing loss in children that 55 children were found to have normal hearing, which was accompanied by an emotional disturbance or "auditory imperception." The number represented 6.8% of the total. The ages ranged from preschool to 16 years, with an average age at the time of first referral of 8.2 years. Barr (1963) reported on 32 cases in a 10-year period, 1952–1962. However, he added that a large number of the milder cases were not recorded as functional. The age range was 9–14 years.

In 1951 a survey of 30 audiology centers was taken to determine the prevalence of functional loss in children (Zwislocki, 1963). The problem was considered negligible by 22 centers. A prevalence of less than 5% was reported by six centers, and a prevalence in excess of 5% was reported by only two centers.

Ten adolescents with functional hearing problems were studied by Lehrer et al. (1964). They ranged in age from 11 years, 3 months to 16 years. The investigators did not refer to a period of time over which the patients were identified. The problem occurs less frequently among school-age children than among the military or among civilian adults (Berger, 1965; Lehrer et al., 1964). The trend may be changing somewhat in recent years, although the percentage of functional problems among children is still nowhere near that among the groups which have received monetary compensation.

A clinical record has been reported in which three daughters from the same family showed both hearing and visual problems that were of "psychic" origin. The hearing problems demonstrated by the two oldest daughters were believed to be "partly simulated." Family conflicts were given as the reason (Lumio et al., 1969).

3. Increase and Decrease

In the 10 years following World War II, functional hearing loss increased significantly among men discharged from the service because of hearing disabilities. Table I is based on numbers given in Johnson et al. (1956). An overall increase from 11 to 45% is shown in the table. The increase is misleading if taken at face value, since the count changed

TABLE I[a]
INCREASE OF FUNCTIONAL
LOSS—WORLD WAR II VETERANS

Year	Percentage of functional loss
1951	11
1952	23
1953	24
1954	45

[a] Percentages are based on more than
10 dB of functional loss (Johnson et al.,
1956).

for reasons other than the fact that more men became functional problems. Over that period of time, testing methods were greatly improved
because of an increased awareness of the condition and the need to
identify it. Consequently, more patients were identified. Some part of
the increase resulted because of the monthly compensation policy. Patients were more highly motivated to receive benefits. Some part of
the increase resulted because of inadequate counseling at the time of
onset.

Functional hearing problems were found in 90% of referrals from
the Veterans Administration who came from a depressed area where
there was serious unemployment (Gibbons, 1962). Large industrial areas
show greater prevalence because of work accidents and compensation
laws. In general, an increase of functional loss is noted during wars,
recessions, and periods when socialized care programs are ignored. Periods of affluence tend to show a decrease in the problem.

Among children, seasonal increases of functional loss have been noted.
Later winter and early spring are times when earache and ear infections
have occurred in the previous months. These times have been related
to times of unusual school pressures. The combination of a "choice"
of the ears as a target with the excess pressure at school creates a
good excuse for lowered performance (Berger, 1965).

D. Causes

The causes of functional hearing loss are, at best, a mystery. Although
the supposed causes will be considered, functional loss, unlike losses
that result from verifiable lesions, is very much an abstraction, an inference. Causes are not well documented.

Although functional hearing loss may show an increase during wars, the increase is "frequently causally unrelated to stresses of combat" (Zwislocki, 1963). By the same token, the man with temporary loss as a result of blast trauma may become functionally deaf if he is not counseled about the gradual return of his hearing (Johnson et al., 1956). Earaches and transient mild, middle-ear pathologies do not cause functional hearing loss. However, emotional stresses that occur at home or in the school may combine with one of those problems to allow the child a choice of a hearing problem to avoid conflict or to excuse his academic performance (Lehrer et al., 1964).

The causes of functional hearing problems may be small in number, yet the ways of manifestation are numerous. The causes may be divided simply into unconscious and conscious. Those in the first category may be a quick and ready adjustment or solution to an emotional situation that the individual is not psychologically strong enough to handle. Those in the second category may begin with the individual's knowledge of what he is doing. At the time he may believe the solution to be efficacious and temporary. The gains may be monetary or psychological. Some individuals continue to know that they are feigning yet will become adapted to the act because they have reached a point of no return. Others may be able to convince themselves that in some way, having been wronged, they have a real hearing problem.

The results of an interdisciplinary study of functional hearing loss (Cohen et al., 1963) provided a number of leads, though the study did not give a complete or definitive explanation of the causes. The investigators concluded that functional loss is due to the subject's lack of cooperation in the test situation. The neurological data suggested that modification of physiological sensory behavior such as hearing loss is a response to psychological stresses and is not conscious. The data suggested that functional loss was present to a greater degree in a wide variety of character and emotional disturbances. Experimental subjects did not differ from control subjects in predisposing factors. Reports of sequelae of head injuries were disproportionate to the extent of injury itself (Cohen et al., 1963). Obviously, experts differ in their opinions about the causes of functional hearing loss; yet there is some common ground.

We may inappropriately label as functional the child or adult whose organic hearing levels are difficult to assess when, in fact, he has poor criteria for listening and/or responding. This inappropriate label is unlikely if inconsistent relations among test responses occur in the majority of procedures. However, in a single test such as Békésy audiometry, the patient with less than strict criteria for listening has free reign (Hopkinson, 1965). Functional problems that do not exceed ±10 dB of disparity among conventional test results may be more accurately labeled "criterial problems." Very few patients are excellent listeners and responders on first encounter with a hearing examination. However, appreciation of the naive listener's plight does not relieve the audiologist of the responsibility to identify and resolve the problem.

II. Identification

Any organic problem is difficult to diagnose or identify if the examiner is not expecting it. On the other hand, the health professional with a mature approach to his work probably should meet every patient with the assumption that he is normal until the examination gives evidence that he is not so. These two statements seem to be contradictory; yet with respect to functional hearing problems they are compatible.

A. Informal Reports and Observations

1. PRETEST BEHAVIOR

Some children and a few adults with functional hearing problems perform without difficulty in an informal conversational situation (Berger, 1965; Campanelli, 1963; Johnson et al., 1956; Lehrer et al., 1964). Yet, when they are put in the formal test situation, they have trouble hearing. The behavior is somewhat naive, which is undoubtedly why it is rarely seen among adults with "confirmed" functional hearing loss.

Gibbons (1962) has stressed that the patient with organic, total bilateral deafness who formerly had normal hearing, invariably demonstrates an eagerness to communicate. The patient tries to get visual cues even if his attempt is only partially successful. On the other hand, the patient with a functional problem may avoid watching lips, or he may behave at the other extreme and exaggerate his attempts to lipread, and still not be able to converse.

In a relatively short period of time, patients with organic, total loss of hearing follow a pattern of deterioration in speech production. The effect shows especially in melody and in the production of clear final consonants (Gibbons, 1962). Patients with functional loss do not show a deterioration in melody or in the production of consonants.

There are a few classical behaviors that have little to do with the act of speaking or hearing. Patients who fail to keep an appointment without canceling are showing poor cooperation, especially if the purpose of the appointment as one of compensation tests is known to patient and clinician (Johnson et al., 1956). Patients who are very late (1 hour) or very early for their appointments suggest poor cooperation, and a need to control the timing of the appointment. Frequently patients who are very early arrive with the excuse that they must leave early, and therefore, hoped they could be rushed through their tests. They seem badly oriented to the concept of time.

The average patient sitting in a waiting area is apt to watch or listen closely to know when he is being called. Patients with a functional problem may be deeply engrossed in a magazine and miss their call. They have thereby stressed the severity of the problem. When these patients do get up to follow the clinician, they behave as though they are badly oriented in space. They may appear not to have noticed in which direction the clinician went or into which room. In some patients, the behavior is exaggerated to such an extent that two "double takes" might follow the clinician's calling of a name.

2. Reports of Onset

Although any of the following reports of onset may result in an organic loss of hearing, any of them also should suggest to the audiologist the possibility of a functional hearing loss. A functional overlay may be present, when the deafness is described as occurring at a time or in a manner that made it an "answer" to an existing problem or that made it a defense of a serious shortcoming.

Patients who are later found to have a functional component often report head injuries, back injuries, and other general injuries about the head, face, or neck. Some patients "blame" a noise trauma. Others report a sudden onset of total bilateral hearing loss (Johnson *et al.*, 1956). Reports of onset sometimes accompany information provided at the time the appointment is made; sometimes the reports are obtained during the case history.

B. Case History

School-age children, whose parents report a large number of general emotional problems that seem out of line with the age of the child, may show some functional hearing loss. The implication is that the child is making adjustments through the expression of emotional or physical problems, not by the direction of energy against the issues themselves. The adult counterpart is the person who answers positively every question in the history that involves health status. His answers sound as if everything is wrong with him. He has every sign and symptom that will make his case look real. Yet, in the final analysis, he has not been selective enough to supply veracity. In any organic condition, a certain set of symptoms tend to define the disorder. Other symptoms confuse the distinction. Too many symptoms cast suspicion on the reality of all of the symptoms.

The patient who dramatizes his answers to questions in the history may have a functional component. He may describe the injury in detail, and embellish occurrences such as flow of blood from the injured ear. Frequently the functional patient's answers to questions are forgotten or omitted. Rarely does the functional patient remember any relatives who had hearing losses or ear conditions. Rarely does he admit to having worked in noise or taken medications unless these are the areas concerning his compensation.

Sometimes the material given on case histories does not match well with other information about the patient. If the audiologist talked with the patient on the phone before the appointment, it is often the case that the patient appeared to converse readily, yet he answered questions concerning the use of the telephone as if he had difficulty. He may report injuries that imply a middle-ear pathology, yet the otological examination shows no evidence of a middle-ear problem. Another patient may fail to report history of early middle-ear infections, yet the otologist finds evidence of old scarring of the tympanic membrane. Obviously every inconsistency cannot be considered here. The examples given should be sufficient from which to generalize.

C. Behavior during Formal Testing

1. RESPONSES AMONG CONVENTIONAL PROCEDURES

Inconsistency of response among repeat tests often is used as an example of nonorganic behavior. There is evidence, however, that pure-tone and speech-reception thresholds may be repeated with a high degree of consistency. Actually, functional patients may be no less or no more consistent than organic patients during repeat measures of threshold (Barr, 1963; Berger, 1965; Campanelli, 1963; Lehrer et al., 1964; Shepherd, 1965; Ventry and Chaiklin, 1965, p. 199).

The comparison of pure-tone and speech-reception thresholds has been an efficient way of identifying patients with functional hearing loss. In a study by Ventry and Chaiklin (1965), 33 of 47 subjects had speech thresholds that were significantly lower than their pure-tone averages. The finding is common in both adults and children (Menzel, 1960; Rintelmann and Harford, 1963).

The relationship between air-conduction and bone-conduction responses is often indicative of poor cooperation. If bone-conduction hearing shows 10 dB or worse hearing than air conduction, the patient may have difficulty making accurate loudness judgments via bone transmission. At the other extreme, when veterans were examined routinely at contract agencies, bone-conduction responses commonly indicated a conductive component. The air-conduction results often indicated a severe loss of hearing, showing a significantly greater air–bone gap than 60 dB. The end result after special tests was that the initial bone-conduction responses represented the organic condition of the sense organ. Sometimes the bone-conduction responses represented the organic level of hearing when the air–bone gap of 60 dB or less was credible. In these cases bone conduction was rarely normal so that the initial functional component represented an overlay on an organic condition of hearing.

a. *Responses to Air-Conduction Tests.* The manner in which a patient responds to pure-tone signals may help to identify him as functional. If the audiologist tries to get his attention, the patient may act as if engrossed in the listening task, to avoid looking at the tester.

The functional patient may respond at one level on an ascending investigation of threshold. If an attempt is made to repeat the response at the same level, the functional patient may not respond until a 5- or 10-dB increment is added. If the same technique is continued, the patient's threshold may have covered another 20 or 30 dB. The higher intensities seem to elicit higher thresholds. Occasionally, a patient who demonstrates very rapid tone decay will perform in a similar manner. The two kinds of responses may be distinguished by using shorter tones, by interrupting the tone presentation more rapidly. The functional patient will continue to behave in the same manner, while the patient with rapid tone decay will "level off," and stabilize quickly at some threshold after brief onset of the tone.

Some patients purposely will respond falsely when a tone is not present. In most instances the behavior is more likely to occur with the patient who is afraid he is hard-of-hearing and is trying hard to hear. On the other hand, if the patient willfully wishes to confuse the examiner, a number of responses given at times when no tone is present will serve the intent. Under these circumstances, changing technique to a descending one may help to distinguish the two kinds of responses.

The audiogram provided by functional patients has been described characteristically by a number of investigators. At one time the "saucer shape" was believed to be the audiogram most indicative of functional loss. However, the trend changed and the audiograms were described as flat (Johnson et al., 1956). The flat audiograms were believed to be the result of listening at most comfortable loudness levels (Barr, 1963; Berger, 1965; Campanelli, 1963; Lehrer et al., 1964). In patients with underlying organic loss, a study showed that neither the saucer shape nor the flat audiogram was characteristic (Ventry and Chaiklin, 1965). The audiologist would be safest in concluding that there is no characteristic pure-tone audiogram for the functional patient.

Studies of audiograms of children with functional loss have shown moderate and moderately severe bilateral loss (Barr, 1963; Berger, 1965). Barr (1963) encountered no losses in high frequencies only.

b. *Responses to Speech Reception Threshold (SRT)*. The nonorganic adult classically responds to spondees by repeating only one-half of the word, while children are not so likely to repeat a part of the word (Berger, 1965). Spondees are presented with equal stress on each syllable. They rise rapidly from 0 to 100% intelligibility (Hudgins *et al.*, 1947). If the patient hears and repeats half of the word, there is no legitimate reason for him not to hear and repeat the other half of the word.

Some patients will repeat no spondee words at one level, yet they will repeat all three words at the next highest level. Frequently, the patient will substitute words for the spondee word that have little likeness to the original. The behavior suggests poor cooperation.

The kinds of errors that functional patients make during speech reception testing have been analyzed. Functional patients show a disproportionate number of no-response errors as well as the types of errors described earlier. A formula for spondee error index has been worked out so that a high score contrasted with a low number of false positive responses during pure tone testing identifies a functional patient (Chaiklin and Ventry, 1965).

c. *Responses to Discrimination Tests*. A large number of no-response errors is frequently a sign that the patient is not cooperating. Some functional patients substitute synonyms and association words. If the same discrimination test is repeated, the patient's consistency of responses may be poor. The patient obtains a similar percent score; however, he misses a different set of words. In some cases he will make errors on the same words, but the errors will be quite different. For example, if the patients errs on the initial consonant in the first test, he may err on the final consonant in the second test.

d. *Responses to Special Tests*. The observations of behavior described so far, involving conventional audiologic procedures, are good indicators for the identification of functional hearing loss. If the use of additional tests is considered a necessity in order to identify functional loss, automatic audiometry may provide further evidence of nonorganic behavior (Jerger and Herer, 1961).

Little is known, at this time, about characteristic responses of functional patients to the standard tone decay test (STDT) or to the short increment sensitivity index (SISI). However, considerable study of responses to Békésy audiometry has followed the finding described as the Type V tracing (Peterson, 1963; Resnick and Burke, 1962; Rintelmann and Harford, 1963; Stein, 1963).

Audiologists who expect patients to display a variety of criteria for listening and responding, generally do not use Békésy audiometry to establish thresholds because the control of signals is in the hands of the listener. Therefore, they have not depended on subject-controlled audiometry for the identification of functional hearing loss. They identify the problem on other bases, and then use tests that aid in the resolution of hearing levels before using Békésy audiometry. If they have seen the characteristic Type V tracing for continuous signals at lower levels than for interrupted signals, they have considered the tracing a sign of poor criteria for listening (Hopkinson, 1965; Price et al., 1965).

At first the Type V tracing was loosely defined, and criteria for validity and reliability were difficult to apply. A more rigid definition was supplied later (Rintelmann and Harford, 1967); yet, some question remains as to whether the patients would have continued to trace the Type V if they had been first exposed to tests in which the signal was under the control of the examiner. According to Melnick (1967) the patient is able to set his own loudness standard when he controls the signal. By inference the patient's opportunity to set his own criteria is disrupted when the signal is under the control of an examiner. Hattler (1968) has shown that the Type V trace can be emphasized among normal subjects by decreasing duty-cycle of the interrupted signal without changing the on-duration. He has attributed the tracing to deficits in loudness memory.

Several studies of the Type V trace have involved children, many of whom are completely naive to automatic audiometry. One study used fixed-frequency audiometry on 61 children who were normals and on 52 children with bilateral sensorineural losses (ages 5–10 years). The results of the study showed that except for ages 5 and 9 years, there was a tendency for children with hearing losses to trace the Type V pattern. The younger children showed greater variability in tracing quality. In either group of children, the Type V pattern was considered the result of learning effects, and did not always indicate a functional hearing loss (Stark, 1966).

The Lombard test is based on the principle that the listener can regulate his own vocal intensity so that he accommodates to the noise in his environment. If the listener hears his voice, he will raise the intensity to compensate for the level of noise.

The Lombard reflex can be measured by having the patient read aloud, while a noise in his earphones is increased. If the Lombard reflex occurs at levels of intensity less than the patient's admitted threshold, the audiologist knows the initial threshold is in error, but he does not know the magnitude of the error (Newby, 1964).

Thus far, only the quality of response has been dealt with. The audiologist has the responsibility of quantifying the organic hearing loss if one is present after he has identified the functional patient. The audiologist will attempt to control response behavior that tends to show wide disparities in conventional procedures. He will help the patient to establish fine criteria for the listening task. When responses are beyond these controls, then the audiologist uses the special procedures with a skill that resolves the inconsistencies sometimes without the functional patient's awareness of the resolution. The experienced, objective clinician rarely has to confront or accuse the patient (Gibbons, 1962).

Identification of a functional hearing problem may be the simplest job for the audiologist to learn, while resolution of hearing levels may be the most difficult.

III. Common Battery of Tests

A. Quantification of Levels—Tests Suitable for Binaural Loss

1. DOERFLER–STEWART TEST

The Doerfler–Stewart (D/S) test depends on a calculated manipulation of speech and noise signals. Normals and patients with organic hearing loss respond to binaural speech signals in the presence of a binaural noise that is 10 dB higher than the speech. Patients with functional components stop responding to speech when the noise is somewhat lower than speech. This behavior was recognized at Deshon Hospital during World War II (Doerfler and Stewart, 1946).

Muth (1952) studied the D/S results on 100 subjects with conductive or sensorineural hearing losses to determine whether the results varied with different organic pathologies. He noted minor differences, involving the noise detection and noise interference measures, between conductives and sensorineurals.

The test was validated on a group of patients that included both organic and nonorganic hearing losses in 1956 by Epstein and Hopkinson. The procedure and the norms were reported that same year in a monograph prepared for the Veterans Administration (Doerfler and Epstein, 1956).

Initially, the D/S test was designed to be given using a sawtooth noise because of the psychological distraction that was caused by the spectrum of the noise with a base frequency of approximately 125 Hz. In the meantime, other noises have been used. One is a complex noise (Ventry and Chaiklin, 1965), and the other is a speech noise (Grason–Stadler Speech Audiometers, 162 and 1701). At 1000 Hz, speech noise is approximately 3 dB down from the output at 125 Hz, and 9 dB down at 2000 Hz. Clinically, speech noise has been as effective as sawtooth noise. The kind of noise does not appear to be critical if it has strong energy components between 125 and 500 Hz.

The speech audiometer must have the same binaural output for speech and noise signals with separate controls over attenuation for each signal. Both speech and noise should be calibrated separately in terms of 0-dB hearing level. Threshold of intelligibility (50% correct) for spondees is used as the reference level for speech.

a. Description. Essentially the test is as follows: During the instructions the patient is *not* told about the noise which is part of the test. Each step of the test must be continuous with the next step so that the patient is not aware of the five separate measures being obtained.

The first speech reception threshold (SRT_1), is obtained in an ascending manner. An additional 4- or 5-dB level above threshold ($SRT_1 + 5$) is allowed so that the patient can easily recognize spondees.

The noise is increased gradually in ascending manner until the patient can no longer repeat words. That level is called noise interference level (NIL). The noise is increased beyond that level so that the patient hears nothing but the noise for a period of time during the procedure. Under the cover of the subjectively loud noise, the clinician continues to say spondees, while he reduces the level of the words. He then reduces the noise until the patient either repeats spondees again at the lower level or until the patient no longer responds and the noise has been removed from the test.

A second speech reception score (SRT_2) is established in the same manner as the first speech threshold. Finally, a separate threshold is obtained for the noise, called noise detection threshold (NDT).

There is an interrelationship among the five measures either because they have measured the same signals, in the same or related context, or they have measured different signals in a threshold context. The first and second speech reception thresholds should relate closely. Speech reception thresholds one and two have a close association with the detection of noise. Noise interference and speech reception above threshold are relevant to one another. Noise detection and noise interference should correlate. The results of these calculations are compared with the norms to provide an overall positive or negative interpretation.

2. GALVANIC SKIN RESPONSE TEST (ELECTRODERMAL RESPONSE)

Auditory sensitivity has been measured by conditioning skin responses to auditory signals since the late 1940s (Bordley *et al.*, 1948). The method and measures have been refined over a period of years so that the validity and reliability of galvanic skin response (GSR) audiometry are widely accepted (Burk, 1958; Doerfler, 1948; Doerfler and McClure, 1954; Giolas and Epstein, 1964; Grings et al., 1959; Hardy and Pauls, 1952; Knapp and Gold, 1950; Meritser and Doerfler, 1954; Stewart, 1954).

a. *Description.* Galvanic skin response is a form of audiometry that is called objective because it does not require a voluntary response from the patient. The classical conditioning paradigm of Pavlov is used in the conventional procedure of GSR to condition responses that are mediated by the autonomic (vegetative) nervous system. The conditioning procedure involves the pairing of an unconditioned stimulus, usually shock, with the conditioned stimulus or tone. Earphones are used to test one ear at a time. Pickup electrodes are affixed to the fingertips of an adult patient and the changes in electrical resistance of the sweat glands of the skin are recorded on apparatus such as an inkwriter. These changes occur when the skin response has been conditioned. The shock electrodes generally are affixed to the forearm of an adult.

b. *Salient Features.* The value of GSR in the diagnosis of functional hearing problems is related to rigidity of the procedure. The cardinal features are as follows:

1. Instructions that sensitize the patient to the conditioning procedure. The word *shock* must be used.
2. The use of a conditioning schedule that combines tone and shock in 40–60% of 10 or 12 presentations before threshold levels are investigated.
3. Conditioning must take place at near-threshold levels as well as at suprathreshold levels.
4. Generally, the frequency at which conditioning is carried out should be one for which the patient admits some hearing.
5. The duration of tone stimulus should not exceed 2 sec.
6. The preferred interval between tone and shock stimuli is 1–2 sec.
7. Duration of the shock should be brief (up to 1 sec).
8. The intensity of shock should be established on a subjective basis so that the patient "feels it." As the conditioning procedure ensues, the level of the shock should be raised slightly at progressive intervals.
9. Following the conditioning procedure, threshold should be investigated in an ascending fashion, beginning at 0 dB hearing level or lower.

10. Reinforcement with the unconditioned stimulus (shock) should be used periodically, approximately 10–20% of the time.

c. Evaluation of Responses. The audiologist rates the conditioning of the patient and the overall reliability of the test. He assigns ratings of good, fair, or poor on the basis of the following criteria:

1. *Judgment of amplitude.* Using an external standard, an amplitude of 5 mm is considered acceptable. However, using the patient as his own standard, the height of amplitude during conditioning should be observed for comparison. Consistency of amplitude is important.
2. *Frequency of response.* Were two successive conditioned responses available at the level interpreted as threshold? Was there only one response? Were two nonsuccessive responses available?
3. *Latency of response.* A latency of 2 sec is average. A latency of 1 sec is too brief to account for physiological latency and a latency of 5 sec is too long. The consistency of latency should be judged using the patient as his own standard.
4. *Generalization of conditioning.* Judgments of generalization of conditioning from frequency to frequency should be recorded as well as generalization from one ear to the other.
5. *Reinforcement.* A percentage of reinforcement should be recorded. The number here should influence the next judgment of extinction.
6. *Extinction.* A rating of slow, average, or rapid extinction can be made by relating this feature to the reinforcement.
7. *Extraneous movement.* A comment should be recorded on whether excessive pen movement caused the clinician to interpret more responses than he would consider average from experience with other patients.
8. Finally the rating of conditioning can be influenced by resistance readings if they are available in the instrumentation used. A measure of electrical skin resistance can be made with some commercially available audiometers. If a reading is taken before the test is begun, a reading that is taken at the end of the test can be compared with it. Classically, the kilo-ohms of resistance should reduce in number from outset to end if the patient was conditioned.

These evaluations allow the audiologist to know how much weight he can attribute to the results of the test. The evaluations may be used to report to referral sources the reasons that the results of GSR were rated as unreliable, if they were so rated.

d. *Present Use.* Although GSR is used less frequently then it once was, many good points remain. In a study of clinical efficiency in compensation audiometry, the incidence of functional loss was reduced by deferring pure tone audiometry, until either speech or GSR tests or both had been administered (Menzel, 1960).

The GSR was used in a study of functional hearing problems among adolescents. In 50% of the patients who took the test, thresholds were within normal limits in at least one ear. Subjective audiograms were obtained immediately following the GSR test with electrodes left in place. Six of seven patients who showed normal GSR audiograms also gave subjective responses within normal limits under the latter condition (Lehrer *et al.*, 1964).

The GSR has been criticized as an ineffective procedure with children who are mentally deficient or cerebral palsied. The effectiveness of the test in these cases may be affected by (1) the loose conditioning procedure used, and (2) the application of an external standard for interpretation of conditioned responses.

The children who bring less than a normal system to the conditioning procedure will be unlikely to meet rigid external criteria for conditioning. Very often, upon seeing the child, the clinician is apt to assume a poor level of conditioning without making a serious attempt to condition him. On the other hand, if the child were used as his own standard, some measure of conditioned responses could be obtained.

Objective audiometric evaluations such as evoked potential audiometry have gained respect in the past several years. These measures will be discussed. In larger clinical departments, evoked response audiometry appears to be in greater use now than galvanic skin response measures.

3. DELAYED AUDITORY FEEDBACK

This test is also known as delayed speech feedback, or as delayed playback or as delayed side tone. The effects of delayed speech feedback were studied before the test was used to investigate auditory sensitivity (Black, 1951; Lee, 1950).

a. *Description.* The subject, wearing earphones, reads a passage into a microphone. The passage is recorded on tape and fed back through the phones at a delayed time. The test can be used in functional hearing problems by controlling the intensity of the feedback to determine at what level the patient hears his voice. When he hears the delayed playback he may hesitate in his reading, he may repeat or stammer. He may only slow his reading time. There are many variations among individuals in response to the feedback.

Features that improve the flexibility of the test when it is used to study hearing levels are as follows: a variety of delay times, a VU-meter for observing changes in vocal intensity, and a stop watch. When delayed feedback techniques depended on the occurrence of extreme disturbances in the patient's reading pattern, criteria for hearing level were too general. The results were of qualitative value only. Procedures have been refined to include timing devices so that more subtle changes in reading time can be measured. Some of the timing devices are as simple as a stopwatch. Others are more complicated and more precise, such as a speech time analyzer (McGranahan et al., 1960).

The patient reads a passage into a microphone without feedback, while the audiologist times his reading. The patient reads the passage several times so that an average of reading times without playback can be obtained as base line for comparison. During successive intensity increases with the delayed-time conditions, the patient continues to read. Although most patients will tend to read more slowly when they hear the feedback, some will speed their reading. At the end of the test an additional reading may be timed without playback. The latter reading provides another standard for comparison of reading time against that for the playback conditions. Threshold of intelligibility (50% correct) should be established for a group of normals on the instrumentation to be used.

When the procedure includes a timing of the readings as well as pre- and postfeedback readings a change in reading rate of +3 sec or greater is significant. The change in rate is significant for a level within +10 dB of threshold of intelligibility. When a speech time analyzer is used, a change of +3.5 sec has been reported as significant for a threshold measure (McGranahan et al., 1960).

A variety of delay times makes possible repeated testing at one level of intensity without adaptation to the effect. The delay time that is usually most effective is 0.18 sec (Hanley and Tiffany, 1954). However, if the delay time is varied from 0.15 to 0.5 sec, and the reading rates are consistent with those obtained at 0.18 sec, it is unlikely that the patient heard the feedback.

The appropriate choice of a reading passage is an important factor. The choice depends on the patient's general level of intelligence and his ability to read. If reading fails for any reason other than the effect of feedback the test becomes inefficient.

Simultaneous feedback may be used to substantiate a change of a few seconds in reading rate at a certain level. At the same level, the patient's reading is fed back without delay, but with amplification. The reading rate obtained in this manner may be compared with the first reading obtained at that level with 0.18-sec delay.

b. Pertinent Studies. Several studies have led to the development of refinements in the procedure so that support for quantitative levels is possible. Early investigators held that the test was effective at high levels of feedback (Tiffany and Hanley, 1952). However, others tried starting without feedback and then increasing the levels until a change in reading rate occurred (McGrahahan *et al.*, 1960). The test has been effective as a binaural or a monaural procedure. If the monaural procedure is used, appropriate contralateral masking is necessary (Gibbons and Winchester, 1957).

The final reading without feedback or amplification became part of the procedure as a result of earlier studies. Hanley and Tiffany (1954) found that subjects seemed to read faster following the experimental readings.

Additional refinements have been made, such as key-tapping in the delayed feedback context. This test will be covered in a section on modifications of the procedure in present use (Section IV,A,4).

B. Tests Suitable for Monaural Loss

1. PURE-TONE STENGER

The pure-tone Stenger test depends on the principle that a relatively loud sound in one ear makes an identical but fainter sound inaudible in the other ear. This test is very effective if a two-channel audiometer with a binaural on–off switch is used to present the same frequency to each ear at different intensities. If the frequencies differ by a few cycles, the patient will hear beats. The beats will identify for the functional patient the fact that both ears are being stimulated. The signals must reach both ears simultaneously so that the functional patient will not recognize that his purportedly poorer ear is being tested. For the same reason, the same rise and decay times are necessary in each ear.

a. Description. The patient is instructed that principally his better ear is being tested. He should raise his hand on the same side as he hears the tone, then lower his hand when the tone goes away. A pure tone is presented at a level 5–10 dB above his threshold for that tone in his better ear. The presentation is repeated several times. Then a high-level tone of the same frequency is presented to the poorer ear simultaneously with the low-level tone in the better ear.

A number of responses to this procedure are possible. Three responses that are most common will be described here.

1. If the patient continues to respond, the lower-level tone is gradually removed (using the interrupter) from the better ear. The signal in the poorer ear may then be reduced until the patient stops responding. A level obtained for the poorer ear in this manner should agree reasonably closely with a "crossover level" obtained without contralateral masking at the same frequency during standard pure-tone audiometry.

2. If the patient continues to respond and indicates that he hears the tone in his poorer ear, the tone gradually may be removed from the better ear. Then the tone in the poorer ear may be reduced until the patient no longer hears it.

Although these two responses are similar, the behavior of the patient in the second case is consciously cooperative. The behavior in the first case is cooperative also, although the patient is less verbal about which ear is being stimulated. The second kind of response also checks against the unmasked response at the same frequency in conventional audiometry.

3. Finally, if the patient does not respond when the high-level tone is presented to the poorer ear, the tone in the poorer ear should be increased. If there is still no response, this means that the patient hears the high-level tone in the poorer ear, that it has interfered with the lower-level tone. The tone in the poorer ear may then be reduced in level until the patient again responds. The response indicates that he again hears the tone in his better ear. The level just above that level of response is the interference level, the response that is considered the classical Stenger effect. These results should be in close agreement with quantitative results on the poorer ear from other tests of functional loss.

Some investigators prefer the technique of initially presenting a tone to the poorer ear about 10–20 dB above that presented to the better ear (Newby, 1964; O'Neill and Oyer, 1966; Zwislocki, 1963). On the other hand, others infer that the number of false positive responses is increased by an ascending presentation of tone to the poorer ear (Gaeth and Norris, 1965). Initial presentation of the tone to the poorer ear at suprathreshold level (one that the patient would identify subjectively as loud) leads to more definitive responses. On the basis of clinical experience the latter case has been true especially when using the pure tone Stenger. There seems to be some surprise element in the initial high-level presentation that causes the patient clearly to respond or not to respond. There is little question about the functional patient's lack of response under these circumstances.

The ideal candidate for the pure-tone Stenger is the patient presenting total unilateral hearing loss (Taylor, 1949). However, the patient with diplacusis may invalidate the test (Zwislocki, 1963). This factor supports the presentation of a loud signal initially to the poorer ear. Once interaural differences in subjectively perceived loudness have passed a critical point, smaller pitch differences should be obscured by the Stenger effect (Chaiklin and Ventry, 1963).

b. Usefulness. The value of the pure-tone Stenger test is unquestionable in the resolution of monaural functional losses. The Stenger has proved its worth over a longer time than other tests of its kind. As a tuning fork method it was used as early as 1907 to discover functional losses. Investigators have found the pure-tone Stenger a useful quantitative tool (Taylor, 1949; Ventry and Chaiklin, 1965; Zwislocki, 1963).

2. SPEECH STENGER

The speech Stenger is a modification of the pure-tone Stenger (Johnson *et al.*, 1956; Taylor, 1949; Watson and Tolan, 1967). It is particularly useful when the loss in the poorer ear is not profound. Since speech is a more complex signal than a pure tone, a lower initial level of signal in the poorer ear is appropriate. False-positive responses can be ruled out more readily by evaluating the appropriateness of the reply to questions.

A two-channel speech audiometer is necessary, so that the speech signal can be presented to both ears simultaneously. The intensity levels in each ear must be controlled independently (Newby, 1964).

The hearing of beats does not occur in the speech Stenger. Diplacusis does not appear to affect the test.

The patient is instructed to raise his hand on the side of the ear in which he hears the words, and to repeat the words. If he hears a simple question, he is to answer the question. The directions are purposely complicated to ensure the patient's attention to the test (Johnson *et al.*, 1956).

Spondaic words are presented by live voice to the patient's better ear at a level 16 dB sensation level (SL). The patient should repeat the words and raise his hand on the side of his better ear each time a word is presented.

A simple question is presented simultaneously to the poorer ear at a level 20 dB above the level being presented to the better ear. Since this is not a subjectively loud level to the patient, the effect of surprise is obtained by substituting a question for a spondee. The patient's responses are interpreted as they were for the pure-tone Stenger, varying the level of signals to the better and the poorer ear. If the patient has been cooperative, the results of this test will relate to the "crossover levels" obtained without contralateral masking during conventional speech testing. If the patient showed the classical Stenger effect, his results can be compared with those of other procedures for testing functional hearing loss. The audiologist also may use the results of the Stenger to identify levels at which to begin other tests or retests of the poorer ear.

3. Story Tests

Although story tests are no longer used frequently, the audiologist may find a variety of story tests to verify a unilateral loss of hearing. A two-channel speech audiometer is necessary with the facility for switching from one ear to the other and to the binaural position.

The story is presented to both ears at the same level. However, the level must be chosen efficiently at the outset so that the intensity is sufficiently above the threshold of the better ear, yet slightly below the hearing levels of the poorer ear. Often these latter levels are not known. A level about 20 dB above the threshold of the better ear may yield the most informative results.

As the audiologist tells the story, parts of it are delivered to the better ear, parts to the poorer ear, and parts to both ears. The story must be designed so that each part of its stands alone as a separate story.

If the patient repeats parts of the story delivered to the poorer ear, then the hearing can be said to be at least as good as that level. If he repeats the major parts of the story delivered only to better ear or to both ears, the hearing level in the poorer ear is probably worse than that level.

To be successful, this test must provide the listener with a sense of continuity. He must not be aware that the story is switched from ear to ear.

The story test may be used to establish a level of hearing for both ears if the level is set below that of the admitted levels for either ear. The level may be set approximately 10 dB lower than the admitted thresholds for the better ear. If the patient does not respond, his hearing levels are probably like the initial thresholds.

The results of each of these tests for functional hearing loss are important only as they relate to the results of all of the common battery of tests. Not one of these tests can be used alone to predict the degree of functional loss or to resolve levels of organic hearing.

IV. Extensions—Present and Future

Tests are means to an end; they are tools to be used by the audiologist to make his decisions more accurate, more contributory. Until this time, at least, tests are only as effective as the persons using them.

The procedures described have been fundamental to the investigation of functional hearing loss. They are basic to the training of audiologists. From these procedures extend modified measurements, employing more refined methods.

A. Modifications and Combinations

1. Speech Measures—GSR

Successful application of classical conditioning to pure-tone signals led to conditioning procedures using speech signals. Two groups of subjects, one with normal hearing and the other with conductive impairments were used in a study validating the procedure (Ruhm and Carhart, 1958). Patients with functional loss were used in a later study of the effectiveness of the test (Ruhm and Menzel, 1959).

The patient is conditioned to a key spondee, presented in a group of spondees. The unconditioned stimulus (shock) is used during the conditioning schedule when the key word is presented. The patient's threshold for intelligibility is established by omitting the shock and presenting words at supposed subthreshold levels.

In the brief series of words, the conditioned stimulus (key word) is always present as one of the words. Other words may cause a small increase in amplitude of the skin response, but only the conditioned word causes a significant increase in amplitude. None of the words causes a change in amplitude when speech is no longer detectable. Threshold is identified as the level at which the amplitude of response differentiates between the spondee that was the conditioned stimulus, and other spondees.

The patient does not make an overt response to the words so the test remains "objective." The clinician must decide whether the criteria for a conditioned response were met.

Chaiklin (1959) reported that speech thresholds using GSR on a group of normals were within ±5 dB of speech thresholds obtained with CID, Auditory Test W-1. The signal was the tape-recorded sentence, "Now you hear me."

2. Instrumental Avoidance Conditioning—GSR

Instrumental avoidance conditioning was compared to classical conditioning in an investigation of pure-tone, electrodermal testing. There were three groups of subjects: normals, patients with sensorineural losses, and patients with functional loss. Essentially, avoidance techniques require a subjective response from the patient if he wishes to avoid a noxious stimulus such as shock. In the comparison of one conditioning procedure to the other, the instrumental avoidance method showed stronger conditioning, greater resistance to extinction, and better discrimination learning than the classical conditioning method in all three groups of subjects (Shepherd, 1964).

3. A COMBINED METHOD

A test was described in 1960 that used instrumental avoidance conditioning to obtain verbal responses to speech signals (Hopkinson et al., 1960). The test takes two practical measurements of speech reception threshold at the same time, the galvanic skin response recording as well as the verbal response of the patient.

In this method, the patient is instructed that he can avoid a shock by repeating the correct word as soon as he hears it. Electrodes are affixed and earphones are placed on the patient as for conventional GSR audiometry. A conditioning schedule incorporates a spondaic word that the patient will have difficulty hearing and repeating so that the unconditioned stimulus (shock) is part of the reinforcement.

A comparison of two conditioning techniques on normal subjects showed that the instrumental avoidance response to speech signals was superior in the following ways: (1) more rapid acquisition of conditioning, (2) greater resistance to extinction, (3) wider intensity generalization, and (4) less appreciable stimulus intensity dynamism (Katz and Connelly, 1964).

4. DELAYED FEEDBACK

Studies of the effects of delayed feedback on other motor types of response than speech have led to an extension of hearing tests using key-tapping methods (Chase et al., 1959; Rapin et al., 1963). Results of studies on the effects of caffeine and alcohol on verbal output under audiofeedback (Forney and Hughes, 1965) suggest that motor responses other than speech may be less readily affected by intake of drugs. Key-tapping is a lower-order motor response that may resist the effects of a variable like alcohol taken in modest amounts. From that point of view, the use of key-tapping as the delayed signal deserves further study.

Normal subjects participated in preliminary investigations of key-tapping that were not concerned primarily with hearing levels. Normal subjects also participated in the earliest investigations concerned with hearing thresholds at low sensation levels (Ruhm and Cooper, 1962).

Ruhm and Cooper (1964) reported the effects of delay on three groups of subjects using pure tones and tapping method. The first group was composed of normally hearing adults whose ears were plugged with acoustic plugs. The second group consisted of patients with organic hearing problems. The third group was made up of patients with functional hearing losses. The investigators tested the validity of the method by comparing the results with those of standard audiometric thresholds with normals and patients with organic loss. They compared thresholds with those of GSR in both organic and functional hearing loss. The investigators concluded that delayed feedback audiometry is valid in assessing the pure-tone thresholds of adults with functional hearing impairment.

Karlovich and Graham (1966) used normals to study modifications of the key-tapping method. A repetitive flashing visual signal was used in addition to the pure-tone audio signal. Pattern and rate were regulated by the visual signal. The pure tones were presented in a synchronous condition of feedback as well as a delayed condition.

The number of tapping errors was too small to compare the results of synchronous with delayed feedback. However, the investigators (Karlovich and Graham 1966) recommended a modified method using both techniques for use with children. Longer delay times were more effective, causing subjects to increase tapping pressure. Tapping pressure was inversely related to sensation level of auditory feedback in both conditions, synchronous and delayed.

5. STENGER

A method has been described in which a patient may be given the Stenger test while tracing his threshold on Békésy audiometry (Watson and Voots, 1964). The method can be accomplished by adding a "simple attenuator arrangement." The examiner controls the intensity of test tone to the poorer ear while the patient traces threshold in his good ear. The investigators believe that approximate measures of threshold can be obtained for the poorer ear.

The fusion at the inferred threshold test (FIT) (Bergman, 1964) is related to the Stenger procedure. Essentially, a tone is presented to the better ear at a level 5 dB SL, while the tone at the test ear (poorer ear) is increased from a subthreshold level until the listener reports a change in the location of the tone. Bergman (1964) reported that for normals conventional and fusion thresholds for pure tones were interchangeable. For patients with conductive, sensorineural or mixed losses, fusion thresholds were repeated consistently within 1–2 dB of the levels shown in the pure-tone audiogram. These results were obtained on patients with unilateral functional loss as well.

6. A LIPREADING TEST

A test of lipreading has been proposed that uses monosyllabic homophenous words to determine hearing levels of patients with functional loss (Falconer, 1966). The face of the examiner is in the patient's view while visual and auditory stimuli are presented simultaneously. The first list of words is presented well above threshold (12 dB). Succeeding lists are presented at reduced intensity levels until only visual stimuli are available to the patient. Falconer stressed that because homophenous words look alike and sound different, they are unlikely to be perceived correctly by lipreading alone.

Suitable lists of words have been tested for use in this method. Speech reception threshold is derived from an articulation gain function. Specific rules have been reported for using the method and for interpreting the results (Falconer, 1966).

A few methods have been described that extend from conventional audiometric studies of functional hearing loss. Further investigation of these kinds of phenomena seems warranted.

B. Advanced Methods

1. IMPEDANCE MEASUREMENTS

Tests of the acoustic reflex have been used for some time to identify patients with functional hearing loss (Jepsen, 1953; Thomsen, 1955). Bilateral contractions of the intraaural muscles occur at 70–90 dB above hearing thresholds when only one ear is stimulated. In the deaf ear, the contractions cannot be elicited. In the ear capable of function, the contractions are elicited.

The bilaterality of the reflex can be accounted for by the fact that the center for the reflex arc is in the pons, probably in the superior olivary nucleus (Jepsen, 1963). Measurement of the reflex is carried out with high level stimulation in the ear contralateral to the test ear.

Jepsen (1953) tested three patients with functional losses. He found the threshold of the stapedial reflex the same as that observed in normal subjects. From the results, he assumed normal function of the cochlea and of the reflex arc. He concluded that the cause of deafness must have been at the level higher than the reflex arc.

Jepsen (1953) wrote that the application of impedance measures presupposed severe impairment of hearing or complete deafness. He noted that recruitment could influence interpretation of the reflex so that normal threshold might be found in many cases of sensorineural loss.

On a patient who claimed complete unilateral loss of hearing, Feldman

(1963) elicited impedance change to the acoustic reflex that was equal in each ear. In general, reflexes recorded from the ipsilateral ear have shown greater impedance change than the reflex from the contralateral ear (Møller, 1961). Although the kind of measurement reported by Feldman suggests the possibility of obtaining quantitative detail, the measure continues to be more reliable as an indicator of functional loss. Terkildsen (1964) stated that if the patient has given subjective thresholds that were poorer than the threshold for the acoustic reflex, the diagnosis is obvious. However, thorough testing with other methods is necessary because other causes than deafness could be responsible for failure of the reflex to occur. Giacomelli and Mozzo (1964) reported failure to elicit the acoustic reflex in cases of brainstem lesion.

In impedance measures on functional patients, recruitment could influence the audiologist to make a false-positive identification of functional loss when, in fact, an organic loss is present. On the other hand, a brain stem lesion could influence the audiologist to make a false-negative identification of a conventional organic loss when, in fact, the organic lesion is not a conventional one of the peripheral system.

2. ELECTRONYSTAGMOGRAPHY

The electronystagmography (ENG) results are helpful in conjunction with the results of an audiologic examination. Evidence of both peripheral vestibular and cochlear lesions indicates that some degree of organic disorder is present, while a normal result on ENG testing only indicates that the peripheral and central vestibular systems are not involved. Organic disorder of the end organ of hearing may be present.

If evidence is available that a lesion of the central vestibular system is present, the behavior exhibited by the patient during audiologic procedures may not be functional, but may be secondary to the central problem. Electronystagmograph examinations can now be carried out on radiotelemetry systems; consequently, the patient would not have to move far from the setting in which the audiologic tests are administered (Osterhammel and Peitersen, 1968).

3. EVOKED RESPONSE AUDIOMETRY

Encephalographic recordings of responses to auditory stimuli were confused with myogenic responses before the use of the vertex electrode in conjunction with computer averaging techniques. The vertex response is mediated by the cochlea and resembles cortical potentials representing the nonspecific sensory system. The amplitude of the response is related to the intensity of the auditory stimulus (Cody and Bickford, 1965).

Advancements in evoked response audiometry (ERA) instrumentation have made it possible to obtain threshold measurements by cortical audiometry for both air and bone conduction. These improvements led to the use of ERA with functional patients (Cody and Bickford, 1965; Cody et al., 1968; McCandless and Lentz, 1968). The consensus of investigations was that ERA evaluates cochlear function. There remained a question as to the reliability of the test in patients with central disturbances of normal brain-wave patterns or with pathology of the auditory pathways (Pollock, 1967).

A study of the validity of ERA using scalp electrodes showed that measures from 12 normal subjects agreed within 5 dB of voluntary thresholds. Other groups with functional hearing loss showed evoked-response thresholds that averaged about 50 dB better than voluntary thresholds. The conclusions of the study were that the test is a valid, objective measure for threshold determinations in patients who give inaccurate behavioral results (McCandless and Lentz, 1968).

Recently, some issue has arisen over whether fine needle electrodes inserted under the scalp provide more definitive data than scalp electrodes. The issue arose in some part because of the concern over whether ERA with scalp electrodes measured myogenic activity instead of auditory sensitivity. Evoked response to auditory stimulation is a small response to visualize; however, computers have enabled the extraction of small potentials from ongoing activity recorded from the intact scalp. Both types of electrodes deserve further study to determine whether superior results are obtained with one than the other.

In addition, reports such as those by Marsh and Worden (1968) and Shimuzu (1968) deserve further investigation. Their studies of evoked potentials in the central auditory pathways and in cases of eighth nerve lesion, respectively, may provide a background of material that will one day be useful in establishing a "site of lesion" for patients who otherwise would be identified as functional.

4. Hypnosis

For years hypnosis has been known as a treatment for functional hearing loss, but it has not been used frequently in diagnosis. The use of hypnosis by experienced hypnotists on a medical center staff has been reported as an aid to diagnosis in the case of a 13-year-old boy (Hallewell et al., 1966). Conventional audiologic procedures were not quantitatively conclusive. The boy showed evidence of emotional disturbance on psychological tests. He had had a progressive loss of hearing for 2 years. His father and a maternal uncle had severe losses of hearing. As a result of the history and the possibility of a severe hearing problem, he was being considered for admission to a school for the deaf. Determination of the loss of hearing was necessary for appropriate placement for educational purposes.

During hypnosis the boy was tested by audiologists for speech reception threshold and pure-tone thresholds. Eventually his threshold of 5 dB hearing level (HL) was obtained for both ears. His pure-tone results were 30–40 dB at 4000 Hz. The boy received psychotherapy and later was placed in a public school. This approach was highly appropriate in this instance.

C. Extensions for Research

1. Delayed Auditory Feedback

An effect of auditory feedback that has not been carefully investigated is the one by which the subject hears his own voice through bone conduction (Lee, 1950). Delayed feedback using speech signals was expected to be effective at levels significantly high enough to dominate the bone-conducted voice.

In contrast to speech signals, pure-tone delayed feedback supposedly allows monitoring only by air conduction (Ruhm and Cooper, 1962). Investigators have expected pure-tone signals to cause a disruptive effect at lower sensation levels than speech because speech must reach levels that override bone-conduction monitoring.

Patients with good bone condition showed alterations in the usual changes in reading time in a study investigating the effects of feedback (Levy, 1958). Good bone conduction in conjunction with a mild or moderate hearing loss postponed the change in duration of reading for 15–25 dB as compared with threshold measures. However, comparatively good bone conduction in conjunction with a hearing loss of 45 dB (ASA, 1951) and higher showed effects of delay 15–25 dB earlier as compared with threshold measures (Levy, 1958). Patients with recruitment react to delayed auditory feedback using speech signals differently than persons with normal hearing (Harford and Jerger, 1959).

The results of such studies stimulate thinking concerning the realm of sensation level, sound pressure level, and level above bone-conduction thresholds. The measures used clinically probably should be modified for appropriate use with different kinds of hearing loss. The implications for thorough study of functional hearing loss or functional overlay are apparent.

2. Receiver Operating Characteristics Curve

In general, automated means of obtaining patient responses are suspect when two conditions exist for the audiologist: (1) He is dealing with a clinical sample in which some percentage of patients show functional hearing loss. (2) He is looking for quantitative data in the test results. However, measures derived from the theory of signal detection can be used to differentiate between two variables that enter into the functional patient's response. One of these variables is the capability of the auditory system for transmitting input information; the other is the criterion which the observer uses for responding to the transmitted information (Clarke, 1964).

The thesis is that patients with organic conditions of hearing will show a lesser ability to transmit auditory information; however, they will have normal criteria for responding. Patients with functional hearing loss will show normal ability to transmit auditory information; however, they will have abnormally conservative criteria for responding to this information. Patients with functional overlay will show both reduced ability to transmit auditory information and abnormally conservative criteria for responding (Clarke, 1964).

Very little data are available on the uses of signal detection to study the responses of patients with functional hearing loss. In this paradigm, hit rate in the form of correct identifications, and correct rejections can be compared with the false alarms and misses (Green and Swets, 1966). Hearing levels can be approximated from the responses to forced choice procedures; consequently, more work in this area should follow.

The study of the behavior of functional patients to auditory stimuli requires methods that provide quantitative resolution of hearing levels. These methods may lead to a better understanding of the nature of functional hearing loss or uncover unknown organic causes. However, patients with functional loss are not available in large numbers for study at the present time, since we seem to be in a period of decrease in prevalence of the disorder.

V. Prevention and Rehabilitation

If preventive measures were effective, diagnostics and rehabilitation would not be necessary. However, by the time the audiologist meets the patient, the possibility of prevention is past. By the same token, treatment and rehabilitation of the functional patient is not within the audiologist's province.

A. Prevention

The audiologist can take some positive action to ensure that he does not contribute to the problem. If he provides competent testing, the "early" functional patient will not be reinforced by behavior that seemed rewarding. The functional patient is assured that he has a serious problem if the audiologist recommends a hearing aid or speech reading lessons when the organic component of the loss does not warrant such a recommendation.

Although a confrontation may not be indicated, the audiologist need not feel compelled to lead further into the functional problem. Children rarely have confirmed conviction of a functional loss. However, the longer the child continues his deafness and the more he is tested, the more strongly he becomes attached to his disability (Barr, 1963).

School pressures, even at the elementary level, are blamed for some percentage of functional behavior in children (Berger, 1965). The possibility of undue or severe requirements as a cause suggests that alleviation of the pressure might serve as a preventive measure.

Industrial hearing programs use baseline audiograms for new workers. Periodically comparison audiograms are taken on employees who work in noise. These measures tend to discourage outright malingering and conscious aggravation for monetary gain (Zwislocki, 1963).

B. Rehabilitation

Generally, treatment and rehabilitation of the functional patient fall to the psychiatrist. Treatment may have its limitations in many instances where a conversion reaction has taken place. Everyone is familiar with the stories told after World War II about patients who were successfully treated for conversion deafness only to transfer their problems to conversion blindness or paraplegia.

The child who is finding the boundaries of what is to be gained by using functional behavior in audiologic procedures can be "treated," so to speak. The audiologist who uses a positive approach to the child, letting him know that a "true" audiogram has not been obtained, will convey the information in such a way that the child has a gracious "out" in the retest (Berger, 1965).

VI. Summary

This chapter deals with the identification of functional hearing loss and with a general description of the tests that are used to measure organic hearing conditions. The tests are divided into two main groups: (1) a conventional, classical battery of procedures, and (2) extensions of the classical battery of procedures. A few advanced methods of testing functional loss are discussed, as are a few suggestions for research.

ACKNOWLEDGMENTS

While this chapter was written the author was supported in part by grants from the National Institutes of Neurological Diseases and Stroke of the United States Public Health Services.

References

American Standards Association. (1951). American National Standards specifications for audiometers for general diagnostic purposes. New York, ANSI Z24.5–1951.

Atkinson, M. (1937). Etiological and clinical types of so-called nerve deafness: psychogenic factors. *Laryngoscope* **47**, 527–531.

Barr, B. (1963). Psychogenic deafness in school-children. *Int. Audiol.* **2**, 125–128.

Beagley, H., and Knight, J. (1968). The Evaluation of suspected non-organic hearing loss. *J. Laryngol. Otol.* **82**, 693–705.

Berger, K. (1965). Nonorganic hearing loss in children. *Laryngoscope* **75**, 447–457.

Bergman, M. (1964). The fit test. *Arch. Otolaryngol.* **80**, 440–449.

Black, J. W. (1951). The effect of delayed side-tone upon vocal rate and intensity. *J. Speech Hearing Dis.* **16**, 56–60.

Bordley, J., Hardy, W., and Richter, C. (1948). Audiometry with the use of galvanic skin-resistance response. *Bull. Johns Hopkins Hosp.* **82**, 569.

Burk, K. W. (1958). Traditional and psychogalvanic skin response audiometry. *J. Speech Hearing Res.* **1**, 275–278.

Campanelli, P. (1963). Simulated hearing losses in school children following identification audiometry. *J. Auditory Res.* **3**, 91–108.

Carhart, R. (1961). Tests for malingering. *Trans. Amer. Acad. Ophthalmol. Otolaryngol.* **65**, 437.

Chaiklin, J. B. (1959). The conditioned GSR auditory speech threshold. *J. Speech Hearing Res.* **2**, 229–236.

Chaiklin, J. B., and Ventry, I. M. (1963). Functional hearing loss. *In* "Modern Developments in Audiology" (J. Jerger, ed.), 1st ed. Ch. 3, pp. 76–125. Academic Press, New York.

Chaiklin, J. B., and Ventry, I. M. (1965). Patient errors during spondee and pure-tone threshold measurement. *J. Auditory Res.* **5**, 219–230.

Chase, R., Harvey, S., Standfast, S., Rapin, I., and Sutton, S. (1959). Comparison of the effects of delayed auditory feedback on speech and keytapping. *Science* **129**, 903–904.

Clarke, F. R. (1964). Comments on the concept of a functional hearing loss. *ASHA* (A) **6**, 403.

Cody, D., and Bickford, R. (1965). Cortical audiometry: An objective method of evaluating auditory acuity in man. *Mayo Clin. Proc.* **40**, 273–287.

Cody, D., Griffing, T., and Taylor, W. (1968). Assessment of the newer tests of auditory function. *Ann. ORL* **77**, 686–705.

Cohen, M., Cohen, S., Levine, M. Maisel, R., Ruhm, H., and Wolfe, R. (1963). Interdisciplinary pilot study of nonorganic hearing loss. *Ann. ORL* **72**, 67–82.

Davis, H., and Fowler, E. P., Jr. (1960). Hearing and deafness. *In* "Hearing and Deafness," (H. Davis, R. Silverman, eds.), (Rev. ed.), chap. 4, pp. 80–124. Holt, New York.

van Dishoeck, H. (1962). Opinions on psychogenic deafness and simulation. *Int. Audiol.* **1**, 112–115.

Doerfler, L. G. (1948). Neurophysiological clues to auditory acuity. *J. Speech Hearing Dis.* **13**, 227–232.

Doerfler, L. G., and Epstein, A. (1956). The Doerfler-Stewart (D-S) test for functional hearing loss. Monograph, Veterans Administration.

Doerfler, L. G., and McClure, C. (1954). The measurement of hearing loss in adults by galvanic skin response. *J. Speech Hearing Dis.* **19**, 184–189.

Doerfler, L. G., and Stewart, K. C. (1946). Malingering and psychogenic deafness. *J. Speech Dis.* **11**, 181–186.

Falconer, G. A. (1966). A Lipreading Test for nonorganic deafness. *J. Speech Hearing Dis.* **31**, 241–247.

Feldman, A. S. (1963). Impedance measurements at the eardrum as an aid to diagnosis. *J. Speech Hearing Res.* **6**, 315–327.

Forney, R., and Hughes, F. (1965). Effect of caffeine and alcohol on performance under stress of audio-feedback. *Quart. J. Stud. Alc.* **26**, 206–212.

Gaeth, J., and Norris, T. (1965). Diplacusis in unilateral high-frequency hearing losses. *J. Speech Hearing Res.* **8**, 63–75.

Giacomelli, F., and Mozzo, W. (1964). An experimental and clinical study on the influence of the brainstem reticular formation on the stapedial reflex. *Int. Audiol.* **3**, 42–43.

Gibbons, E. (1962). Aspects of traumatic and military psychogenic deafness and simulation. *Int. Audiol.* **1**, 151–154.

Gibbons, E., and Winchester, R. (1957). A delayed side-tone test for detecting uniaural functional deafness. *Arch. Otolaryngol.* **66**, 70–78.

Giolas, M., and Epstein, A. (1964). Intensity generalization in EDR audiometry. *J. Speech Hearing Res.* **7**, 47–53.

Goldstein, R. (1966). Pseudohypacusis. *J. Speech Hearing Dis.* **31**, 341–352.

Green, D. M., and Swets, J. A. (1966). "Signal Detection Theory and Psychophysics." Wiley, New York.

Grings, W., Lowell, E. L., and Rushford, G. (1959). Role of conditioning in GSR audiometry with children. *J. Speech Hearing Dis.* **24**, 380–390.

Hallewell, J., Goetzinger, C., Allen, M., and Proud, G. (1966). The use of hypnosis in audiologic assessment. *Acta Oto-Laryngol.* **61**, 205–208.

Hanley, C. N., and Tiffany, W. (1954). An investigation into the use of electro-mechanically delayed side tone in auditory testing. *J. Speech Hearing Dis.* **19**, 367–374.

Hardy, W., and Pauls, M. (1952). The test situation in PGSR audiometry. *J. Speech Hearing Dis.* **17**, 13–24.

Harford, E., and Jerger, J. (1959). Effect of loudness recruitment on delayed speech feedback. *J. Speech Hearing Res.* **2**, 361–368.

Hattler, K. W. (1968). The Type V. Békésy pattern: The effects of loudness memory. *J. Speech Hearing Res.* **11**, 567–575.

Heston, L. (1970). The genetics of schizophrenia and schizoid disease. *Science* **167**, 249–256.

Hopkinson, N. T., Katz, J., and Schill, H. (1960). Instrumental avoidance galvanic skin response audiometry. *J. Speech Hearing Dis.* **25**, 349–357.

Hopkinson, N. T. (1965). Type V. Békésy audiograms: Specification and clinical utility. *J. Speech Hearing Dis.* **30**, 243–251.

Hopkinson, N. T. (1967). Comment on "Pseudohypacusis." *J. Speech Hearing Dis.* (L). **32**, 293–294.

Hudgins, C. V., Hawkins, J. E., Jr., Karlin, J. E., and Stevens, S. S. (1947). The development of recorded auditory tests for measuring hearing loss for speech. *Laryngoscope* **57**, 57–89.

Hurst, A. (1940). A discussion on functional deafness. *Proc. Roy. Soc. Med.* **33**, 463–470.

Jepsen, O. (1953). Intratympanic muscle reflexes in psychogenic deafness (impedance measurement). *Acta Oto-laryngol. Suppl.* **109**, 61–69.

Jepsen, O. (1963). Middle-ear muscle reflexes in man. *In* "Modern Developments in Audiology " (J. Jerger, ed.) 1st ed., Chap. 6. Academic Press, New York.

Jerger, J., and Herer, G. (1961). An unexpected dividend in Békésy audiometry. *J. Speech Hearing Dis.* **26**, 390–391.

Johnson, K. R., Work, W., and McCoy, G. (1956). Functional deafness. *Ann. of ORL* **65**, 154–170.

Karlovich, R., and Graham, J. T. (1966). Effects of pure tone synchronous and delayed auditory feedback on keytapping performance to a programmed visual stimulus, *J. Speech Hearing Res.* **9**, 596–603.

Katz, J., and Connelly, R. (1964). Instrumental avoidance vs. classical conditioning in GSR speech audiometry. *J. Auditory Res.* **4**, 171–179.

Knapp, P., and Gold, B. (1950). The galvanic skin responses and the diagnosis of hearing disorders. *Psychosom. Med.* **12**, 6–22.

Lee, B. S. (1950). Some effects of sidetone delay. *J. Acoust. Soc. Amer.* **22**, 639–640.

Lehrer, N., Hirschenfang, S., Miller, M., and Radpour, S. (1964). Nonorganic hearing problems in adolescents. *Laryngoscope* **74**, 64–70.

Levy, E. (1958). Some relations between delayed auditory feedback and auditory threshold obtained in a clinical situation. Unpublished M.S. thesis, Univ. of Pittsburgh.

Lumio, J., Tapani, J., and Gelhar, K. (1969). Three cases of functional deafness in the same family. *J. Laryngol. Otol.* **83**, 299–304.

Maran, A. (1966). The causes of deafness in children. *J. Laryngol. Otol.* **80**, 495–505.

Marsh, J., and Worden, F. (1968). Sound evoked frequency-following responses in the central auditory pathway. *Laryngoscope* **78**, 1149–1163.

Martin, N. (1946). Psychogenic deafness. *Ann. ORL* **55**, 81–89.

McCandless, G., and Lentz, W. (1968). Evoked response audiometry in nonorganic hearing loss. *Arch Otolaryngol.* **87**, 123–128.

McGranahan, L., Causey, D., and Studebaker, G. A. (1960). Delayed sidetone audiometry. *ASHA* (A) **2**, 357.

Melnick, W. (1967). Comfort level and loudness matching for continuous and interrupted signals. *J. Speech Hearing Res.* **10**, 99–109.

Meltzer, H. (1968). Creatine kinase and aldolase in serum: Abnormality common to acute psychoses. *Science* **159**, 1368–1370.

Menzel, O. (1960). Clinical efficiency in compensation audiometry. *J. Speech Hearing Dis.* **25**, 49–54.

Meritser, C., and Doerfler, L. G. (1954). The conditioned galvanic skin response under two modes of reinforcement. *J. Speech Hearing Dis.* **19**, 350–359.

Møller, A. R. (1961). Bilateral contraction of the tympanic muscles in man. *Ann. ORL* **70**, 735–752.

Muth, E. B. (1952). An attempt to standardize the D-S test for malingering and psychogenic deafness. Unpublished M.A. thesis, Univ. of Maryland.

Newby, H. A. (1964). "Audiology," (Rev. Ed.). Appleton New York.

O'Neill, J., and Oyer, H. J. (1966). "Applied Audiometry, " Ch. 9. Dodd, Mead, New York.

Osterhammel, P., and Peitersen, E. (1968). Telemetry system for nystagmus recording. *Acta Oto-Laryngol.* **65**, 527–532.

Pauling, L., (1968). Orthomolecular psychiatry. *Science* **160**, 265–271.

Peterson, J. L. (1963). Nonorganic hearing loss in children and Békésy audiometry, *J. Speech Hearing Dis.* **28**, 153–158.

Pollock, K. C. (1967). Electroencephalic audiometry by cortical conditioning. *J. Speech Hearing Res.* **10**, 706–716.

Price, L., Sheperd, D. C., and Goldstein, R. (1965). Abnormal Békésy tracings in normal ears. *J. Speech Hearing Dis.* **30**, 139–144.

Rapin, I., Costa, L., Mandel, I., and Fromowitz, A. (1963). Effect of varying delays in auditory feedback on key-tapping of children. *Percept. Motor Skills* **16**, 489–500.

Resnick, D. M. and Burke, K. S. (1962). Békésy audiometry in nonorganic auditory problems. *Arch. Otolaryngol.* **76**, 38–41.

Rintelmann, W., and Harford, E. (1963). The detection and assessment of pseudo-hypoacusis among school-age children. *J. Speech Hearing Dis.* **28**, 141–152

Rintelmann, W., and Harford, E. (1967). Type V. Békésy pattern: Interpretation and clinical utility. *J. Speech Hearing Res.* **10**, 733–744.

Rosenthal, D. and Kety, S. (eds.) (1968). "The Transmission of Schizophrenia," Pergamon, Oxford.

Ruhm, H., and Carhart, R. (1958). Objective speech audiometry: A new method based on electrodermal responses. *J. Speech Hearing Res.* **1**, 169–178.

Ruhm, H., and Cooper, W., Jr. (1962). Low sensation level effects of pure-tone delayed auditory feedback. *J. Speech Hearing Res.* **5**, 185–193.

Ruhm, H., and Cooper, W. Jr. (1964). Delayed feedback audiometry. *J. Speech Hearing Dis.* **29**, 448–455.

Ruhm, H., and Menzel, O. (1959). Objective speech audiometry in cases of non-organic hearing loss. *Arch. Otolaryngol.* **69**, 212–219.

Shepherd, D. C. (1964). Instrumental avoidance conditioning vs. classical conditioning in electrodermal audiometry. *J. Speech Hearing Res.* **7**, 55–70.

Shepherd, D. C. (1965). Non-organic hearing loss and the consistency of behavioral auditory responses. *J. Speech Hearing Res.* **8**, 149–163.

Shimuzu, H. (1968) Evoked response in VIIIth nerve lesions *Laryngoscope* **78**, 2140–2152.

Stark, E. (1966). Jerger types in fixed-frequency Békésy audiometry with normal and hypacusic children. *J. Auditory Res.* **6**, 135–140.

Stein, L. (1963). Some observations on type V Bekesy tracings. *J. Speech Hearing Res.* **6**, 339–348.

Stewart, K. C. (1954). Some basic considerations in applying the GSR technique to the measurement of auditory sensitivity. *J. Speech Hearing Dis.* **19**, 174–183.

Taylor, G. J. (1949). An experimental study of tests for the detection of auditory malingering. *J. Speech Hearing Dis.* **14**, 119–130.

Terkildsen, K. (1964). Clinical application of impedance measurements with a fixed frequency technique. *Int. Audiol.* **3**, 147–155.

Thomsen, K. A. (1955). Case of psychogenic deafness demonstrated by measuring impedance. *Acta Oto-Laryngol.* **45**, 82–85.

Tiffany, W., and Hanley, C. N. (1952). Delayed speech feedback as a test for auditory malingering. *Science* **115**, 59–60.

Ventry, I. M. and Chaiklin, J. B. (1962). Functional hearing loss: A problem in terminology. *ASHA* **4**, 251–254.

Ventry, I. M. and Chaiklin, J. B. (1965). The efficiency of audiometric measures used to identify functional hearing loss. *J. Auditory Res.* **5**, 196–211.

Watson, J., and Voots, R. (1964). A report on the use of the Békésy audiometer in the performance of the Stenger test. *J. Speech Hearing Dis.* **29**, 36–46.

Watson, L., and Tolan, T. (1967). "Hearing Tests and Hearing Instruments" (Facsimile of the 1949 Ed.). Hafner, New York.

Wood, K. S. (1957). Terminology and nomenclature. *In* "Handbook of Speech Pathology" (L. Travis, ed.), Ch. 2. Appleton, New York.

Zwislocki, J. (ed.) (1963). Critical evaluation of methods of testing and measurement of nonorganic hearing impairment. Report of Working Group 36, NAS-NRC Committee on Hearing, Bioacoustics and Biomechanics.

Chapter 7

Aural Rehabilitation

JOHN J. O'NEILL

University of Illinois

HERBERT J. OYER

Michigan State University

212   JOHN J. O'NEILL AND HERBERT J. OYER

I. Introduction

Aural rehabilitation is a practical science, the principal objective of which is to deal with communication problems that frequently accompany a loss of hearing. One of the first tasks of aural rehabilitation is determining the nature and extent of a patient's handicap in order to describe and isolate those factors that contribute significantly to the hearing handicap. A systematic and orderly attempt should be made to obtain data on how the patient's hearing loss affects his speech, self-image, social relations, and his academic or vocational success. Combined with organic factors, this information can be used to draw a profile of the handicap, and the client's habilitation or rehabilitation can be planned accordingly.

Rehabilitation of the auditorally handicapped has been a concern of society for hundreds of years. Early records show that the first attempts in teaching the deaf to speak were made during the sixteenth century. This work had been delayed for many years because of the mistaken idea that those who were congenitally deaf were incapable of speaking due to a physical relationship between deafness and the organs used for speech. Serious consideration of the need for aural rehabilitation has led to the construction of residential schools for the deaf in which total educational needs are considered. It has also led to the formulation of special programs within existing school environments for children, and in educational programs for adults. Many individuals in agencies, clinics, and centers throughout the United States and other countries have seen the need for aural rehabilitation of the hearing handicapped, and have provided for specialized personnel, equipment, and programming.

There are no figures available on the percentage of hearing-impaired individuals who need the services of an aural rehabilitation program. While a survey of the entire population is impossible, a relatively refined survey sampling procedure could be used that would yield a good estimate of those who sustain hearing loss and those who are in need of aural rehabilitation in the total population. With such information at hand, it would then be possible to plan comprehensively to meet the nation's aural rehabilitation needs.

The purpose of this chapter is to give the reader a close look at that area of audiology called aural rehabilitation, or by some, "rehabilitative audiology." In so doing we shall attempt to define the area of aural rehabilitation, review its historical development, and set forth some major aims and concerns of those dealing with the habilitation or rehabilitation processes. Additionally, the relevance of certain diagnostic procedures to the various aspects of aural rehabilitation will be discussed. Research findings and needs will be emphasized, particularly in the areas of visual and auditory communication. Finally, future directions will be suggested toward which clinical scientists must move in order to one day attain a greater degree of specificity and success in the aural rehabilitation process.

II. Definition of Aural Rehabilitation

Aural rehabilitation in the broadest sense of the term implies the application of certain principles and techniques of management to individuals with hearing impairments. The techniques usually include lipreading, auditory training, and speech conservation.

The first formal programs of aural rehabilitation, which were developed during World War II in military settings, had a very broad orientation. They placed emphasis upon the reconstitution of the personality of the hearing-impaired person. Lederer (1946) described the goals of one such program as, "the psychophysical reconditioning of a person to the point where he is a healthfully functioning person." In essence, the emphasis was upon the total person who was being taught how to live a complete, full, economically and socially sufficient life in a normal-hearing world.

A broad definition, but a meaningful one, could be adapted from Hirsh's (1951) description of audiology, "the modification of the stimulus, the modification of the organism and the modification of the experience and learning of the organism." Such a definition takes into account training with amplified sound (individual hearing aid or auditory training unit), the rehabilitation of the subject (lipreading, auditory training, and speech conservation), and the educational, psychological, and vocational management of the individual. Under these three broad rubrics it is possible to offer the following definitions of each of the areas.

A. Lipreading

Lipreading, in its early history, was descriptive of what appeared to be the basic concern—the translation of lip movements into meaningful communication. However, in the 1950s a more general term, speechreading, came into use. It was felt that this term described what was happening—the interest was in the observation of the person speaking and an understanding of the communicative process—rather than just the observation of the lips. Mason (1943) broadened this concept with her advocacy of the concept of visual hearing which she felt was more descriptive. She considered this process to consist of phonetic and mental elements. A more recent viewpoint (O'Neill and Oyer, 1961) stresses the concept of visual communication or the correct identification of thoughts transmitted via the visual components of oral discourse.

B. Auditory Training

The earliest use of the term auditory training implied the stimulation or education of the hearing mechanism. The concept was advanced to define a process by which the aurally handicapped learned to take advantage of all of the acoustic cues still available to them. Such a definition implied that the hearing impaired were to become alert to sounds about them and that they should be able to discriminate adequately between sounds with highly similar acoustic characteristics. A further broadening occurred with the development of the concept that auditory training was a special kind of training given to the acoustically handicapped which resulted in more effective speech perception and production, which in turn affected language development. The most recent concept relates to the broad one of auditory communication—the development of as adequate a reception of speech and the understanding of language as is possible (Oyer, 1966).

C. Conservation of Speech

The major focus is upon retaining speech and language abilities which might deteriorate because of the hearing impairment. Also, the focus is upon assuring that both speech and language develop as they should. More recently, the argument has been raised that there is no need for speech conservation. It is claimed that what is being undertaken is an improvement of deteriorated speech and voice patterns rather than dealing with a deteriorated ability (Bergman, 1964).

In essence, when we speak of aural rehabilitation we should be focusing our attention upon the following: the improvement of existing input systems (auditory and visual), the expansion of unused or slightly used input systems, the combination or integration of all input systems, and the insurance and retaining of adequate output (linguistic and vocal).

III. Historical Aspects of Aural Rehabilitation

It was not until the 1940s that aural rehabilitation received attention as an entity. Prior to that time attention was paid to auditory training and lipreading as separate rather than concurrent rehabilitative entities.

The earliest presentation of material relative to lipreading occurred in 1620 when Bonet published his text on methods of teaching the deaf. The first scientific effort to develop residual hearing was undertaken in 1802 by Itard. Prior to the 20th century, the references to lipreading and auditory training appeared in publications which described training methods that were employed with the deaf.

The most meaningful approach to the historical aspects of auditory training and lipreading is to review research efforts in these areas rather than reviewing "schools of thought" or describing existing "cookbook" approaches.

A. Auditory Training

In 1888 Urbantschitsch initiated a program of training in the recognition of musical sounds produced by special signal units, the Urbantschitsch whistles. Vowel, consonant, word, and sentence discrimination were also taught with some success. In the late 1800s Alexander Graham Bell, in the United States suggested the use of the telephone in auditory training and under his leadership the Clarke School for the Deaf initiated such a program. Goldstein, in 1895, after a year's training under Urbantschitsch, introduced auditory training at the Central Institute of the Deaf. In 1939 he published his book, *The Acoustic Method*. His training program made extensive use of hearing tubes in the training of discrimination with musical tones.

Very little research was reported between 1917 and 1948. Some five studies were published. The results of four of these studies were not too conclusive, in terms of indicating that auditory training led to improvements in auditory reception (Wright, 1917; Forrester, 1928; Ballenger, 1936; and Goodfellow, 1942). The results of the other study indicated that auditory training resulted in some improvement in terms of retention of a drill vocabulary (Johnson, 1939, 1948).

The first comprehensive study of an auditory training program involved 472 servicemen who had been fitted with hearing aids (DiCarlo,

1948). The servicemen were enrolled in an 8-week auditory training program at one of the military-sponsored aural rehabilitation centers. The training resulted in the improvement of consonant recognition at increased distances. Larsen (1950) reported on the effects auditory training had upon the recognition of consonants. A series of studies evaluated the effects auditory training had upon the recognition of phonetically balanced (PB) words. The results of these studies were quite positive in that auditory training produced a significant improvement in discrimination performance (Hudgins, 1953; Miller, 1952; Numbers and Hudgins, 1948; Wedenberg, 1951). Silverman (1947) found that auditory training allowed individuals to improve their tolerance for pure tones to an appreciable degree. Training with a group hearing aid improved the capacity of a group of deaf school-aged children to comprehend speech in a study reported by Clarke (1957). The greatest improvement occurred when hearing was combined with lipreading. The results, which were presented in terms of pre- and posttest scores obtained from a locally developed test indicated that there was very little improvement by hearing alone.

In looking over the research completed prior to 1960 it is obvious that the results were rather inconclusive. One obvious deficiency is the lack of standardized tests to be used in evaluating the efficiency of an auditory training program. As a result, there is no common "yardstick" that can be used to interpret the results. It is interesting to note that while the importance of auditory training is verbally supported, very little research has been undertaken and apparently very little systematic record-keeping was done by persons conducting auditory training programs. As a result, there are no reports of population studies which pool the results from several installations that were undertaking auditory training programs.

One of the basic problems then is the lack of data that would allow analysis of research results in auditory training. In the studies that have been cited, three approaches were used: subjective evaluation, improvement in threshold sensitivity, and improvement in discrimination as measured by standardized or locally developed tests.

B. Lipreading

While there was some interest in the results of auditory training and little interest in the development of testing instruments and an evaluation of the processes underlying auditory perception, the situation is reversed when research in the area of lipreading is reviewed. Here the major attention is focused upon a study of the lipreader and the testing of his ability, with hardly any attention being paid to the results of training programs. Investigators apparently assumed that they understood the processes involved in auditory training and that it was a group phenomenon. On the other hand, they appeared to view lipreading as an individual phenomenon which they needed to study to discover what processes underlay this phenomenon.

A rather complete review of early and present-day research in lipreading can be found in Section VI. Perusal of this material will indicate that major concentration has been placed upon the development of lipreading tests (face-to-face and filmed tests). Also, there has been considerable study of the aptitudes and abilities that possibly could relate to skill in lipreading. These include the role characteristics of the sender play in the transmission of visual information and the effects the code itself as well as the environment have upon lipreading performance.

As was the case with the review of the experimental studies of auditory training, the results of lipreading studies were not too conclusive. It is not possible to offer too many statements about the attributes of a good lipreader. The nature of the stimulus used and the characteristics of the speaker apparently have some effect upon lipreading. Of greater interest is the lack of any studies of organized training programs in lipreading. This lack may be attributed to the absence of reliable and valid tests of lipreading and a vagueness as to what processes are important in teaching lipreading.

At the beginning of 1960 there was very little research evidence that supported the extensive use of auditory training and lipreading. Also, there was very little documented, clinical record-keeping that was available for study.

IV. Aims and Concerns

The aims and concerns of aural rehabilitation are not the same for every individual. Each person, depending upon his age, education, nature and severity of the hearing handicap, the roles he fulfills, etc., will receive from the alert rehabilitative audiologist a "tailored approach" that meets his needs in a very specific way. Although this is true, the needs of the hearing handicapped are classifiable, thus making possible a statement of general aims and concerns.

A. Identification

One of the abiding concerns of the rehabilitative audiologist is the identification of those who are handicapped because of hearing loss. In some school systems there have been, and continue to be, surveys of hearing. Some surveys are carried out for the purpose of identifying those children with hearing losses that can be reversed medically. Others purport to identify hearing losses that are significant from both medical and educational standpoints. Except for selected school programs serving hearing-handicapped children, the writers know of no standardized procedures being employed in schools (as in pure-tone audiometric screening) that attempt to quantify handicaps associated with hearing loss. Certainly such a set of procedures could be developed.

Far too little is being done for the school child in this area, and there are virtually no organized programs for identification of the hearing-handicapped preschool child except for a few programs of infant screening. Likewise, there is little effort to locate adults who sustain hearing loss and handicap. Ideally, there should be routine screening of all infants, preschool children, schoolchildren, and adults.

B. Sensitization to Communication Process

One of the aims of aural rehabilitation is to sensitize the hearing-handicapped person to the communication process, and to show how the process is affected by his deficit and the uniqueness of his surrounds. He must understand the importance of his speech intelligibility and learn to appreciate the importance of factors that interfere with it. He also must be cognizant of the probabilities that are associated with successful message reception. These aims can be met through rather direct and objective means with adults. With children, however, the approach is not as direct, but can be accomplished indirectly through play. Unless sensitization to the dynamics of the total communication loop is accomplished, the chances for optimal performance by the hearing-handicapped individual are reduced.

C. Utilization of Residual Hearing and Environmental Clues

Still another major aim of the rehabilitative audiologist is to assist the hearing handicapped in using his residual hearing. This can occur in two ways, namely, by amplification of sounds and by training in sound discrimination.

Closely coupled with the aim of better utilization of residual hearing is that of making maximal use of other contextual clues. Since many of these are visual, the context might provide meaningful clues appropriate to other sensory channels. The effective rehabilitative audiologist trains the hearing-handicapped person to be aware of the texture of his environment, to utilize those aspects that enhance successful communication, and to synthesize the clues. The client is made aware of the many visual clues available to him through emphasis on lipreading and other aspects of visual communication.

D. Evaluation of Handicap

Another major aim of aural rehabilitation is to provide the hearing-handicapped individual with sufficient information about his effectiveness as a communicator and to help him develop the insights necessary for understanding his attitudes and those of others concerning his handicap. Unless the dynamics of social situations are understood, they can serve to increase the handicap. Realistic evaluation of his condition by the hearing-handicapped person is a vital aspect of the rehabilitative process. It is the foundation upon which good adjustment and progress are built.

E. Interpretation of Implications of Hearing Handicap

It is important to assist the handicapped individual to view his problem objectively, but of no less importance is interpreting to parents, siblings, spouses, teachers, etc., the implications of hearing loss.

It is extremely important for the parents in particular to know of the social penalties that frequently accompany hearing handicaps. Just as important is the interpretation that must be made to parents and teachers concerning the effects that hearing loss can have upon academic achievement, and the steps that must be taken to assure maximum success in the school years.

Adults sustaining hearing handicaps also frequently need help in interpreting their problems to those with whom they live, socialize, and work. Frequently tensions arise that are related to the handicap (turning the TV up too high, not answering questions directed from another room, missing a ringing telephone, etc.) that could be substantially reduced if only those persons near the hearing handicapped could realize that the mate, friend, or employee was not really trying to be difficult, but that his behavior was to be expected in light of his handicap. A pioneering study in this area revealed that husbands of hearing-handicapped homemakers exhibited significantly more marital tension than the comparison group of husbands whose wives had normal hearing (Oyer and Paolucci 1970). The rehabilitative audiologist cannot consider his responsibilities fulfilled if he has not determined the extent to which he should interpret the communication problems of his clients to others with whom they must interact, and proceed to make interpretations as required.

F. Assessment and Evaluation

It is indeed laudable to develop and adhere to a set of clearly defined aims for aural rehabilitation, and much good work has been accomplished through past years when this has occurred. However, to continue to do this without measuring the changes that have taken place in the behavior of the hearing-handicapped client, and evaluating those changes in light of a meaningful frame of reference, serves little to advance the practical science of aural rehabilitation. This is not to imply that scientific studies have not been attempted that relate to the aural rehabilitation process, for they have been made in various settings. However, it is imperative that efforts continue to be made to answer the many questions concerning effectiveness of training and counseling procedures. New approaches must be devised that provide new knowledge concerning the social consequences of hearing handicaps if we hope to counsel those who suffer hearing handicaps and significant "others" who suffer along with them.

V. Relevance of Diagnostic Procedures to Aural Rehabilitation

A major problem that needs to be considered is the determination of the purpose of the diagnostic procedures. Is the diagnostic procedure to be used to classify individuals and to assign them for rehabilitative management or is the purpose of the examination to determine communicative efficiency and to tailor management procedures in terms of discovered strengths and weaknesses? Both of these approaches are used and will be described below.

A. Audiometric Data

Basic pure-tone audiometric testing will yield threshold data for both ears. For the purposes of this discussion, categories of hearing loss will be described in terms of the average hearing loss at 500, 1000, and 2000 Hz for the better ear (ISO values). A slight loss would be on the order of 27–40 dB, a moderate loss from 41 to 55 dB, a marked hearing loss from 56 to 70 dB, a severe hearing loss from 71 to 90 dB, and an extreme loss 91 dB or more. One school of thought would recommend traditional therapy approaches in terms of the degree of loss as indicated below (Illinois Commission on Children, 1968).

1. SLIGHT HEARING LOSS

Child should be reported to school principal. May benefit from a hearing aid as loss approaches 40 dB. May need attention to vocabulary development. Needs favorable seating and lighting. May need lipreading instructions. May need speech therapy.

2. MILD HEARING LOSS

Child should be referred to special education for educational follow-up. Individual hearing aid by evaluation and training in its use. Favorable seating and possible special class placement, especially for primary children. Attention to vocabulary and reading. Instruction in lipreading and speech conservation and correction, if indicated.

3. MARKED HEARING LOSS

Child should be referred to special education for educational follow-up. Resource teacher or special class. Special help in language skills: vocabulary development, usage, reading, writing, grammar, etc. Individual hearing aid by evaluation and auditory training. Lipreading instruction, speech conservation and correction, and attention to auditory and visual situations at all times.

The suggestions for the severe and extreme hearing losses will not be discussed because the major interest of this chapter is the hard of hearing.

B. Audiometric Data and Therapy Approaches

Another approach which is based on audiometric results has been described by O'Neill (1964). This approach is related to specific goals of therapy which are described in Table I. Only three categories of loss are described in keeping with our interest in the hard of hearing and not the deaf.

C. Educational Approach

If we utilize the concept of aural deficiency which Blair (1966) has defined as, "A group of diverse problems in which the auditory system

TABLE I
Suggested Therapy Approaches

Therapy goals	Therapy approaches	Degree of hearing loss[a]		
		Slight	Mild	Marked
Auditory awareness (relating to auditory environment)	Listening practice	1	3	2
Understanding of communicative processes	Counseling	1	1	1
Development of communicative intake	Visual communication	1	1	1
	Auditory communication	2	1	1
	Combined practice		3	1
Adjustment to own communicative system	Counseling		3	1

[a] 1 equals first choice, 2 equals second choice, and 3 equals third choice.

is incapable of normally providing the child with acoustic information to the detriment of his speech, language and in some cases cognitive development," then we need to investigate such concepts as sensory modalities, sensory channels, and sensory capacity. Also, we will need to answer the question, "what type of communicative skill do we want to develop?"

Two basic areas need to be evaluated—channel efficiency and information processing. The following could be evaluated under each of the above areas. Some of the tests are presently available, some tests used for other purposes can be modified, and in some instances tests will have to be developed.

1. CHANNEL EFFICIENCY

a. Visual. This will include the phonetic (tests of visual reception of phonetic elements and single words) and meaning (tests of visual reception of contextual materials—phrases and sentences).

b. Auditory. This will include the phonetic (tests of auditory reception of phonetic elements and single words) and meaning (tests of auditory reception of contextual materials—phrases and sentences).

c. Tactual. Tests of abilities to utilize skin as sensory channel.

d. Information Processing. Will include evaluation of reading ability and language facility.

e. Cognitive Abilities. Will evaluate the following areas: use of reduced cues, synthetic ability, abstracting ability, and stored information.

In using such an evaluation we would have to assume that the significance of our findings will vary with the age of the individual being tested. Specifically, is major interest to be directed toward the development of speech or language or will the major interest be in the development of everyday communication? In essence, is the interest directed toward habilitation or rehabilitation?

If the third type of approach is utilized it will ensure a better understanding of the effects hearing impairment may have upon the communicative behavior of individuals with hearing losses. The idea of prescriptive therapy is of importance in today's society in that more and more demands are being made upon audiologists to outline techniques to be utilized to modify behavior of individuals with hearing impairment. Audiologists need to move away from the idea of merely being sources for suggestions of what types of evaluations need to be done after audiometric testing is concluded. They should be doing a majority of the evaluations if they are to be honest with their clients.

Evaluation is important not only as a determinant of the effects of hearing impairment upon an individual's communicative behavior, it can also be used to assist in the evaluation of habilitative and rehabilitative procedures. This statement implies a pre- and posttest situation. Data that tell us something about a person's level of performance will have been gathered. If the same tests are administered after a period of therapy it should be possible to obtain some quantifiable estimate of improvement.

VI. Visual Communication

A. Definition

The broadest definition that can be offered is, "visual communication is a learned form of linguistic behavior." A more specific definition provided by O'Neill and Oyer (1961) and cited earlier is as follows, "the correct identification of thoughts transmitted via the visual components of oral discourse."

The development of skill in visual communication will depend upon the attitude and motivation of the individual being taught. However, of prime importance is the reason for teaching an individual to utilize visual communication. There appear to be, in an operational sense, four reasons for attempting to develop such a skill. These are:

1. The development of communicative efficiency. The visual channel can serve as an auxiliary communicative channel, a helping channel, or as a single, input channel.

2. To assist in the development of speech. The visual channel will serve to develop speech awareness and be of primary importance in the acquisition of speech.

3. To assist in the development of language through the medium of the visual channel, thus allowing the child to develop facility in language and experience in language usage.

4. To assist in educational, social, and vocational management.

To implement such a viewpoint it will be necessary to revise the usual diagnostic approach used with children and adults (see Section V). Suggestions for approaches to be used in educational, social, and vocational management will be obtained, when indicated, through the use of intelligence and aptitude tests, projective personality tests, and tests of social functioning.

B. Research Findings

Since there have not been sustained programs of research in lipreading, an examination of the literature reveals that the research has been rather diversified. Even so, however, it can be classified under five general categories: (1) tests of lipreading ability, (2) the sender, (3) the code, (4) the transmission link, channel, or environment, and (5) the receiver or lipreader.

1. TESTS OF LIPREADING

The early tests of lipreading were essentially the same as the more recent ones in that they were constructed in order to obtain a measure of lipreading performance by using a restricted number of items for testing. Some of the early tests were filmed and others carried out face-to-face. The developers of these tests were located in a variety of settings that included schools for the deaf, clinics, and university programs (Cavender, 1949; Conklin, 1917; Day et al., 1928; Heider and Heider, 1940; Kelly, 1959; Lowell, 1957; Mason, 1943; Morkovin, 1947; Moser, et al., 1960; Nitchie, 1913; Posthove, 1962; Reid, 1947; Utley, 1946). Many of the tests have good reliability as test instruments but they still leave much to be desired. The outstanding difference between the earlier tests and the later ones is in the degree of refinement offered by the later tests.

2. THE SENDER

Early studies of the sender revealed some very interesting findings, namely, that more intelligible speakers were more lipreadable (O'Neill, 1951a). Also it was found that normal lip movement, unsmiling expression, and full torso exposure cause a lipreader to be understood more readily (Stone, 1957). Some have thought that by slowing the rate of speaking the speaker would be more lipreadable. This was not found to be true by investigation (Byers and Lieberman, 1959). However, Mulligan (1954) found that the slower the speed of projection, the better the recognition of filmed materials.

Some of the later studies of the sender have examined other factors. Several have examined the question of voicing and whispering in the lipreading training session. One investigation found that there was appreciable visible difference between voiced and unvoiced words insofar as size and/or amount of lip opening, mouth width, jaw movements, and mouth and teeth areas were concerned. There was also an appreciable difference found in the percentage of time that both the tongue and the teeth were visible in voiced and unvoiced words. This was an exploratory study and thus not completely conclusive. It does point in a particular direction, however, namely, that there was more exaggeration occurring in movement when the words were not voiced. The analyses were made of filmed speakers analyzed frame-by-frame (Fulton, 1964).

Facial movements of males and females were later examined while producing common expressions and sentences by voice and by whisper in order to learn whether or not any appreciable differences among three measures of facial movement existed when common expressions and sentences were voiced or whispered. The measurements of the facial movements that were obtained on each speaker were made by attaching a mercury strain gauge to the speaker's face. These attachments were led from each led of the gauge to the input of a plethysmograph and fed to a polygraph. The stimulus material consisted of a list of 31 common expressions and sentences from Form A of the Utley Lipreading Test. There were ten speaker subjects used in the investigation; five females and five males.

Measures of (1) a total duration of movement, (2) amount of maximum movement, and (3) a time-to-amount of maximum movement were obtained. These three measures were made for each sentence and common expression produced by each speaker. In all, there were 93 voiced measures and 93 whispered measures for each speaker over the stimulus material.

These data revealed that there were no significant differences in the amount of time taken for maximum movement to occur for certain facial movements between males and females when voicing and then whispering common expressions and sentences, and that there was no significant difference between males and females in the amount of maximum movement occurring for certain facial movements when producing common expressions and sentences by voice and then by whisper. It was also found that no significant differences existed between males and females in the duration of certain facial movements when producing common expressions and sentences by voice and then by whisper, and that there were no significant differences in the amount of time taken for maximum movement to occur, the amount of maximum movement, and the duration of certain facial movements between voicing and whispering common expressions and sentences when produced by males or females.

A contribution made by this investigation was the development of a refined means of exploring the facial movements of speakers, an area in need of further investigation (Leonard, 1968).

3. THE CODE

Perhaps more investigations have been made in the area of code than in any other single area within lipreading. One early study showed that there was definite decrease in lipreading performance as the length of sentences increased, and that when words were surrounded by long sentences they were much more difficult to understand than when they were placed within a short sentence. However, the lipreadability of a sentence was not significantly influenced by its position within a group of sentences, and the position of the groups of sentences had no noticeable effect upon lipreading performance (Morris, 1944).

Some years later research showed that lipreading performance was affected by the number of syllables and words in a sentence, the number of vowels and consonants, and the length of the words that were spoken (Taafee and Wong, 1957).

At about this same period the code was studied to determine the contribution of vision to intelligibility. It was found that vision contributed 29.5% to the recognition of vowels; 57% to the recognition of consonants; 38.6% to the recognition of words and 17.4% for phrases (O'Neill, 1954).

Other investigators found that the visual contribution to speech intelligibility was substantially increased as the speech-to-noise ratio was decreased (Sumby and Pollack, 1954).

A third study showed essentially the same kinds of results as the two previous ones cited, (O'Neill, 1954; Sumby and Pollack, 1954), that when visual cues were added to auditory cues, the intelligibility of the speech was increased by about 20% (Neely, 1956).

There is disagreement as to the effects of place of articulation and effects on lipreading performance. One investigator suggests that articulatory differences are not noticeable and that other variables must be studied (Woodward, 1957). Other research results showed that the visual identification of words was directly related to the place of articulation (Brannon and Kodman, 1959).

Homophenous words have been studied to determine the ability of viewers to identify them correctly when given in isolation on a silent film. Viewers indicated their responses on a multiple-choice test form. Viewers were able to select correctly the homophenous words more frequently than would be expected by chance alone. The results indicate that homophenous words, even though highly similar, are not produced exactly alike on the lips (Roback, 1961).

Another research was carried out to determine the time it took speakers to say homophenous words. Results revealed that the differences in time required for uttering homophenous words within each group considered in the study were not statistically significant. This study was exploratory in nature and the data collected and analyzed suggested further exploration in this area (Jorgenson, 1962).

About the same time another research was carried out to determine the effects of visual stimuli fractionation on the lipreading performance of trained subjects. Twelve females who had normal hearing and vision and no formal training in lipreading served as subjects. Silent motion-picture films were made of a speaker saying the first 25 words in Voelker's list of most frequently spoken words. Subjects were trained on specially prepared films until they recognized the minimum of 90% of the vocabulary. Films were prepared in such a way that on one film 15% of the visual signals were made nonvisible, on the second film 30.5% were made nonvisible, and on the third 45% were made nonvisible. This was accomplished by blacking out at random portions of the filmed stimulus.

The findings of the study indicate that lipreading performance of trained subjects does not differ significantly as they are deprived of 15, 30, or even 45% of the visual stimuli (Subar, 1963).

A study was made of the ability of skilled lipreaders in determining the accented syllable of polysyllabic words. Thirty unskilled lipreaders and two talkers were employed in the study. One talker was filmed while speaking 60 three-syllable nonsense words that were especially designed for the study. The 60 three-syllable nonsense words comprised a test of visual accent placement. Statistical analysis of the data showed that it is possible for unskilled lipreaders to lipread accent placement in polysyllabic words and to obtain a score greater than would be expected by chance occurrence alone (Greene, 1963).

Franks and Oyer (1967) reported on the investigation of the influence of the known-vowel consonant stems of monosyllabic words on the identification by lipreading of the initial consonants of the words. The basic hypothesis tested was that the same consonant united with different stems would be identified with different degrees of accuracy when the stems were known by the subjects. It was found that knowledge of the vowel-consonant stems resulted in differences in accuracy of identification of the initial consonants by lipreading. The number and familiarity of the rhyming alternative words seemed to be contributing factors that influenced the correct identification of consonants, but familiarity of the stimulus words themselves was not a significant factor in influencing identification.

The effects of redundancy on visual recognition of frequently spoken words was studied by Nielsen (1966), who hypothesized that immediate repetition of a word will improve the visual intelligibility of that word. She found that the mean scores for lipreadability after one utterance were 30.6%, after two successive utterances 29.4%, after three successive utterances 33.3%, after four successive utterances 31.3%, and after five succesive utterances 31.8%. This would seem to suggest that if a person is going to perceive a word from the lips of a speaker, he is going to recognize it without having to have it repeated.

Lloyd (1964) investigated the relationship between sentence familiarity and sentence lipreading difficulty. He used 52 normal-hearing college students as subjects. The 60 sentences that he employed were taken from the filmed test of lipreading by Taaffe. There were 52 judges who rated each of the 60 sentences on a five-point scale of familiarity. The familiarity ratings were then compared with data on the difficulty of each sentence in lipreading from an earlier study by Taafee and Wong in 1957. He found a weak correlation (0.31) between difficulty and familiarity of each sentence. He did find, however, a significant difference between the six most familiar and the six least familiar sentences.

Sahlstrom (1967), through the use of a strain gauge, carried out a study to determine the effect of a speaker's sex upon the amount and pattern of movement occurring on certain areas of the face while speaking selected groups of homophenous words. In addition, he studied differences in certain facial movements among selected phonemes in the English language that were thought to be homophenous, and examined the effect of the position of the phoneme within a word upon certain facial movements that accompanied a production of the word. He found that the male speakers presented greater intensity of facial movement over the total duration of a word than female speakers across all consonant sounds and word positions, and that /p/ and /b/ consonants were consistently associated with greater intensity of facial movement, more changes in pattern of facial movement, and greater elapsed time in facial movement than was the case with the /m/.

In a confusion study of visually perceived consonants, Fisher (1968) compared the classical listing of nonlabial homophenous and consonant phonemes and the Woodward and Barber lists as they were visually perceived by normal-hearing subjects. His results support the Woodward and Barber list more than classical listings. The concept of homophenous sounds was supported.

4. The Transmission Link, Channel, or Environment

An early study by Mulligan (1954) was among the first to investigate the effects of distance on lipreading performance. She found of the four distances she studied, 5 feet, 10 feet, 15 feet, and 20 feet from the screen, that 10 feet was apparently the most favorable viewing distance, but not significantly different from the others.

Room illumination has been studied in an effort to determine the effects of various room lighting conditions on the lipreading efficiency of subjects. Viewer subjects in this study were ten men and ten women screened for visual acuity at 20–30. Thomas (1962) found that lipreading efficiency of trained subjects tends to decrease, but not significantly so, as intensity of room illumination decreases. In other words, there was no significant difference between 30 foot-candles of light, which is normal room lighting, and 16, 8, 4, and 0.5 foot candles when the subjects were trained. This study suggests that those who are familiar with the content of messages and who are given some training, do very well even in very poor lighting conditions.

Leonard (1962) also was interested in the effect of environmental factors upon lipreading and studied effects of select continuous auditory distractors. His findings indicate that selected continuous auditory distractors significantly affected lipreading performance. In quiet, the subjects achieved 92.7% correct response; with white noise, 59.7%; with speech, 61.0%; and, with music, 62.3%. There was a significant difference between the quiet condition and the experimental conditions, but no significant differences among the experimental conditions.

Oyer (1961) carried out a study dealing specifically with the channel as regards the teaching of lipreading. The purpose of the study was to determine whether students participating in televised lipreading lessons can significantly upgrade their proficiency for that task. The results showed that individuals can be upgraded in lipreading performance when taught by way of television. The study also showed that there was no significant difference between the group that was receiving the lesson face-to-face and the group that was receiving the same lesson simultaneously by way of television. In other words, this study shows that lipreading training can occur as well in two dimensions as in three dimensions.

Greenberg and Bode (1968) carried out a study to determine the ability of viewers to discriminate two conditions of facial exposure and found that the mean percent of consonants differentiated under lips-only condition was 56.4%, but for full face condition was 59.2%.

Keil (1968) explored the effects of peripheral visual stimuli on lipreading performance. In order to accomplish this purpose, a black-and-white 16-mm motion picture experimental test film was developed. The test film was viewed against four different backgrounds: (1) blank gray background, (2) two photos of girls alongside the speaker, (3) a photograph of a building, car, trees, and (4) a moving background of a busy street corner. Keil found that the peripheral visual stimuli, as employed in this study, had no significant effect upon the lipreading performance of scores of subjects. It appears that persons confronted with a visual task are able to select the relevant information and filter out the irrelevant peripheral visual stimuli.

5. The Receiver or Lipreader

Some of the early effort in studying lipreading was directed toward factors of intelligence, behavioral patterns, and visual skills. Pintner (1929) found no significant correlation between the lipreading scores obtained by deaf students and levels that they obtained on the Pintner Nonlanguage Mental Test.

Likewise, Heider and Heider (1940) using their filmed test of lipreading found no significant relationship between lipreading performance and achievement in school.

Studies by Davidson and O'Neill (1956) and also one by Simmons (1959) determined that there were no significant relationships between lipreading performance and intelligence.

Attention has also been paid to particular behavioral patterns that characterize good and poor lipreaders. It can be said at this point in time that the findings are scattered and sometimes in disagreement.

Personal relations and emotional stability are personality dimensions that appear to be important in lipreading, as well as reasoning, ideational fluency, spontaneous flexibility, and associational fluency (Wong and Taafee, 1958).

Additionally, performance on the Digit Symbol, Picture Arrangement and Block Design subtests of the Wechsler–Bellevue Test have been found to correlate significantly with lipreading performance, as does the ability to extract key words in the Iowa Reading Test (Simmons, 1959). Simmons also found visual memory span, rhythm, and synthetic ability to be important.

Both Gault (1927–1928) and Johnson (1963) have found that tactual stimulation increases lipreading performance.

Tatoul and Davidson (1961) found good lipreaders not to be significantly better letter predictors than the poor lipreaders.

Kitchen (1968) examined the relationship of visual synthesis to lipreading performance. The major purpose of his study was to design a test of visual synthetic ability and further to assess the relationship of this instrument to lipreading ability. The results showed that two of the synthesis subtests (dotted outlines and scattered letters) and the total synthesis score were correlated significantly with the ability to lipread words, stories, and with the total lipreading score. Dotted outlines and scattered letters were thought to be closure-type tasks which involved arranging disparate elements to form a meaningful whole. These same subtests were thought also to require speed of visual perception. None of the synthesis variables correlated significantly with the ability to lipread sentences.

In a thorough analysis of optometric tests and their relationship to lipreading, it was found that only visual acuity related significantly to lipreading test performance (Hardick *et al.*, 1970).

C. New Directions

Although past research has been, in the main, somewhat less conclusive than one might have hoped for, this does not mean that the areas investigated should be abandoned or that the approaches made are in need of drastic change. Even though positive findings are few in lipreading, much effective work has been carried out clinically. Research should continue to be aimed at determining the (1) attributes of successful and unsuccessful lipreaders, (2) effects of code, environment, etc., on lipreading, and (3) characteristics of speaker lipreadability. More effort should be made to design studies involving pattern analysis. Additionally, larger groups should be used, and wherever possible and appropriate, hearing handicapped should serve as subjects.

There must also be an attempt made to quantify stimuli that are employed in visual language and nonverbal communication.

Another area in need of research is the tactile as it relates to stimulus reception by the hearing handicapped. Geldard and Steward are undertaking basic work on tactile stimulation at Princeton University's Department of Psychology. Investigation of verbal–tactile stimuli has been initiated and is an area currently emphasized in several laboratories.

The need for programs of research in the area of visual communication is great, for much of the work has apparently been short term and restricted in scope. Not until there is a far greater understanding of the physical, neurological, and psychological correlates of visual communication can habilitative and rehabilitative procedures be based upon scientific facts.

At some time in the future, training in visual communication for the hearing handicapped should be "prescriptive" and should be based upon evidence that permits prediction of levels of success. The evidence will include items found to be significantly positively correlated with success in visual performance. The in-depth assessment of the hearing-handicapped individual and his visual proficiency will enable a clinician to design a program to increase that proficiency.

VII. Auditory Communication

A. Definition

Auditory communication can be defined as the communication that occurs when acoustic events, verbal or nonverbal, are received, perceived, and assigned meanings by the auditor. This process might or might not be facilitated by amplification or use of collateral sensory stimuli. If there is facilitation by other sensory stimuli, the question arises as to the relative importance of their contributions and whether or not the communication that has occurred can rightfully be attributed to auditory processing of acoustic events. This is a reasonable question and the answer to it is that auditory communication occurs when the correct assignment of meaning can be attributed to acoustic events on the basis of audition alone irrespective of other supporting or facilitating sensory stimuli.

If one accepts this definition of auditory communication, then evaluative procedures must assure the isolation of the acoustic stimulus when testing adults or children and also provide for a means of assessing the contributions of collateral sensory stimuli. Likewise, habilitative and rehabilitative procedures must be employed that make optimal use of the residual hearing of the handicapped individual. In some instances auditory stimuli alone will be employed whereas in other instances these will be coupled with stimuli to other sensory pathways. Not all agree with the simultaneous use of multiple stimuli. There is much more to be learned about such an approach.

B. Research Findings

Experimental studies dealing with auditory perception have been carried out for many years. Some of the earliest laboratory work was carried out at Harvard and later in other installations throughout the country during the time of World War II. Too few experimental studies have been carried out in the area of auditory communication of the hearing impaired.

1. VERBOTONAL METHOD

One of the more recent and more controversial approaches to auditory training is the verbotonal or Guberina method. The basic approach is an auditory one, with band-passed speech sounds being used to determine auditory threshold of detection and identification. The results are expressed in terms of octave steps through the frequency range of hearing. The training program is based upon having the hard-of-hearing child use the determined residual hearing for the perception and discrimination of the elements of speech (including the phonemes themselves, rhythm, intonation, and pause). The approach utilizes especially constructed amplification equipment. Of interest is the fact that the intensity of the amplified sound is often not much above the level of normal conversation.

In a study at the Metropolitan Toronto School for the Deaf, Roberts

(1969) reported that after a 13-month training period (verbotonal and regular program children), speech was significantly more intelligible when lipreading was allowed and the usual form of amplification was provided than when lipreading was not provided. However, it was felt that a longer period of training must be allowed before a realistic evaluation can be made of the verbotonal method. Black (1968) has provided a discussion of the theoretical basis of Guberina's method as well as descriptions of the specialized equipment and the results of several research studies. Of the conclusions Black presented, the following seemed to be the most interesting: the verbotonal system of audiometry should not be considered as an important part of the system; speakers who are already familiar with language can learn to perceive distorted linguistic signals and improve their perception of such signals.

2. Frequency Transposition

The use of amplified sound with the hearing-impaired, especially the deaf, appears to have gained increased attention during the past few years. This interest is the result of developments in instrumentation that allow for certain manipulations of the auditory signal. One approach that has received considerable attention involves the shifting of speech downward into the lower frequencies which are more sensitive to sound for hearing-impaired individuals. Bennett and Byers (1967) indicate that two methods are employed in such shifting of the frequency of speech. One is a proportionate method which preserves the harmonic relations between the frequency components of speech, and a disproportionate method which does not maintain such a relationship. The authors cite as examples of the disproportionate method the frequency transposer and the frequency converter, while the proportionate method is represented by slow-played speech. Other approaches, not cited by Bennett and Byers, include coding procedures such as the vocoder, speech compression, bandwidth compression, and artificial speech spectra.

The frequency transposer, which consists of an amplifier, an amplitude compression unit, and low- and high-pass filters, modulates inaudible speech sounds from high-frequency ranges into low-frequency ranges that are audible to the hearing-impaired. In essence the hearing-impaired individual is presented with a new hearing pattern (Johansson, 1961). Wedenberg (1961) has indicated that individuals can learn to recognize elements in this new pattern with a resulting improvement in the discrimination of speech.

Ling (1968, 1969) in a series of studies which utilized the Johansson transposing equipment and the Ling–Druz Vocoder, and hearing aids with low-frequency response and aids with a standard response, found that the use of the specialized equipment with deaf children led to only marginal improvement in auditory discrimination. He indicated that transposition did not appear to be advantageous either as an alternative or as a supplement to linear amplification.

Bandwidth compression of synthetic speech produced by a vocoder had been described by Piminow (1968). This procedure involved the transmission of an analogous form of speech which has been compressed or reduced in bandwidth without loss of the information that is important to speech perception. This technique has not been used, as yet, in a formal auditory training program. However, as a result of some pilot studies, the author reports that training can bring about improvement in the understanding of individual words. Piminow does indicate that the system has not produced, in the instance of deaf subjects, the type of results that were anticipated. Another approach using coded or synthetic speech has been reported by Guttman and Nelson (1968) who developed equipment which generated low-frequency coded cues for phonetic elements that normally have only high-frequency energy (ficative and fricativelike sounds). Experimental evaluation of the system is now in process.

Raymond and Proud (1962) using a frequency converter which shifted all speech sounds down in frequency to the extent to which two radio frequency carrier waves were separated found that discrimination scores were improved but that scores did not approach those for conventionally amplified speech.

Another approach involves the shifting in frequency of speech by tape playback at slower speeds than those employed in the original recording of the speech. Bennett (1963) and Bennett and Byers (1967) have investigated this particular approach. Bennett's study, which involved normal-hearing subjects was encouraging enough to suggest the use of the technique with hard-of-hearing subjects. Such a population was used in the study by Bennett and Byers whose results indicated that discrimination improved at a playback speed of 80% while there was a decrease in discrimination scores at playback speeds of 60 and 70%.

A technique which utilized bandwidth compression but did not require an actual synthesis of low-frequency speech signals was developed by Stover (1967). The method does not utilize synthetic speech as does the method used by Piminow. This technique has not been tested with hearing-impaired individuals.

2. Time-Compressed Speech

Auditory signals have also been modified through the use of time-compressed speech. The most widely used method is the sampling method in which brief segments of speech are periodically discarded and the resulting gaps are closed. Zemlin (1966) reported the results of some pilot work that utilized bandwidth time-compressed speech with a group of hearing-handicapped children. He reported that his results were quite similar to the results obtained in studies that utilized slow-played speech—the children were able to exhibit some learning in terms of improvement in discrimination scores. Furthermore, he offered the following conclusions: recognition of speech material is dependent upon frequency pattern rather than frequency distribution per se. Also, restoration of time in bandwidth-compressed speech at least partly overcomes distortion effects. Finally, frequency shifts beyond a certain amount, regardless of time restoration, seem to transcend a listener's previous language experiences and his common experience of human speech.

The indefinite nature of the results obtained in the above studies has led the majority of experimenters to suggest that there must be further studies in order to obtain more basic information. For example, there is a need to explore training interference effects due to the difference between natural speech and synthetic speech. Other suggestions that have been made are that there should be a fuller evaluation of transposing instruments as practical auditory training devices for training with children. When experimental studies are undertaken, control groups should be run so that training procedures are identical to transposer training but no transposing is employed. Also, there should be sufficient training for each subject before any experimental study is evaluated. A sufficient level of training is defined as the point where there is little or no increase in discrimination scores with increased training.

3. EVALUATION OF EQUIPMENT

A very basic but meaningful study which was undertaken in California involved an evaluation of commercial auditory training units and a survey of the use of such equipment. The study presented a survey of nine different makes of auditory training systems and twenty-seven different models of auditory training units. The equipment was submitted to acoustical analyses and quality control studies. The results of the analyses are presented in the report by Griffing and Hayes (1968) Matkin and Olsen (1968–1969) in an evaluation of loop amplifying systems in use in classrooms found that there was no appreciable acoustic superiority of hearing aid outputs when instruments were activated by a loop amplifying system as compared to the same hearing aids used in a conventional manner. Also, when comparisons were made between several different induction loop amplifying systems, they found a great deal of variability in the acoustic outputs of the systems. It appeared that the amplification, in several instances, was unsatisfactory for children with extreme losses of hearing.

4. RESULTS OF TRAINING

It is in this area that there is a noticeable dearth of information concerning the effects of training upon subsequent performance of the hearing handicapped. Several studies have been made to measure the effects of specific approaches. Saleh (1965) reports the attempts made to structure an auditory training program for young, deaf children. Six primary-level filmstrips were constructed which showed familiar scenes and were accompanied by sound recordings. These materials were tested with the children and were shown to increase the correct responses by a factor of approximately 50%.

Bode and Oyer (1970) in a study of speech discrimination as a function of concentrated auditory training with 32 adults with sensorineural losses elicited significant changes in speech discrimination as shown by testing with the W-22 and Rhyme Tests. In addition, it was found that as age, sensation level of training materials, and intelligence increased, there was an increase in speech discrimination scores.

Another instance in which aural training showed positive results was reported by Lang et al. (1962) who studied preschool children. Audiometric checks were made using pure tones in a free field and the peepshow technique. This was followed by 12–18 months of auditory training. They also utilized a control group of normal-hearing children. Findings revealed that the control group was virtually unchanged at the end of the period, whereas the experimental group of hard-of-hearing preschoolers showed improved hearing level and speech development. The results of this study are supportive of the DiCarlo (1958) study that showed increased performance by children after they received auditory training. Lichtenberg (1966) in a comparison of speech sound discrimination ability among three groups of (1) normal hearing and speaking children, (2) normal hearing, speech-defective children, and (3) children with sensorineural or mixed losses, found that intensive auditory training caused a significant change in speech discrimination for both the normal hearing–normal speaking group and for the hard-of-hearing group.

C. New Directions

Research must continue in many of the directions it has gone in the past and is going at present, although there are some new directions that also should be considered. Fundamentally there should be continued research work in auditory perception of speech and nonspeech sounds, by those with various types of hearing impairments, and long-range studies of academic achievement and vocational adjustment correlated with programs of auditory training.

In view of the sophisticated electronic gear that is available, it is imperative that we obtain a better estimate of how sound is perceived by those with hearing impairments. With this information at hand it will be possible to compensate for the distortion that occurs in the human system. Then we can also plan programs of training that are focused squarely on a true measure of the deficit, not relying solely upon pure tone measures and speech reception thresholds and discrimination scores.

Additionally, another point of emphasis should be in determining to what measure the individual with impaired hearing is assisted in his auditory communication by supplementation through a multiple input channel approach. Geldard (1960) points up some additional possibilities for communication. He suggests that audition is the great spatial sense but that mechanical vibration to the skin offer a realistic supplemental pathway for communication. Brown and Hopkins (1967) in their study of interaction of sensory modalities within the frame of detection theory suggest that there is no apparent interaction between the auditory and visual sensory information processing networks. Karlovich (1968), on the other hand, in his investigation of sensory interaction studied loudness perception during stimulation and reports that visual stimulation presented in synchrony with an auditory stimulus can influence the perception of the magnitude of the auditory stimulus. In a study of unimodal and bimodal sensory stimulation, Costello and Purcell (1968) determined that the combined normal auditory and defective visual presentation was not superior to the normal auditory method alone (their defective auditory and visual methods were created through a filtering process in which information was deleted from their sound film). However, superior to both the single modality presentations of the defective stimuli was the combined presentation of defective auditory and defective visual presentations. Perhaps sensory interaction is dependent upon the nature and amount of information that is being processed simultaneously.

Yet another direction that should be pursued in depth is that of the use of manual language via finger-spelling, signs, and cued speech as adjuncts to aural communication. Some basic work has been accomplished in determining the intelligibility of finger-spelling as a function of distance from the source (Moser et al., 1961). A system for cued speech has been devised and published by Cornett (1967). Real contributions are yet to be made in using these forms of communication in conjunction with auditory cues that can be made available to the hearing handicapped. In a study directed toward combining auditory and visual cues in oral communication, it was concluded that rehabilitation programs for hearing-impaired persons should include auditory training and lipreading (U. of Oklahoma, no date).

Quigley (1969) reports, in his study of the use of finger-spelling and its effects upon other facets of the development of the child, that when finger-spelling is used in conjunction with oral techniques, there need not be any adverse effects upon the acquisition of good oral skills.

VIII. Hearing Aids and Aural Rehabilitation

The review of research in this area will concentrate on those studies that have implications for aural rehabilitation. No effort has been made to make this an inclusive review. Rather, an effort has been made to include those studies that represent trends in research or research that is in an ongoing, continuing state.

A. Evaluation of Characteristics of Hearing Aids

Several research installations have evidenced an interest in experimental study of the effectiveness of hearing aids. In a study completed by Jerger (1968), attention was directed to the relationship between speech understanding and the electroacoustic parameters of frequency response, effective bandwidth, and harmonic distortion in a sample of 20 commercially available hearing aids. The findings of the study were as follows: the use of especially constructed sentence identification tests with competing messages was recommended as a starting point for hearing aid evaluation. The observed relationship between physical characteristics of hearing aids and discrimination of speech was found to be dependent upon the nature of the speech task. Also, the response irregularity of the hearing aids being tested appeared to be the best indicator of differences in the responses of hearing aids while the slope of the hearing loss was the most important factor in evaluating hearing aids.

Carhart and Olsen (1967–1968, 1968–1969) at Northwestern University reported that hearing-impaired individuals experienced more difficulty than did normal-hearing individuals in understanding speech when speech and competing stimuli were amplified to appropriate levels. Also, such difficult listening situations helped to differentiate between different hearing aids in terms of performance on speech discrimination tests. They indicated that the bandwidth of a hearing aid seemed to be the most important physical performance characteristic that was related to speech discrimination. The hearing aid having the widest frequency response provided the best performance while the poorest performance was attained with the hearing aid having the narrowest bandwidth. Also, the results appeared to indicate that even marked harmonic and inter-modulation distortion did not seriously disrupt speech intelligibility for monosyllabic words in quiet or in competition with other auditory signals.

B. Hearing Aid Selection

The variability of the gain control potentiometers of two groups of hearing aids which had been selected in terms of their average gain was investigated by Kasten and Lotterman (1969). They not only found a large variability among the various aids but they also found there was much less change in gain with rotation in the upper half than in the lower half of the control. Also, they indicated that the gain control of an aid will almost always have less range in decibels than the gain of the aid. Kasten *et al.* (1967) indicated that audiologists should be cautious in their interpretation of hearing aid response curves provided by the manufacturers of the aids. This caution was the result of their evaluations of full-on gain vs. frequency response from 150 hearing aids representing ten different models. In another investigation Lotterman, *et al.* (1967) evaluated the difference between average acoustic gain in a 2-cc coupler and improvement in sensitivity for spondee words. The gain settings were the result of subjects setting the aids to a com-fortable listening level. There was a moderate relationship between acoustic gain and threshold improvement. The improvement provided by the aids was approximately 10 dB less than the measured acoustic gain.

A new approach to setting the gain of a hearing aid during evaluations was investigated by Markle and Zaner (1966). This approach utilized the unaided most comfortable loudness level instead of adjusting the acoustic gain of the hearing aid to the unaided speech reception thresh-old. The investigators concluded that gain requirements should be related directly to unaided most comfortable listening level rather than to speech reception levels and that the new method was a more efficient one for individuals with auditory recruitment. These results were similar to those obtained by Loftiss and O'Neill (1964) who utilized an experimental method that was somewhat similar to the method used by Markle and Zaner. The method resulted in better "fitting" of hearing aids, in terms of improved discrimination and social adequacy measures. Discrimina-tion scores were higher and more reliable when the presentation levels were within the range of comfortable listening. These results indicated that discrimination scores should be obtained at levels relative to measures of comfortable loudness rather than at levels relative to the speech reception threshold and that the use of the speech reception threshold did not result in as adequate a measure of sensitivity for various gain settings.

The concept of selective frequency amplification was put to test by Reddell and Calvert (1966). They utilized experimental hearing aids which had been custom adjusted for each of 24 individuals with high-frequency hearing losses. Mean speech reception thresholds and discrimination scores were slightly superior for the experimental aids. When subjects rated the performance of the aids, they preponderantly preferred the experimental aid. The authors indicated that if a "slope of amplification curve" concept was employed in place of a "selective frequency amplification" concept, selective frequency amplification had value as a technique for hearing aid selection.

C. Hearing Aids and Unilateral Hearing Loss

Within the past few years attention has been directed toward the use of hearing aids by persons with unilateral hearing losses. The use of the CROS hearing aid has been evaluated by Harford and colleagues at Northwestern University. In the initial study Harford and Barry (1965) found that when the CROS aid was used by subjects with a slight impairment of hearing throughout the speech range or a loss in the high frequencies in the better ear that there was a pronounced improvement in discrimination scores (23% increase in score). A follow-up survey some 8 months after the initial testing indicated that individuals who had purchased a CROS aid appeared to be satisfied with its performance. Forty-five individuals who had been recommended for fitting with the CROS aid were evaluated by Harford and Dodds (1966). The results of this study led to the recommendation that until more sensitive auditory tests were developed, the most meaningful approach to determining the value of the CROS aid is a trial period of actual use of the aid in everyday activities. A followup study by Dodds and Harford (1968) indicated that those individuals who utilized an open earmold with the CROS hearing aid obtained more meaningful results than did individuals who used a standard or vented earmold with the CROS aid. Discrimination performance was improved for patients with high-frequency hearing losses and normal or near normal hearing in the lower frequencies. For persons with a bilateral loss of hearing and one unaidable ear it was recommended that they try the BICROS hearing aid. With this aid, signals originating on either side of the head are picked up by two hearing aid microphones, one on each side of the head, are mixed and amplified and fed to an earphone in the better (usable) ear. Harford (1967) reports that such an aid has definite clinical value in that it improves the person's ability to hear sounds on the unaidable side as well as reducing the patient's tension.

D. Earmold Characteristics

Several investigators have studied the effect modifications of conventional earmolds have upon hearing aid performance. Harrison (1969) found that speech discrimination performance was improved through the use of modified earmolds. Also, a majority of the individuals preferred the quality of amplification produced by the use of a special mold. The effectiveness of vented earmolds in improving discrimination in noise was investigated by McClellan (1967). He found that when discrimination performance for vented and unvented earmolds was compared, the vented mold provided a mean gain of 15.2% in discrimination scores for individuals with high-frequency losses. Such a finding was attributed to a change in acoustic impedance. Green and Ross (1968) found that the nonoccluding CROS type of ear mold reduced the amplification for low-frequency sounds. An open earmold was found by Dodds and Harford (1968) to give greater improvement in discrimination performance than did a standard earmold for 35 individuals with a high-frequency hearing loss. The use of a nonoccluding earmold on the same side of the head upon which the hearing aid had been placed was evaluated by Green (1969). He referred to such an arrangement as the IROS mode (ipsilateral routing of signal). The results of a study of four individuals indicated that such an arrangement was of value to individuals with marked bilateral high-frequency hearing losses in that they received a high-frequency emphasis from the nonoccluding earmold without appreciable feedback.

E. Effectiveness of Hearing Aids

In a study of 134 hard-of-hearing children, Gaeth and Lounsbury (1966) reported that the parents of 120 of the children who wore hearing aids were poorly informed about the hearing aid and its usage. Also, only 44 of the children arrived for initial evaluation with hearing aids that were functioning properly. Forty eight percent of these children were wearing hearing aids which provided adequate gain. The use of ear-level hearing aids by individuals who would not ordinarily be considered as candidates for hearing aids (hearing losses were less than 30 dB for the better ear) was investigated by Ross et al. (1966). Nearly all of the subjects reported that the advantages of wearing the aid outweighed the possible disadvantages. Also, the results would appear to indicate that amplification per se was an important factor in such performance. The effects of the wearing of a hearing aid upon hearing acuity was investigated by Ross and Lerman (1967) who found that there was no significant correlation between the relative shift in hearing acuity and the maximum power output of the hearing aid. Bentzen *et al.* (1969) investigated the use of binaural hearing aids by individuals with presbyacusis. A followup study of 50 patients who had been fitted with binaural ear-level hearing aids indicated that 55.2% used their aids full time while 75% indicated they used their aids at least 6 hours a day.

This summary of research which has been undertaken during the past 5 years points out that investigators are beginning to concentrate on more meaningful research which is focused upon a determination of how hearing aids process speech rather than how they process pure-tone stimuli. Also, they are exhibiting more attention to factors that contribute to difficulties in the reception of speech, and they are exploring techniques for the evaluation of hearing aids which relate to listening tasks that are relevant to the type of listening the hard-of-hearing individual is exposed to in his daily activities. One area that has not aroused comparable research interest is the contributions that hearing aids make to organized programs of aural rehabilitation.

IX. Tests and Followup Evaluation

Evaluative measures are needed, not only to determine the extent of the problem but to determine the value of the suggested rehabilitative procedures. With such an approach it will be possible to have a quantified record of the results of rehabilitative procedures. There are three major test areas that will be considered—visual, auditory, and combined.

A. Visual Tests

One area of visual tests involves tests of speech reading while a second involves the broad area of visual perception.

There are basically two types of tests of speech reading. The first is the face-to-face test and the second is the motion-picture test. The Mason and Utley motion-picture tests are the most frequently used. For the clinical situation where a projector may not be available, the Kelly test may be used. This is a relatively simple face-to-face test which employs lists of letters, multiple-choice word lists, and sentences. Kelly (1954) reported a high test–retest reliability.

Tests of visual perception would include figural and symbolic elements. Examples of such tests would be the Progressive Matrices, the Case and Ruch Survey of Space Relations Ability, the Graham–Kendall Memory for Designs Test, the Frostig Development Test of Visual

Perception, the Developmental Test of Visual–Motor Integration, the visual subtests of the revised Illinois Test of Psycholinguistic Ability, the Southern California Figure–Ground Visual Perception Test, and tests of visual acuity, ocular motility, and other visual skills.

There is a definite need to develop a more meaningful test of the comprehension of visual speech. Many factors go into the development of such a test; populations to be tested, format of the test, selection of test items, testing conditions, and scoring procedures. In the realm of visual perception many tests are being developed, especially in relation to language usage and reading. Considerable research needs to be undertaken to determine the significance of such tests, especially in terms of visual communication and language learning.

B. Auditory Tests

In describing auditory tests we can use a modification of Hardy's (1956) steps for language acquisition. The first three steps are concerned with sensitivity and the second three steps with auding–listening. Sensitivity, in this instance, would involve basic auditory measures (pure tone and speech reception), discrimination, and perception as measured by phrases, sentences, or longer passages of connected discourse. Auding or listening could be evaluated by means of the following tests: Cooperative Sequential Tests of Educational Progress-Listening, Brown-Carlson Listening Comprehension Test and the Harvard Sentence Tests. However, the results of a rather comprehensive study by Dreyer (1969) cause questions to be raised in regard to the validity of the use of such tests with hearing-impaired individuals. The main reason for such questioning is that these tests were developed under the assumption that they would be administered to individuals with normal reading ability and normal hearing. Also, other tests that could be used would include tests of auditory memory and recognition of auditory patterns and other tests of auditory storage ability. Tests of listening could be administered under difficult conditions (noise background, white noise masking, and environmental noise). In regard to this particular area it is of interest to note that quite a few audiological evaluations never involve the testing of discrimination or perception, even when the referring complaint was an inability to understand speech.

There are several basic problems in this area, such as the need for meaningful tests of speech reception and speech discrimination and tests for the determination of basic auditory abilities. Efforts are being made to improve speech reception and discrimination tests. Tillman and Carhart (1966) have developed a test (N.U. Auditory Test No. 6) which has a high reliability and good interlist equivalence. Speaks and Jerger

(1965) have developed synthetic sentences which have a linguistic pattern but little meaning. The Modified Rhyme Test has been developed by House *et al.* (1963) for the evaluation of speech discrimination. These efforts reflect dissatisfaction with present tests. However, very little research effort has been directed toward a study of parameters that affect the perception of speech. This type of research is needed if meaningful efforts are to be made in terms of relating the results of auditory tests to needed rehabilitative procedures. Some efforts have been made in this direction by Jerger and Speaks (1968) who utilized the Synthetic Sentence Identification Test to evaluate the extent to which speech discrimination performance could be improved by auditory training procedures that utilized alternate forms of the test. Their results indicated that the test provides a promising approach to the evaluation of success in auditory training procedures.

C. Combined Tests

Very little research has been reported in this area. There is one commercially available test which has some utility, but there has been very little comprehensive evaluation of it. This test was developed by Hutton *et al.* (1959). It is a multiple-choice test which is suitable for testing auditory, visual, and combined auditory–visual intelligibility in aural rehabilitation. In developing the test consideration was given to the phonetic occurrences of sounds, word familiarity, and phonetic contrasts. The investigators found the test to be sensitive to different types of hearing loss. Another test which utilized letters of the alphabet was developed by Kelly (1959) to test auditory, visual, and combined reception. Preliminary research indicated that the test was reliable and that it could provide a measure of improvement in performance. There is a need to utilize one or both of these tests in an organized program of research.

The area of listening is of prime importance. However, most of the research literature deals with techniques without an undergirding of a paradigm that is related to basic auditory abilities. Three investigators (Hanley, 1956; Harris, 1957; Peters, 1960) have provided us with some information re basic auditory abilities. Such material has not been given serious attention in terms of applied usage. Also, there are other important areas such as the developmental nature of listening. When we touch upon the area of listening we get into speech perception, second language learning, and language for the deaf. It points out that we have based our diagnostic procedures in audiology upon the phonology of the language when it appears that the basic problem for aural rehabilitation is one of psycholinguistics. Our major interest may center around the effects of amplified sound, but we need to understand some basics before we start worrying about problems introduced by amplification.

D. Other Areas

An area that has received very little attention is that of social-behavioral and vocational evaluation of the hard of hearing. In the minds of some individuals, the most important outcome of a program of aural rehabilitation is the behavioral and attitudinal changes such a program brings about. Nett (1960) developed measures of social–psychological–vocational handicap and related these to the degree of hearing loss. Her findings have significance in terms of rehabilitative programs. Two of the more significant findings were as follows: the kind of social–psychological–vocational handicaps reported were a function of associations between the hard-of-hearing individual and persons in different role relationships to him, the size and function of the group, and the frequency of auditory failure. Also, the degree of handicap as measured by ratings was a function of the knowledge that the rater had of facts about the hearing loss and the life situation of the individual with the loss.

Another scale of hearing handicap developed by High *et al.* (1964) provides for an evaluation of changes in psychosocial status. The authors report a significant correlation between scores on the scale and all measures of auditory sensitivity for the subject's better ears. Oyer and Haas (1969) have reported on the development of a scale which includes assessment of receptive and expressive language participation and social involvement by way of effectiveness of communication.

X. Summary

This chapter has presented the historical development of aural rehabilitation, and a discussion of some of the aims and concerns of those who work with the hearing-handicapped. Visual and auditory communication have been defined and a review has been made of past research and modern developments. Tests constructed to aid in assessment of the problems of the aurally handicapped have been described.

A. Present Situation

The present situation can be characterized as one in which many good programs of aural rehabilitation and habilitation exist throughout the country, and one in which there has been some research in lipreading and far too little in auditory training. In both areas of lipreading and auditory training research has lagged for a number of reasons. Perhaps the paramount reason for the dearth of research has been a lack of interest on the part of audiologists and others who deal with the hearing-impaired. Probably an equally important factor is the lack of research preparation of many who have been engaged in aural rehabilitation. Difficulty involved in the isolation and adequate control of variables has also played a role in discouraging the development of research. Because of these reasons, too few good test instruments for handicap measurement have been developed.

B. Future Directions

One of the future directions in aural rehabilitation research should be the elaboration of a conceptual framework to describe the process. Through this should emerge the constructs that are supported by extant scientific data and, likewise, the constructs that are not supported by scientific data. With orderly conceptualizations of the process, future researches should bear a more meaningful relationship to each other and permit theory construction. At the time of this writing there is a project underway on conceptual framework development in aural rehabilitation at Michigan State University supported by a contract with the Health Services and Mental Health Administration of the U.S. Department of Health, Education, and Welfare (Oyer, 1970).

Another direction for future research should be the shift in approach from one of primarily lipreading and auditory training to a much broader approach that embraces language development, the social ramifications of hearing loss, and also vocational aspects.

Still another direction that should be a part of future work is the undertaking of longitudinal studies of individuals suffering hearing loss and the long-term effects of aural rehabilitation procedures on self and social adjustment.

An important step we must take is that of assisting in the development of specifications for amplification systems, rather than attempting to adapt to the specifications set by commercial sources.

Appropriate tools must be developed to carry out research. It is only through the development of adequate tools that we will one day come to a better understanding of what we have chosen to call hearing handicap and the development of a means of altering factors that cause the handicap. Not until we have at hand the research tools, and have used them to discover facts concerning the communication disability that accompanies hearing loss, will we be able to prescribe with greater accuracy or specificity the procedures that will one day ameliorate the handicap of hearing loss.

References

Ballenger, H. C. (1936). The 'aural or acoustic' method of treating deafness: Further investigation. *Ann. Otol. Rhinol. Laryngol.* **45**, 632–637.

Bennett, D. (1963). A study of slow-play distortion and its influence on speech intelligibility under low-pass filter conditions. Unpublished doctoral dissertation, University of Washington.

Bennett, D., and Byers, V. W. (1967). Increased intelligibility in the hypacusic by slow-play frequency transportation. *J. Auditory Res.* **7**, 107–118.

Bentzen, O., Frost, E., and Skaftason, S. (1969). Treatment with binaural-hearing aids in Presbyacusis. *Int. Audiol.* **8**, 529–534.

Bergman, M. (1964). The present status of auditory training and speech conservation. Auditory Rehabilitation in Adults, 85–93. Cleveland Speech and Hearing Center and Western Reserve University.

Black, J. W. (1968). Perception of altered acoustic stimuli by the deaf. Final Report, R. F. Project 1688, Ohio State Univ. Research Foundation, Columbus, Ohio.

Blair, F. X. (1966). Problems in the habilitation of aural deficiency. "Aural Rehabilitation of Aural Deficiency." 1–22. Michigan State Univ., East Lansing, Michigan.

Bode, D. L., and Oyer, H. J. (1970). Auditory training and speech discrimination. *J. Speech Hearing Res.* **13**, 839–855.

Brannon, J. B., Jr., and Kodman, F. Jr. (1959). The perceptual process in speech reading. *Arch. Otolaryngol.* **70**, 114–119.

Brown, A. E., and Hopkins, H. K. (1967). Interaction of the auditory and visual sensory modalities. *J. Acoust. Soc. Amer.* **41**, 1–6.

Byers, V. W., and Lieberman, L. (1959). Lipreading performance and the rate of the speaker. *J. Speech Hearing Res.* **2**, 271–276.

Carhart, R., and Olsen, W. O. (1967–68, 1968–69). Annual report of the Auditory Research Laboratories. Northwestern Univ., Evanston-Chicago.

Cavender, B. J. (1949). The construction and investigation of a test of lipreading ability and a study of factors assumed to affect the results. Unpublished Master's Thesis, Indiana Univ.

Clarke, F. R. (1957). *In* "Educational Guidance and the Deaf Child" (A. W. G. Ewing, ed.), Ch. 6. Manchester Univ. Press, Manchester.

Conklin, E. J. (1917). A method for the determination of relative skill in lipreading. *Volta Rev.* **19**, 216–220.

Cornett, R. O. (1967). Cued speech. *Amer. Ann. Deaf.* **112**, 3–13.

Costello, M. R., and Purcell, G. (1968). Perception of defective visual and acoustic verbal patterns. *Int. Audiol.* **7**, 5–8.

Davidson, J. L., and O'Neill, J. J. (1956). Relationship between lipreading ability and five psychological factors. *J. Speech Hearing Dis.* **21**, 478–481.

Day, H. E., Fusfeld, I. S., and Pintner, R. (1928). The value of individual hearing aids for hard of hearing children. National Research Council, Washington, D.C.

DiCarlo, L. M. (1948). Auditory training for the adult. *Volta Rev.* **50**, 490–496.

DiCarlo, L. M. (1958). An educational program for children with impaired hearing. *Elementary School J.* **48**, 160–167.

Dodds, E., and Harford, E. (1968). Modified earpieces and CROS for high frequency hearing losses. *J. Speech Hearing Res.* **11**, 204–218.

Dreyer, D. E., (1969). Listening performance related to selected academic and psychological measures. Unpublished doctoral dissertation, Michigan State Univ.

Fisher, C. G. (1968). Confusions among visually perceived consonants. *J. Speech Hearing Res.* **11**, 796–804.

Forrester, C. R. (1928). Residual hearing and its bearing on oral training. *Amer. Ann. Deaf.* **73**, 147–155.

Franks, J. R., and Oyer, H. J. (1967). Factors influencing the identification of English sounds in lipreading. *J. Speech Hearing Res.,* **10**, 757–767.

Fulton, R. M. (1964). Comparative assessment of visible difference between voiced and unvoiced words. Unpublished Master's thesis, Michigan State Univ.

Gaeth, J., and Lounsbury, E. (1966). Hearing aids and children in elementary schools. *J. Speech Hearing Dis.* **31**, 283–289.

Gault, R. (1927–28). On the identification of certain vowel and consonant elements in words by their tactual qualities and by their visual qualities as seen by lipreading. *J. Abnormal. Psychol.* **22**, 33–39.

Geldard, F. A. (1960). Some neglected possibilities of communication. *Science* **131**, 1583–1588.

Goldstein, M. A. (1939). "The Acoustic Method." Laryngoscope Press, St. Louis.

Goodfellow, L. D. (1942). The re-education of defective hearing. *J. Psychol.* **14**, 53–58.

Green, D. S. (1969). Non-occluding earmolds with CROS and IROS hearing aids. *Arch. Otolaryngol.* **89**, 512–522.

Green, D. S., and Ross, M. (1968). The effect of a conventional versus a nonoccluding (CROS-Type) earmold upon the frequency response of a hearing aid. *J. Speech Hearing Res.* **11**, 638–647.

Greene, J. D. (1963). An investigation of the ability of unskilled lipreaders to determine the accented syllable of polysyllabic words. Unpublished Master's thesis, Michigan State Univ.

Greenberg, H. J., and Bode, D. L. (1968). Visual discrimination of consonants. *J. Speech Hearing Res.* **11**, 869–874.

Griffing, B. L., and Hayes, G. M. (1968). Educational amplification response study. EARS Monograph 1, San Diego Speech and Hearing Center.

Guttman, N., and Nelson, J. R. (1968). An instrument that creates some artificial speech spectra for the severely hard of hearing. *Amer. Ann. Deaf* **113**, 295–302.

Hanley, C. N. (1956). Factorial analysis of speech perception. *J. Speech Hearing Dis.* **21**, 76–87.

Hardick, E., Oyer, H. J., and Irion, P. E. (1970). Lipreading performance as related to measurements of vision. *J. Speech Hearing Res.* **13**, 92–100.

Hardy, W. (1956). Problems of audition, perception and understanding. *Volta Rev.* **58**, 289–300 and 309.

Harford, E. (1967). Bilateral CROS: Two-sided listening with one hearing aid. *Arch. Otolaryngol.* **84**, 426–432.

Harford, E., and Barry, J. (1965). A rehabilitative approach to the problem of unilateral hearing impairment: The contralateral routing of signals (CROS). *J. Speech Hearing Dis.* **30**, 121–138.

Harford, E., and Dodds, E. (1966). The clinical application of CROS. *Arch. Otolaryngol.* **83**, 455–464.

Harris, J. D. (1957). A search toward the primary auditory abilities. Med. Res. Lab., U.S. Naval Submarine Base, New London, Conn. Memo. Rep. No. 57–4.

Harrison, A. (1969). Clinical use of earmold modifications in supplying amplification to a presbyacusic population. *Int. Audiol.* **8**, 509–516.

Heider, F. K., and Heider, G. M. (1940). An experimental investigation of lipreading. *Psychol. Monographs,* **52,** 1–153.

High, W. S., Fairbanks, G., and Glorig, A. (1964). Scale for self-assessment of hearing handicap. *J. Speech Hearing Dis.* **29,** 215–230.

Hirsh, I. J. (1951). Audiology and the basic sciences. *Acta Oto-Laryngol.* **40,** 42–50.

House, A. S., Williams, C. E., Hecker, M. H. L., and Kryter, K. D. (1963). Psychoacoustic speech tests: A modified rhyme test. Electronic Systems Division, Air Force Systems Command, Hanson Field, Technical Documentary Report ESD-TDR-63-403.

Hudgins, C. V. (1953). The responses of profoundly deaf children to auditory training. *J. Speech Hearing Dis.* **18,** 273–288.

Hutton, C., Curry, E. T., and Armstrong, M. B. (1959). Semidiagnostic test materials for aural rehabilitation. *J. Speech Hearing Dis.* **24,** 319–329.

Illinois Commission on Children (1968). A comprehensive plan for hearing impaired children in Illinois, Springfield, Illinois.

Jerger, J. (1968). Effects of electro-acoustic characteristics of hearing aids on speech understanding. Progress Report on Research Conducted for Prosthetics and Sensory Aids Service Veterans Administration, Houston Speech and Hearing Center. Tex. Med. Center, Houston, Texas.

Jerger, J., and Speaks, C. (1968). Speech identification as a measure of discrimination loss. Houston Speech and Hearing Center, Final Report VRA Project No. RD 1904.

Johansson, B. (1961). A new coding amplifier system for the severely hard of hearing. *Proc. 3rd Int. Congr. Acoustics,* **2,** 655–657.

Johnson, E. H. (1939). Testing results of acoustic training. *Amer. Ann. Deaf* **84,** 223–233.

Johnson, E. H. (1948). The ability of pupils in a school for the deaf to understand various methods of communication, II. *Amer. Ann. Deaf* **93,** 280–314.

Johnson, G. F. (1963). The effect of cutaneous stimulation by speech on lipreading performance. Unpublished Doctoral Dissertation, Michigan State Univ.

Jorgenson, A. (1962). The measurement of homophenous words. Unpublished Master's thesis, Michigan State Univ.

Karlovich, R. S. (1968). Sensory interaction: Perception of loudness during visual stimulation. *J. Acoust. Sco. Amer.* **44,** 570–575.

Kasten, R. N., and Lotterman, S. H. (1969). The influence of hearing aid gain control rotation on acoustic gain. *J. Auditory Res.* **9,** 35–39.

Kasten, R. N., Lotterman, S. H., and Revoile, S. G. (1967). Variability of gain versus frequency characteristics in hearing aids. *J. Speech Hearing Res.* **10,** 373–376.

Keil, J. M. (1968). The effects of peripheral visual stimuli on lipreading performance. Unpublished Doctoral Dissertation, Michigan State Univ.

Kelly, J. C. (1954). A summer residential program in hearing education, *J. Speech Hearing Dis.* **19,** 17–27.

Kelly, J. C. (1959). "Audio-Visual Speech Reading." Univ. of Illinois, Urbana.

Kitchen, D. W. (1968). The relationship of visual synthesis to lipreading performance. Unpublished Doctoral Dissertation. Michigan State Univ.

Lang, J., Orbán, L., Palatás, G., Mérei, V., and Csányi, Y. (1962). Audiological consequences of auditory training in early childhood. *Int. Audiol.* **2,** 198–201.

Larsen, L. L. (1950). "Consonant Sound Discrimination." Indiana Univ. Press, Bloomington.

Lederer, F. L. (1946). Hearing and speech rehabilitation. *U.S. Nav. Med. Bull. Suppl.* 183–249.

Leonard, R. (1962). The effects of selected continuous auditory distractions on lipreading performance. Unpublished Master's thesis, Michigan State Univ.

Leonard, R. (1968). Facial movements of males and females while producing common expressions and sentences by voice and by whisper. Unpublished Doctoral Dissertation, Michigan State Univ.

Lichtenberg, F. S. (1966). A comparison of children's ability to make speech sound discriminations. *Volta Rev.* 68, 426–434.

Ling, D. (1968). Three experiments on frequency transposition. *Amer. Ann. Deaf* 113, 283–294.

Ling, D. (1969). Speech discrimination by profoundly deaf children using linear and coding amplifiers. *IEEE Trans. Audio Electroacoustics* AU-17, 298–303.

Lloyd, L. L. (1964). Sentence familiarity as a factor in visual speech reception (lipreading). *J. Speech Hearing Dis.* 29, 409–413.

Loftiss, E. W., and O'Neill, J. J. (1964). Estimation of acoustic gain in fitting of hearing aids. Summary Report, N.I.H. Grant NB 04307-01, Univ. of Illinois, Urbana, Illinois.

Lotterman, S. H., Kasten, R. N., and Revoile, S. G. (1967). Acoustic gain and threshold improvement in hearing aid selection. *J. Speech Hearing Res.* 10, 856–858.

Lowell, E. L. (1957). A film test of lipreading. *John Tracy Research Papers,* II.

Markle, D. M., and Zaner, A. (1966). The determination of "gain requirements" of hearing aids: A new method. *J. Auditory Res.* 6, 371–377.

Mason, M. (1943). A cinematographic technique for testing visual speech comprehension. *J. Speech Dis.* 8, 271–278.

Matkin, N. D., and Olsen, W. O. (1968–69). Evaluation of auditory training units. *Annual Report of the Auditory Research Laboratories,* Evanston-Chicago, Illinois.

McClellan, M. E. (1967). Aided speech discrimination in noise with vented and unvented earmolds, *J. Auditory Res.* 7, 93–99.

Miller, J. D. (1952). An analytical evaluation of speech discrimination scores prior to and following an auditory training program. Unpublished Master's thesis, Univ. of Maryland.

Morkovin, B. V. (1947). Rehabilitation of the aurally handicapped through the study of speech reading in life situations. *J. Speech Dis.* 12, 363–368.

Morris, D. M. (1944). A study of some of the factors involved in lipreading. Unpublished Master's thesis, Smith College.

Moser, H. M., Oyer, H. J., O'Neill, J. J., and Gardner, H. J. (1960). Selection of items for testing skill and visual recognition of one syllable words. Ohio State Univ. Development Fund Proj. 5818.

Moser, H. M., O'Neill, J. J., Oyer, H. J., Abernathy, E., and Showe, B. Jr. (1961). Distance and finger spelling. *J. Speech Hearing Res.* 4, 61–71.

Mulligan, M. J. (1954). Variables in the reception of visual speech from motion pictures. Unpublished Master's thesis, Ohio State Univ.

Neely, K. K. (1956). Effect of visual factors on the intelligibility of speech. *J. Acoust. Soc. Amer.* 28, 1275–1277.

Nett, E. M. (1960). The relationship between audiological measures and handicap. Univ. of Pittsburgh School of Medicine and Office of Vocational Rehabilitation, U.S. Dept. Health, Education and Welfare.

Nielsen, K. M. (1966). The effect of redundancy on the visual recognition of frequently employed words. Unpublished Doctoral Dissertation, Michigan State Univ.

Nitchie, E. B. (1913). Moving pictures applied to lip-reading. *Volta Rev.* 15, 117–125.

Numbers, M. E., and Hudgins, C. V. (1948). Speech perception in present day education of the deaf. *Volta Rev.* 50, 449–456.

O'Neill, J. J. (1951a). Contributions of the visual components of oral symbols to the speech comprehension of listeners with normal hearing. Unpublished Doctoral Dissertation, Ohio State Univ.

O'Neill, J. J. (1951b). An exploratory investigation of lipreading ability among normal hearing students. *Speech Monogr.* 18, 309–311.

O'Neill, J. J. (1954). Contributions of the visual components of oral symbols to speech comprehension, *J. Speech Hearing Dis.* 19, 429–439.

O'Neill, J. J. (1964). "Hard of Hearing." Prentice Hall, Englewood Cliffs, New Jersey.

O'Neill, J. J., and Oyer, H. J. (1961). "Visual Communication for the Hard of Hearing." Prentice-Hall, Englewood Cliffs, New Jersey.

Oyer, E. J., and Paolucci, B. (1970). Homemakers hearing losses and family integration. *J. Home Econ.* 62, 257–262.

Oyer, H. J. (1961). Teaching lipreading by television. *Volta Rev.* 63, 131–132.

Oyer, H. J. (1966). "Auditory Communication for the Hard of Hearing." Prentice-Hall, Englewood Cliffs, New Jersey.

Oyer, H. J. (1970). *A Study and Evaluation of the Aural Rehabilitation Process.* Health Services and Mental Health Administration, Division of Chronic Diseases Programs, Neurological and Sensory Disease Control Program, U.S. Department of Health, Education and Welfare, Washington, D.C., Contract No. HSM 110-69-222.

Oyer, H. J., and Haas, W. (1969). Paper presented at 4th Annual Meeting of Academy of Rehabilitative Audiology.

Peters, R. W. (1960). Research on psychological parameters of sound. Aerosp. Med. Lab., Wright Patterson Air Force Base, Ohio, WAD Techn. Rep. 60–249.

Piminow, L. (1968). Technical and physiological problems in the application of synthetic speech to aural rehabilitation. *Amer. Ann. Deaf.* 113, 275–282.

Pintner, R. (1929). Speech and speechreading tests for the deaf. *J. Appl. Psychol.* 13, 220–225.

Postove, M. J. (1962). Selection of items for a speechreading test by means of scalogram analysis. *J. Speech Hearing Dis.* 27, 71–75.

Quigley, S. P. (1969). The influence of fingerspelling on the development of language, communication and educational achievement in deaf children. Inst. Research on Exceptional Children, Univ. of Illinois, Urbana, Illinois.

Raymond, T., and Proud, G. (1962). Audio frequency conversion—an aid for rehabilitation in neurosurgery hearing loss. *Arch. Otolaryngol.* 76, 436–446.

Reddell, R. C., and Calvert, D. R. (1966). Selecting a hearing aid by interpreting audiological data. *J. Auditory Res.* 6, 445–452.

Reid, G. (1947). A preliminary investigation in the testing of lipreading achievement. *J. Speech Dis.* 12, 77–82.

Roback, I. M. (1961). Homonphenous words. Unpublished Master's thesis, Michigan State Univ.

Roberts, L. (1969). The verbotonal and regular programmes in the Metropolitan Toronto School for the deaf: A descriptive study. Research Department, Metropolitan Toronto School Board, Toronto.

Ross, M., and Lerman, J. (1967). Hearing-aid usage and its effect upon residual hearing. *Arch. Otolaryngol.* **86**, 639–644.

Ross, M, Barrett, L. S., and Trier, T. R. (1966). Ear level hearing aids for motivated patients with minimal hearing losses. *Laryngoscope* **76**, 1555–1561.

Sahlstrom, L. J. (1967). Objective measurement of certain facial movements during production of homophenous words. Unpublished Doctoral Dissertation, Michigan State Univ.

Saleh, H. (1965). Sights and sounds. An auditory training program for young deaf children. *Amer. Ann. Deaf* **110**, 528–534.

Silverman, S. R. (1947). Tolerance for pure tones and speech in normal and defective hearing. *Ann. Otol. Rhinol. Laryngol.* **56**, 658–677.

Simmons, A. A. (1959). Factors related to lipreading. *J. Speech Hearing Res.* **2**, 340–352.

Speaks, C., and Jerger, J. (1965). Method for measurement of speech identification. *J. Speech Hearing Res.* **8**, 185–194.

Stone, L. (1957). Facial cues of context in lipreading. *John Tracy Clinic Research Papers,* V.

Stover, W. R. (1967). Electronic speech processing methods for the hearing impaired. *J. Auditory Res.* **7**, 313–325.

Subar, B. E. (1963). The effect of visual deprivation on lipreading performance. Unpublished Master's thesis, Michigan State Univ.

Sumby, W. H., and Pollack, I. (1954). Visual contribution to speech intelligibility in noise. *J. Acoust. Soc. Amer.* **26**, 212–215.

Taafee, G., and Wong, W. (1957). Studies of variables in lip reading stimulus materials. *John Tracy Clinic Research Papers,* III.

Tatoul, C. M., and Davidson, G. D. (1961). Lipreading and letter predictions. *J. Speech Hearing Res.* **4**, 171–181.

Thomas, S. (1962). Lipreading performance as a function of light levels. Unpublished Master's thesis, Michigan State Univ.

Tillman, T. W., and Carhart, R. (1966). An expanded test for speech discrimination utilizing CNC monosyllabic words (Northwestern University Auditory Test No. 6). USAF School of Aerospace Medicine, Aerosp. Med. Div. (AFSC), Brooks Air Force Base, Texas, Technical Report SAM-TR-66-55.

University of Oklahoma Research Institute (no date). Effects and interactions of auditory and visual cues in oral communication. Submitted to U.S.O.E. department of H.E.W.

Utley, J. (1946). A test of lipreading ability. *J. Speech Dis.* **11**, 109–117.

Wedenberg, E. (1951). Auditory training of deaf and hard of hearing children. *Acta Oto-Laryngol. Suppl.* **94**, 1–129.

Wedenberg, E. (1961). Auditory training of the severely hard of hearing using a coding amplifier. *Proc. 3rd Int. Congr. Acoustics,* 658–660.

Wong, W., and Taaffe, G. (1958). Relationships between selected aptitude and personality tests and lipreading ability. *John Tracy Clinic Research Papers,* VII.

Woodward, M. F. (1957). Linguistic methodology and lipreading research. *John Tracy Clinic Research Papers,* IV.

Wright, J. D. (1917). Auricular education of deaf children. *Med. Rec.* **92**, 241–242.

Zemlin, W. R. (1966). The use of bandwidth and time compression for the hearing handicapped. *Proc. Louisville Conf. on Time Compressed Speech,* Center for Rate Controlled Recordings, Univ. of Louisville.

Chapter 8

Psychoacoustic Instrumentation

WILLIAM MELNICK

Ohio State University

I. Introduction

The material in the remainder of this book gives excellent testimony to the importance of instrumentation in auditory investigation. All of the data were in some way connected with an instrument or a series of instruments and, of necessity, reflect the properties and limitations of this equipment. Auditory measurement was given a tremendous boost by the development of electronic devices for signal production, control, and measurement. The electronic waveform generators, amplifiers, microphones, headphones, meters, oscilloscopes, etc., have been and will continue to be used in accumulating and refining information about the auditory system. Development of psychoacoustic instrumentation has

253

paralleled that of electronics. Their electronic nature is irrefutable. The scope of this chapter does not include discussion of electronic principles and techniques, although knowledge of basic electricity and electronics would facilitate understanding the instruments, their operation, and restrictions which they impose on the data. This chapter is not an exhaustive catalog of instruments available, but rather an overview of the devices which form a core of equipment for auditory investigation and some of the principles and problems which accompany their use.

A. Instrument Function

Instruments used in investigation of audition belong to the much broader realm of "greater instrumentation." The field of instrumentation encompasses knowledge necessary for development and design of the myriad of instruments used in scientific, technical, and industrial observation, measurement, and control. Several guiding principles have been set forth in the instrumentation area: These include the following points: (1) Eliminate all variables by reducing them to measurables. (2) Isolate each measurable. (3) Whatever is to be controlled must first be measured. (4) If something can be measured, its effects can be controlled. (5) If an instrument can be controlled by hand, it can be controlled automatically (Behar, 1951). These principles can assist the instrument user as well as the developer.

Instruments extend the range of the human senses, which are semiquantitative at best. They supplement our senses by permitting measurables to be quantified, thereby providing data suitable for mathematical manipulation. Instruments can measure quantities for which there are no sensory receptors. They can transform energy from one form to another which is more amenable to transfer and control.

Any instrument or instrumentation scheme has certain attributes. The variable being sampled and measured by the instrument must be effectively isolated. If the effects of sound are to be investigated, it must be certain that the instruments primarily demonstrate the effects of sound and not some other variable. The measuring system should not influence the system being measured. There should be effective isolation of the system whose behavior is being measured, a difficult task with living systems.

B. Error

The accuracy of information from any investigation requiring instrumentation depends directly on the accuracy of the instruments and the error introduced by the investigator in using them. Accuracy is the resultant of all the measuring properties that play a part in the instrumentation scheme. An instrument must be capable of accuracy commensurate with the description of experimental results. It must have a range of measurement or performance sufficient to cover that anticipated for the investigation. It should not interfere with the system so as to alter the measured values nor should it introduce signals extraneous to the data.

Instrument errors may come from any of several sources. The design, construction, workmanship, and grade of manufacture may be responsible for functional errors. The mechanism of the instrument might produce inaccuracies through nonlinearity of electronic components, unusual play in levers, backlash in gears, change in the elasticity of springs, etc. Errors might result from the scale used for a meter. The notation may be difficult to read with precision or the scale units may be too large to permit the degree of accuracy required. The instrument may be sensitive to environmental conditions such as temperature, humidity, and barometric pressure. Errors may arise from the pointer-scale-reader relationship when a meter is read, as in the case of parallax. The arrangement of the mechanical inertial, elastic, and frictional elements and/or the analogous electrical components of inductance, capacitance, and resistance may induce damped harmonic oscillation which could affect the frequency response of the instrument and meter ballistics. These elements may also produce phase and amplitude distortion (Stacy, 1960).

Measurement errors may be systematic or they may be random. Systematic errors usually involve the magnitude of all measurements. This type of problem would occur if there were a change in the sensitivity of the instrument. Random errors refer to fluctuations not related to experimental conditions. Random fluctuation, or noise, influences the accuracy of an instrument when it is a significant fraction of the signal, that is, when the signal-to-noise ratio is relatively small.

The accuracy of a measurement is the relation between the "true" value of the magnitude and the obtained value of a quantity. Error is equal to the difference between the observed and the "true" value. The intrinsic accuracy of the instrument is the extent to which the instrument readings approach the "true" values under calibration conditions—conditions under which errors can be determined and "true values" may be known. A "true" value operationally is simply the measure of a quantity obtained by a more accurate instrument (Behar, 1951).

Manufacturers usually specify instrument accuracy. Unfortunately, new instruments do not always meet nominal accuracy or other specifications. Furthermore, instrument accuracy and performance is not permanently fixed. The only way to ensure that instruments perform accurately and appropriately is by initial and subsequent periodic checks of their essential characteristics, that is, by regular calibration.

II. Psychoacoustic Instrumentation

Psychoacoustic instrumentation includes all the elements of an audio system together with instruments which monitor performance of the system and record responses from the subjects. An audio system is composed of all devices and networks that exist between the sound source (or its electrical equivalent) and its point of final reproduction (Bernstein, 1966). Microphones, headphones, amplifiers, filters, etc., are system elements, and the number and type of elements within a system determine its operating characteristics.

An audio system is a cascade of instruments through which a signal passes from source to load arranged to provide the specific characteristics for the overall system. Audio systems involve at least one and frequently two transducers, one at the source end (input) and the other at the load (output). Instruments between the input and the output may raise or lower signal amplitudes, match impedances, limit bandwidth, determine frequency response, combine inputs from several sources, distribute the signal to several loads, define the temporal rate and signal sequence, alter phase relations, and so on.

To understand a system of instruments used in auditory investigation, it is important to know the operating characteristics of each component and the effects of interaction. For the present these instruments will be categorized according to their primary function as sound sources, electroacoustic transducers, signal control devices, monitoring devices, and finally tape recorders and computers, which are multipurpose instruments.

A. Sound Sources

A familiar psychoacoustic instrument is the electronic waveform generator. For the most part these devices consist of an electronic oscillator and a wave-forming network. An oscillator produces an output signal that is repetitive with time. Oscillator circuits can produce sine waves, square waves, sawtooth waves, triangular waves, and other kinds of periodic waveform, some of which are illustrated in Figure 1. There are many applications for oscillators. They may serve as sources for simple and complex signals. They can provide carriers for high-frequency transmission systems. Sine, square, and sawtooth oscillators can be used for timing, triggering, and gating of events in instruments and as test

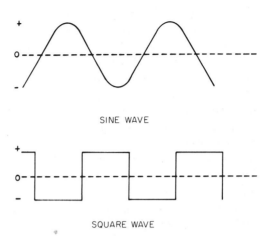

SINE WAVE

Fig. 1. Periodic waveforms
which can be produced by an
electronic waveform generator.

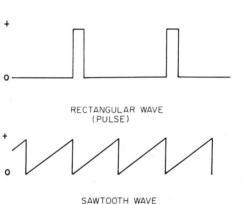

SQUARE WAVE

RECTANGULAR WAVE
(PULSE)

SAWTOOTH WAVE

signals for other electronic equipment. Although these devices serve many
functions, they shall be considered here as electronic signal sources.

1. SINE-WAVE OSCILLATORS

A basic piece of equipment for auditory investigation is the sine-wave
audiooscillator. This instrument can generate a relatively pure sine wave
over a range of 20–20,000 Hz. One type of oscillator generates sine waves
using the principles of electronic feedback, positive and negative, and
the resulting self-oscillation of the vacuum tube or transistor arrangement. The device is basically an amplifier with an electronically tuned
wave-forming system whose output is returned, in phase, to the input
of the amplifier section. This positive feedback, if of the proper magnitude, will lead to self-oscillation at the frequency dictated by the wave-
forming circuit. Negative feedback introduces the output of some later

stage in the amplifying circuit back to the input, but 180° out of phase and has the effect of reducing the noise level and stabilizing the amplified output.

For audiofrequencies the wave-forming network usually is composed of a tuned-bridge circuit using variable combinations of resistance and capacitance (RC oscillator). The RC network controls the frequency of oscillation by means of a dial connected to a variable capacitor. With this system it is possible to tune a wide range of frequencies but, unfortunately, not all audiofrequencies because of practical limitations in the range of variable capacitors. The frequency range can be changed by switching different resistances into the circuit so that ultimately any audible frequency would be available.

A second major type of audiooscillator employs the beat-frequency (BFO) principle (Tremaine, 1959). In operation, the outputs from two high-frequency oscillators, one fixed and one variable, interact and produce a difference frequency in the audio range which is detected, filtered, and amplified and becomes the final output of the oscillator. When the dial of the BFO which is connected to the variable oscillator is rotated, its frequency is changed by varying the beat-frequency output. A comparatively small change of the variable oscillator will produce a relatively large change in the audiofrequency output. The chief advantage of this oscillator is that it may be swept over the entire audio spectrum in one revolution or less of the dial.

Beat-frequency oscillators have the disadvantage of drifting when cold and should be warmed up at least 15 minutes before using. Each time the oscillator is shut off or allowed to cool it must be recalibrated. Since the BFO requires frequent calibration during its use, it often has some sort of frequency calibrating circuit. The calibration procedure usually involves beating the output of the BFO with the 60-cycle line frequency and is indicated by fluctuations of the meter pointer. The oscillator is adjusted until fluctuations of less than one per second are achieved.

2. SQUARE-WAVE GENERATORS

A periodic signal in the form of pulses assumes a rectangular waveform. When the widths of the positive and negative half cycles are identical, the waveform is called a square wave. A Fourier analysis of the square wave shows this wave to be composed of the fundamental frequency and an infinite number of odd harmonics, all in phase. The square wave is useful as a complex sound source, as an electrical signal for testing other electronic devices, and in electronic switching circuitry.

Square waves may be produced in a number of ways. The output of a sine-wave oscillator may be clipped and squared electronically or the output of a multivibrator circuit may be used.

3. SAWTOOTH GENERATORS

The sawtooth waveform has been used as a source of low-frequency noise. It contains all the harmonics, with amplitude decreasing as the frequency of the harmonic increases so that the sound energy is "weighted" in favor of the lower frequencies. The sawtooth-waveform generator is more frequently used as a time-base generator. In connection with other electronic circuitry, the sawtooth wave can be employed to change duration of the "on" and "off" time in an electronic switch. With pulse generators, it can be used to affect the timing and duration of pulses to produce rectangular waveforms. Sawtooth waveforms may be generated in several ways. Most of the methods take advantage of charging and discharging characteristics of capacitors.

4. COMPLEX-FUNCTION GENERATORS

Waveform generators are available commercially which generate sine, square, sawtooth, and triangular waves. The frequency ranges of these generators include not only the audio frequencies but also subsonic and ultrasonic frequencies. In addition to those functions stated earlier, these devices can be used as complex noise sources, for testing servosystems, and for driving frequency modulation circuits.

5. RANDOM-NOISE GENERATORS

The properties of random noise make it particularly useful in psychoacoustic investigation. The equal-energy spectrum has proven important in studies of masking. The statistical properties of random noise make it an excellent background noise for experiments in signal detection.

A random-noise generator typically involves a gas-discharge tube or a noisy crystal diode. The noise source is operated in a magnetic field which serves to suppress unwanted oscillation. The noise is then amplified and shaped to the desired spectrum. The noise is further amplified and is usually coupled to an output attenuator. A meter may be provided to measure the output voltage. When the noise spectrum is uniform over a wide frequency band, it is referred to as white noise because it is analogous to white light. The noise output can be filtered, providing bandwidths of an octave, $\frac{1}{3}$ octave, and narrower.

B. Electroacoustic Transducers

A transducer converts one form of energy to another. In psychoacoustics the transducers are microphones, which change sound into electrical signals, and loudspeakers, headphones, and bone vibrators which turn electrical energy into sound energy. There are many kinds of electroacoustic transducers. Knowledge of their operating principles and the advantages and disadvantages of these transducers is a must in psychoacoustics.

1. MICROPHONES

The essential features of a microphone include its frequency response, output, sensitivity, distortion, internal noise, directivity, dynamic range, impedance, environmental stability, and size. There are several types of microphone. The most common include the carbon, the crystal, the dynamic, the condenser, and the ribbon microphone. Figure 2 displays diagrammatically the operation of these five types of microphone. The carbon and ribbon microphones are not commonly used in studies of audition.

a. Crystal Microphone. The crystal microphone depends on the piezoelectric effect of Rochelle salt, ammonium dehydrogen phosphate (ADP), or lithium sulfate crystals for its operation. The motion of the diaphragm deforms the crystal and results in the generation of voltage between the electrodes on the crystal surface (see Figure 2b).

Crystal microphones are generally nondirectional. The frequency response depends on construction and quality. Typical responses may extend from 80 to 6500 Hz, but these microphones can respond up to 16,000 Hz. The output voltage is fairly high, on the order of —50 dB referred to 1 volt (1 V) per dyne cm^{-2} (Bogert and Peterson, 1957). These microphones present high output impedances in the range of 60,000–100,000 ohms. Because of the high impedance, a crystal microphone should not be separated too far from the input of the amplifier, the maximum distance being in the neighborhood of 50 feet. The crystal microphone is affected by temperature and humidity but should operate effectively under normal laboratory conditions.

The ceramic microphone, which employs a barium titanate slab, operates in the same way as the crystal microphone. The ceramic material is made piezoelectric by being permanently polarized with a high, electrostatic potential for a period of time. This type of microphone also has a high impedance but seldom exceeds 20,000 ohms. It can be operated under conditions of higher temperature and humidity than the crystal microphone (Tremaine, 1959).

b. Dynamic Microphone. In the dynamic microphone, movement of a coil in a strong magnetic field generates a voltage across the terminals of the coil. The coil is attached to a diaphragm and the voltage developed is proportional to the displacement of this diaphragm (Figure 2c). The

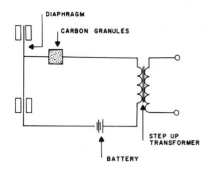

(a) CARBON MICROPHONE

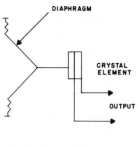

(b) CRYSTAL MICROPHONE

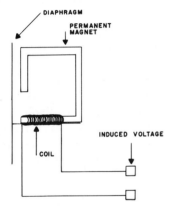

(c) DYNAMIC MICROPHONE

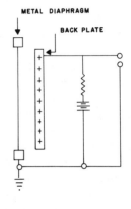

(d) CONDENSER MICROPHONE

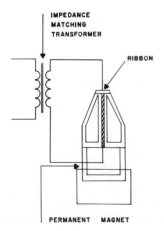

(e) RIBBON MICROPHONE

FIG. 2. Operational diagram of five common types of microphones.

261

electrical impedance is about 20 ohms so it may be operated with long cables and other apparatus without any undue effect. The field pattern is essentially nondirectional or circular (Figure 3a). The frequency response may be uniform to 10,000 Hz although sensitivity starts to decrease approximately at 8000 Hz. Distortion and internal noise are relatively low. The open-circuit sensitivity of this type of microphone is on the order of −85 dB referred to 1 V per dyne cm^{-2} (Bogert and Peterson, 1957). These microphones can be constructed to operate in sound fields of 140 dB or greater, depending on the spectrum. They are affected by variations in temperature and pressure. Alternating magnetic fields in the vicinity can induce large voltages in the coil. The dynamic microphone is sturdy and can resist rough handling and is generally a useful microphone in communication circuits.

   c. *Condenser Microphones.* The condenser microphone has found considerable use in the field of psychoacoustics because of a flat frequency response over a relatively wide range and low internal noise. The operating principle is illustrated in Figure 2d. The diaphragm of the microphone is a thin, stretched metallic membrane which acts as the plate of a condenser. The backplate is insulated from the diaphragm and serves as the second capacitive plate. Sound waves striking the diaphragm cause it to vibrate, varying the capacitance between the two plates. When a source of high, direct-current (dc) polarizing voltage is applied to the capacitor plate through a high resistance, the variation in capacitance created by diaphragm displacement will cause a proportional voltage variation across the resistance (Beranek, 1949). Condenser

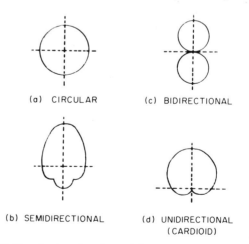

(a) CIRCULAR   (c) BIDIRECTIONAL

(b) SEMIDIRECTIONAL   (d) UNIDIRECTIONAL
                                          (CARDIOID)

Fig. 3. Four basic microphone field patterns of sensitivity.

microphones are used in laboratories when an accurate and quantitative reproduction of acoustic waveform is required. It has been the microphone of choice for calibration of other transducers and for sound field analyzers.

These microphones can be small ($\frac{1}{4}$ inch in diameter) and as a result, can be used without greatly distorting a sound field. Generally as the size of the microphone decreases, the range of flat, frequency response increases and the sensitivity decreases. Half-inch condenser microphones are available with flat frequency response, ± 1 dB, from 20 to 20,000 cycles and with an open-circuit sensitivity -58 dB re 1 V per dyne cm^{-2} (Hewlett-Packard, 1968). The microphone is nondirectional. Half-inch microphones can be used in sound fields greater than 180 dB with less than 4% harmonic distortion.

The condenser microphone is sensitive to ambient pressure, temperature, and humidity changes. The chief disadvantage, however, arises from the high impedance of the microphone, which is often in the range of 30 megohms. It must therefore be operated within a few inches of the amplifier input. Generally the microphone and the amplifier are assembled as a unit. The amplifier usually is a cathode follower, an electronic circuit useful for matching high to low impedances.

A condenser-microphone circuit may be used to modulate a high-frequency carrier. This type of operation requires a relatively low polarizing voltage and can extend the low-frequency response down to 0 Hz.

d. Ribbon Microphone. The ribbon microphone uses a light metallic ribbon suspended in a strong magnetic field as shown in Figure 2e. Sound waves cause the ribbon to vibrate in the magnetic field, generating a voltage corresponding to the particle velocity of the wave. This microphone is, in fact, a special case of the dynamic microphone responsive to particle velocity instead of sound pressure. It is generally bidirectional (Figure 3c) with a null sensitivity in the plane of the ribbon, but can be designed to be unidirectional (Figure 3d) or cardioid. The internal impedance is low (less than 1 ohm) therefore it must be used in conjunction with an impedance-matching transformer in order to match the line impedance.

e. Carbon Microphone. Carbon microphones (Figure 2a) are relatively simple and have good sensitivity. These devices have many problems which dictate use in systems with limited fidelity. They are nonlinear and produce amplitude, harmonic, and intermodulation distortion. The frequency range is limited. The carbon microphone generates considerable internal noise. These microphones are used most extensively in telephones.

f. Microphone Calibration. The most widely used method for absolute calibration of microphones is the reciprocity method, described in detail in U.S.A. Standard S 1.10-1966. The calibration may be conducted under free-field conditions, usually an anechoic chamber, or more conveniently as a pressure calibration using a small enclosed cavity, or coupler. Both methods require two microphones and an independent sound source. At least one of the microphones must be reciprocal and able to function as a microphone and a loudspeaker. In this procedure, the unknown or unmeasurable quantities cancel each other out and only the measures of the physical properties and the electrical quantities remain. Calibration is simplified if both microphones are the same type. Differences between the sound field and the pressure calibration in a coupler arise chiefly because of the geometry of the microphone and the obstacle effect which the microphone introduces to the sound field (Hewlett-Packard, 1968).

A relative calibration of microphones can be made using a sound field (not necessarily anechoic) or in a coupler. This method involves the use of a standard, calibrated microphone to measure sound pressure first. Then the unknown microphone is substituted and the results from the two measurements are compared (Tremaine, 1959).

2. LOUDSPEAKERS

Most loudspeakers use the dynamic or moving-coil mechanism. These loudspeakers may be of the direct-radiator type or of the horn type. A cross-sectional diagram of a direct-radiator dynamic speaker is shown in Figure 4. A voice coil acts in a strong magnetic field. This voice coil is attached to the apex of a diaphragm. Audio frequencies applied to the voice coil cause it to react in the permanent magnetic field, resulting in motion of the cone which in turn forms sound waves. The horn type of loudspeaker couples the loudspeaker diaphragm to the air by means of a horn, generally with an exponential shape starting with a small throat and expanding to a large bell. The horn serves to match the impedance of the loudspeaker to the air medium (Beranek, 1954).

The principal advantages of the director–radiator type of speaker are small size, low cost, and a satisfactory response over a comparatively wide frequency range. The disadvantages are low efficiency and a narrow directivity at high frequencies. The horn speaker has a higher efficiency of radiation but also has a greater cost and larger size than the direct–radiator type.

Loudspeakers are not optimum as standard sources of sound. Sound fields generated by speakers will vary over a range of many decibels as a function of observation point. This nonuniformity arises from three

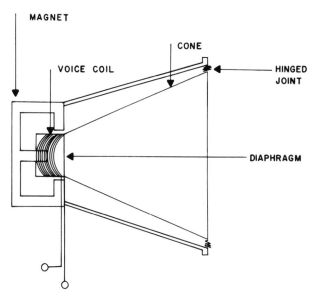

Fig. 4. Cross-sectional diagram of a direct-radiator type of dynamic loudspeaker.

sources: breakup of the diaphragm into higher orders of vibration, radiation patterns of the diaphragm, and combination of direct waves with waves refracted from the loudspeaker housing. When an investigation is carried out in a sound field, great care should be taken to specify as accurately as possible the sound energy at the point of measurement.

The impedance of a speaker is generally low and is frequency dependent. At the low-frequency resonant point and at high frequencies the voice-coil impedance is several times that of the mid-frequencies. The rated impedance is really nominal, being measured at one point—generally at 400 Hz.

Speakers should be operated with a baffle which serves to isolate the sound emanating from the front of the loudspeaker from that coming from the rear. Frequency response of the speaker system may be altered significantly by mounting it in an enclosure. Enclosures often are used to enhance the low-frequency response of the system (Tremaine, 1959).

Loudspeaker performance usually is measured in an anechoic chamber with an accurately calibrated microphone system. The system also can be measured in the unobstructed outdoor environment. Frequency response measurements specify speaker sound-pressure output, at a particular distance, under constant input. Measurements of harmonic distortion require the use of a wave analyzer in conjunction with the microphone system. These are the usual measures of interest to an investigator, but, to be fully specified, other measures of a speaker must be obtained: the directional characteristics, impedances, power handling capacity, and transient properties.

3. EARPHONES

There are several kinds of earphones available but earphones used in psychoacoustics have been most frequently one of three types: (1) dynamic, (2) crystal, and (3) condenser. Electromagnetic earphones have more distortion and a narrow frequency range and find their main use in telephones. The operating principles of the earphones are reciprocally related to those illustrated for the same types af microphones in Figure 2.

a. Dynamic Earphones. These devices operate in the same way as the dynamic loudspeaker. The moving-coil earphone produces uniform sound pressure over a wider range of frequencies than does the magnetic earphone. Changes in acoustic impedance of the ear to which the earphone is coupled have relatively minor effects on acoustic output. The nonlinear harmonic distortion produced by the dynamic earphone is less than that of a magnetic earphone for comparable constant power.

The impedance is usually low, in the neighborhood of 10–600 ohms and is usually specified for a particular frequency as in the case for loudspeakers. Impedance of the energy source should be matched to that of the earphone.

The dynamic earphone has a relatively good transient response. The response is well damped with just a slight oscillation occurring at the onset and termination of a pulsed input.

b. Crystal Earphone. The crystal earphone is constructed similarly to the crystal microphone. Audiofrequency current is applied to the crystal and because of the piezoelectric effect the crystal bends or twists. This movement is transmitted to the diaphragm by a mechanical linkage. These earphones are high-impedance devices, in the range of 10,000 ohms, and consequently are coupled to the output amplifier by an impedance-matching transformer. Because of the high internal impedance, the output may be sensitive to changes in impedance of the load presented by the ear.

The frequency response of the crystal earphone is as wide, if not wider, than the dynamic earphone. However, for a comparable input voltage, the crystal produces less output. Crystal earphones are also sensitive to changes in humidity and temperature.

c. Condenser Earphone. Condenser microphones are sometimes used as wide-range earphones. A half-inch microphone can produce a uniform output up to 20,000 Hz. This kind of transducer has been used in high-frequency threshold measurements (Zislis and Fletcher, 1966). Maximum outputs in a closed, rigid cavity for 1-inch, $\frac{1}{2}$-inch, and $\frac{1}{4}$-inch microphones have been found to be 120, 100, and 75 dB, respectively. When operating at these maximum levels harmonic distortions of 1% or less can be obtained (Molnar et al., 1968).

d. Earphone Calibration. Earphone function may be measured using real ears or acoustic couplers of the type shown in Figure 5. Of the two methods, the use of a coupler has had increasing acceptance.

Using real ears the response of the earphone can be measured in at least three ways: eardrum-pressure method, the outer ear canal method, and the equal-loudness method. In the eardrum-pressure method, the sound pressure produced by the earphone is measured in the vicinity of the drum by means of a flexible probe tube coupled to a calibrated, pressure microphone and a sound measuring system. Because of the danger of possible damage to the ear, the outer canal method is em-

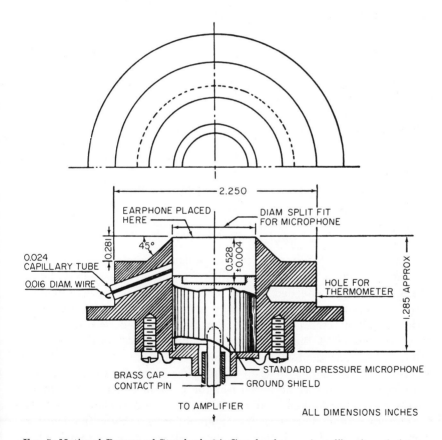

FIG. 5. National Bureau of Standards 9A Coupler for use in calibration of air-conduction earphones.

ployed. Sound pressure is measured at some point in the ear canal and converted to pressure at the drum. The equal-loudness method makes a determination of the pressure in a sound field (or standard earphone) which will produce the same loudness at the ear of a subject as perceived with an earphone for a given electrical input.

The frequency response of the earphone is affected by the method for coupling the earphone to the ear. Whether the earphone is circumaural or supraural, the volume of air enclosed under the earphone cap, the effective seal of the earphone to the head or pinna, and the coupling force all influence the earphone response to some degree (Shaw, 1966). If the input signal to the ear is to be specified accurately, the effect of these factors must be considered.

The American standard method for the coupler calibration of earphones is specified in U.S.A. Standard A 24.9-1949. This method employs an acoustic cavity to couple the test earphone to a standard pressure microphone. A specified signal is applied to the earphone. The electrical response of the standard microphone is measured with appropriate and calibrated instruments for measuring electrical output. A possible equipment arrangement for a coupler earphone calibration system appears in Figure 6 as a block diagram.

C. Signal Control Devices

Once the signal has been generated or has been transduced from sound waves to electrical waveforms, another class of instruments becomes involved. These instruments control and modify the signal to meet the desired purpose.

1. AMPLIFIERS

Any electronic device or circuit in which the output signal exceeds the input signal is called an amplifier. Amplifiers are usually labeled according to their intended use or functions, such as voltage amplifier, current amplifier, power amplifier, preamplifier, line amplifier, differential amplifier, etc. They might also be designated according to the coupling method of the input to the amplifier, such as direct-coupled (DC) or resistance and capacitance coupled (RC). They may be labeled according to the action of their amplifying elements, vacuum tube or transistor, and the specific pattern of the plate or collector current into classes designated alphabetically as class A, class AB, class B and class C. The important characteristics of amplifiers are gain, frequency response, linearity, phase distortion, noise output, power output, and the impedance, both input and output.

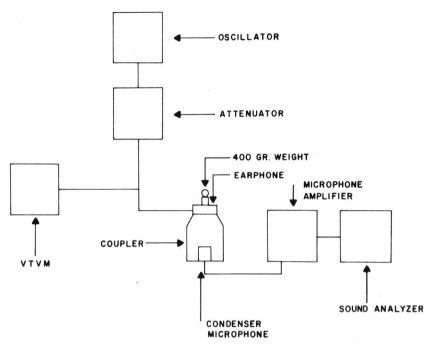

FIG. 6. Block diagram of an equipment arrangement for earphone calibration using an acoustic coupler.

a. Voltage Amplifier. This type of amplifier is used when voltage output is more important than power. All amplifiers produce power but in the voltage amplifier the power output is in the ½-watt range. These amplifiers usually have a high output impedance. They may act as booster amplifiers to compensate for equipment insertion losses which occur in the circuit.

b. Power Amplifier. The power amplifier delivers a sizable amount of current to the load. The output impedance, as a rule, is low, 16 ohms or less. Power amplifiers may be designed to deliver up to several hundred watts and are sometimes known as current amplifiers.

c. Preamplifier. The output from some signal generators or transducers is very low level and must be amplified before being transmitted further in the system. Preamplifiers serve this function. They are used any place where a 30–50-dB gain is required with a low-level output. Preamplifiers are designed for extremely low internal noise and distortion.

d. Direct-Current Amplifier. The direct-current or direct-coupled amplifier permits amplification at very low frequencies approaching 0 Hz. These amplifiers are slow acting and tend to drift, leading to instability. They are not normally used in psychoacoustic operations except when biological potentials are indicators of auditory response as with the electroencepholograph or evoked cortical response.

e. Differential Amplifiers. The operation of an amplifier is sometimes used to reduce system and ambient noise. In this device there are two input terminals, both above ground, which are subject to the same ambient environmental noise sources about 180° out of phase. One of the inputs comes from the point of measurement. The potential difference between the two inputs is amplified while the common noise is cancelled or greatly reduced as a result of destructive interference from phase inversion. This type of amplifier also has its chief application with biological potentials.

f. Operational Amplifiers. These amplifiers find use in computers, calculators, and experimental programming. They are high-gain direct-coupled amplifiers especially designed for versatility and stability. By varying the input and feedback impedances these devices can be designed to perform many mathematical functions (Stacy, 1960).

g. Amplifier Distortion. Amplifier nonlinearity may produce harmonic, intermodulation, and phase distortion. Amplifiers should be operated within specified input and output limitations. If operated at rated power, amplifiers will generally have less than 2% harmonic distortion. Whenever possible the output capabilities of an amplifier should be 6–10 dB higher than the working level. When a wide frequency range is necessary, with low distortion and flat uniform response, the amplifier should be able to handle a bandwidth 7–10 times that to be used. Amplifier phase distortion is important in the reproduction of pulses, square waves, and other abrupt, transient waveforms. The phase shift is frequency dependent. If this phase shift is a nonlinear function of frequency, the shape of the waveform will be distorted.

2. ATTENUATORS

An attenuator is an arrangement of noninductive resistors with the primary purpose of reducing, with minimal distortion, the magnitude of the electrical signal and consequently the intensity of the sound resulting from transduction of the electrical signal. The resultant decrease in signal is measured most frequently in decibels. Attenuators may be fixed or variable in value. They may be manually or motor driven.

The fixed attenuator is known as a pad. These attenuators may be used to introduce a fixed loss to the circuit or they may be used as a method for matching the impedance of two components. A pad can serve to isolate two pieces of equipment to prevent undesirable interaction.

A pad designed to match circuits of unequal impedance brings with it a loss in the signal being transmitted. The minimum loss is dependent on the impedance ratio of the two circuits, increasing as the impedance mismatch increases. The insertion loss may be more than this minimum loss but never less (Tremaine, 1959).

Variable attenuators are generally designed to reduce the signal logarithmically and are calibrated in decibels. For laboratory use these attenuators often use the decade principle. Several attenuators, each having units of attenuation ten times as great as the preceding attenuator, are connected in tandem. If impedances are matched at the input and output of the tandem, the total attenuation is the sum of the losses of individual attenuators. Variable attenuators also introduce a minimum loss which is determined by the ratio of impedance of the input and output devices.

3. Mixers and Splitters

Psychoacoustic investigations may require the combination of signals from several different sources as, for example, in masking studies. On the other hand, it may be necessary to have the same signal source feed two loads, as in binaural investigations. In both of these cases it may be necessary to manipulate one component without any effect on the others. To perform these functions, resistive networks are designed so that changing the level of any signal source or any output has no effect on the other circuits. The networks are called mixers when used to combine signals, and splitters when used to divide a single source into several. These devices, as with attenuators, can be designed for use with any impedance. They can be used reciprocally, that is, a resistive network designed as a mixer can be reversed and used as a splitter (Bernstein, 1966).

4. Wave Filters

Wave filters are networks of electronic reactive elements, inductance and capacitance (LC), used for attenuating or removing a given band of frequencies from the transmitted waveform. The frequencies which are transmitted are called the pass band while those which are attenuated are stop bands. The network may be passive, one which is simply acted on by an external source, or active and supply power to the circuit.

A filter is classified according to its action on the electrical wave. A high-pass filter attenuates all frequencies below a predetermined frequency called a cutoff. A low-pass filter attenuates frequencies above a cutoff frequency. A band-pass filter transmits only a predetermined band of frequencies, reducing those frequencies above and below the band, while a band-rejection filter removes a band of frequencies and transmits the rest of the signal. The cutoff point of the filter is defined as the half-power point or the point 3 dB less than the level in the pass band. The bandwidth of a filter is the number of cycles between the upper and lower limiting frequencies. Figure 7 shows simple filter circuits together with their transmission characteristics. Simple filter circuits such as these produce an attenuation of 6 dB per octave for frequencies outside the cutoff frequency. Steeper filter slopes are produced by combining several of these simple networks; for example, two of them would give a slope of 12 dB, for three, 18 dB, etc. The pass band of a filter is frequently specified by its center frequency which is defined as the geometric mean of the low and high cutoff frequencies.

Filters may be fixed or they may be variable. A fixed filter might be used to prevent line noises from entering the power supply and causing noise in amplifier systems by being inserted in the power line at the primary of a power transformer. Most frequently the filters used in psychoacoustics are variable and may function as high-pass, low-pass, band-pass filters, or band-rejection filters. The important characteristics are the bandwidth, the frequency range, transient response, the accuracy of cutoff frequency calibration, the insertion loss, the attenuation slopes, maximum attenuation, impedances, input and output power limits, distortion, and internally generated noise.

Filters will produce a phase shift in the input signal. Maximum phase shift occurs outside the pass band with both high-pass and low-pass sections contributing to the shift. The phase of the output for frequencies below the low cutoff may lead the input by as much as 360°, while above the high cutoff, the output may lag the input by the same amount. Phase shifts also occur for frequencies within the pass band but approach 0° at mid-frequency.

5. Electronic Switches and Timers

In psychoacoustics, signal duration and repetition rate are significant variables. These temporal factors may well be the independent variables of an experiment and should be precisely controlled. Electronic timing and switching circuits which permit the necessary precision are available.

If timing involves fairly long intervals, of the magnitude of seconds or minutes, and the precision of the time sequencing can afford errors of a few seconds without appreciably affecting the results, then a simple clock mechanism and manual, mechanical switches can be employed. However, in many instances this is not the case. Frequently the investigator is interested in the micro and millisecond time domain for the signal and subjective response. These circumstances dictate the use of electronic switches and timers.

Electronic switches depend on the fact that vacuum-tube or transistor

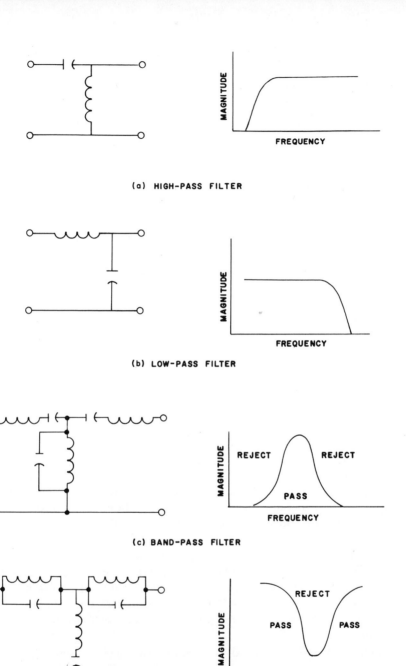

(a) HIGH-PASS FILTER

(b) LOW-PASS FILTER

(c) BAND-PASS FILTER

(d) REJECTION FILTER

FIG. 7. Electronic diagrams of four simple filter circuits shown with their transmission characteristics.

amplification elements can be operated in much the same way as an electromagnetic relay switch. Circuits have been designed which cause these electronic elements to function at their cutoff point or at the saturation point, depending on a biasing voltage. The bias voltage therefore, can dictate whether the device is "on" or "off" (Malmstadt et al., 1962).

An electronic switch is commonly operated in conjunction with a timing circuit. This circuit might be an integral part of the electronic switch or it may be separate in the form of another instrument. The timing can be provided in several ways. If the time intervals are relatively short (milliseconds to a few seconds) and if the signal sequence is to be repetitive as in the case of a tone-pulse train, then the timer could be a square or rectangular wave generator.

The timing generator may be in the form of a multivibrator (Malmstadt et al., 1962). Multivibrators are two-stage devices, that is, these circuits use two tubes or transistors. They operate in one of two stable states of conduction. When one stage is conducting, the other stage is in the cutoff state and vice versa. The transition between states is rapid and the time interval between transitions is determined by the time constants of resistors and capacitors in the timing circuit. Multivibrators may be astable or "free running," periodically changing states without external triggering. They may be bistable or monostable devices. The bistable multivibrator (flip flop) is forced into another state by an external trigger pulse. The Schmitt trigger, a well-known switching circuit used to convert sine waves to square waves, is a modification of a bistable multivibrator. A monostable multivibrator will change states when triggered by a pulse, return to its original state after a specified time period, and remain in that state until triggered again. This "one-shot" multivibrator is a hybrid of the bistable and astable devices.

A preset counter can be employed for timing longer intervals. Briefly, this device employs an oscillator and electronic counting circuits which can be set to deliver a pulse after a fixed number of events have been counted. This pulse, in turn, can be used to trigger either a bistable or a monostable multivibrator which will operate an electronic switching circuit.

When an auditory signal is abruptly switched on and off, transient sound energy is introduced in the form of an audible click. To minimize this form of transient distortion, an electronic network may be incorporated in the switch for varying the rise and decay times of the signal pulses. Rise and decay times in the range of 25–100 msec are suitable for click reduction but other rise and decay times may be available, particularly for use with short tone pulses.

The gain of the two sections of an electronic switch, the on an off sections (A and B sections), must be balanced. If they are in a state of imbalance, a square or rectangular wave having a frequency dictated by the switching period will be introduced. Since switches are prone to drift, the switch sections should be checked and adjusted for balance periodically. This may be done by listening to the output of the switch or by using the oscilloscope for signal display.

The important characteristics of a switch are the range and accuracy of timing periods. Since switches make use of amplifying circuits, they are subject to the same distortion problems as other amplifiers. The operating characteristics must be viewed from the aspect of minimizing distortion products. In addition, the consumer should be aware of the degree of isolation between channels and the on-to-off ratio.

Switches may be controlled from external electronic timers permitting more flexibility. In repetitive signal presentation, the period and duty cycle need not be fixed at discrete values, but can be varied over a continuous time range. External timers also permit switching at varying phases of the input signal.

Electronic circuits are available which depend on inputs from two or more circuits for their switching operation (Malmstadt et al., 1962). Devices which require simultaneous input pulses from more than one source to switch are coincidence circuits known as AND gates. Other circuits, NAND gates, perform in just the opposite way and inhibit transmission of pulses which occur simultaneously. Circuits which operate when signals from either of several inputs occur are called OR gates, while those which will inhibit when a signal is received from any of the inputs are known as NOR gates. These circuits are extremely useful in programming experimental sequences, in altering experimental conditions, and in recording conditional responses.

There are certainly other timing and switching methods which might be useful. Synchronous motors similar to those used in electric clocks may provide the time base and operate with electromagnetic relay switches. Perforated paper tape and a tape transport system could be used to operate mechanical switches. The important point is that the user be familiar with the advantages and limitations of the various methods.

D. Monitoring Devices

If subjective responses to auditory signals are to have meaning, the signal must be defined and controlled as precisely as possible. Uncontrolled changes in instrument operation, in the signal, and in the auditory environment would seriously affect the results of an investigation, leading to completely useless data or, worse, to erroneous decisions.

1. Meters

To test the operational characteristics of an instrument or to trouble-shoot, it is necessary to measure accurately voltage, current, resistance, phase angle, and frequency. These measurements usually involve meters of one kind or another.

Meters which measure electrical quantities most frequently are moving coil devices similar to that shown in Figure 8. A fine-wire coil is mounted between the poles of a permanent magnet. An indicating pointer is attached to the coil assembly together with springs which return the needle to a fixed point. Current flowing through the coil creates a magnetic field which interacts with the permanent magnetic field and forces the coil to rotate. The magnitude of pointer deflection is proportional to the current. Most electrical measuring instruments are current sensitive. Instruments for measuring other electrical properties such as voltage or resistance must be designed so deflection of the pointer will be proportional to the variable to be measured.

In selecting a meter, the concern must be with its range, its impedance, frequency limitations, the accuracy of the instrument, its stability, and

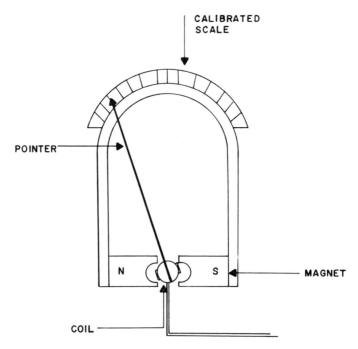

Fig. 8. Diagram of the common moving-coil meter mechanism.

its measuring properties, that is, whether it is a peak meter, average meter, or true root-mean-square (rms) meter. The accuracy rating is usually expressed as a percentage of the full-scale reading of the instrument. Accuracy may be affected by temperature, external magnetic fields, and by the voltage and frequency of the measured signal. If the value being measured varies in magnitude sufficiently to cause the pointer to fluctuate perceptibly, it is impossible to assign a definite value to the reading within the stated accuracy. The sensitivity and accuracy of a meter can be determined by calibration with standard current sources.

The most familiar meter in a psychoacoustic laboratory is the voltmeter. Although other types of voltmeters are available, a high-quality, vacuum tube voltmeter (VTVM) which reads the true root-mean-square (rms) value is the most desirable. Root-mean-square measurements are of fundamental importance in psychoacoustics because electric power and acoustic intensity are directly proportional to this measurement value. True root-mean-square circuits can be used with complex signals as well as sinusoids without affecting the accuracy of the meter. Average-reading voltmeters with scales calibrated to read rms will measure 1 dB less than a true rms meter for complex signals. Vacuum-tube voltmeters have high values of input impedance, therefore errors in circuit voltage measurement resulting from the resistance values of the voltmeter itself are reduced to insignificance (Beranek, 1949). Voltage measurement determines the potential difference between two points in a circuit. The potential difference is measured by connecting the two voltmeter leads to these points or in parallel with the measured circuit.

The VU meter is a special form of voltmeter used particularly in speech-transmitting circuits (Bernstein, 1966). It is calibrated in decibels referred to the power of 1 milliwatt (1 mW) through 600 ohms. Readings from the meter are expressed as VU to avoid confusion with other meters calibrated in decibels with respect to another reference. The VU meter was designed to indicate power levels which avoid distortion from amplifiers in the circuit and overload of the transmission system, to indicate losses or gains in the transmission, to give some indication of the loudness of the output when transduced to sound, and to provide a measurement of sine-wave transmission.

The multimeter (VOM) measures volts, resistance, or current. By switching and proper selection of probe jacks it can be a direct current or an alternating current voltmeter, a direct current milliammeter, or an ohmmeter. These devices are particularly useful in repairing and maintaining electronic equipment.

Sometimes electrical events are too rapid for human recording and observation, or it is necessary that the investigator be free for other more fruitful activities. As a result, measuring instruments which record in some permanent form have been developed. These records are inscribed on strip charts with ink pens, optical devices, or heated styli. With these recorders, time is represented on the horizontal axis. The strip-chart drive system has controlled speeds with distance calibrated in time. The measuring system is similar to the moving-coil meter described earlier, but larger in size. The meter mechanism requires stronger springs, magnet, a larger coil, and a motor drive to overcome the frictional force of the writing implement with the surface of the chart. The frequency range of events to be measured dictates the type of writing method; frequencies from 0 to 60 Hz use the ink pen; frequencies up to 2000–3000 Hz, an optical recording system; higher frequencies, an oscilloscope (Stacy, 1960). Multichannel recorders make use of several measuring and pen drawing systems with the same strip chart for simultaneous recording of several phenomena.

Graphic level recorders are used in conjunction with sound analyzers to produce curves of amplitude as a function of time or as a function of frequency. In addition to the requirements of the other recording measuring devices, it is desirable that the graphic record be logarithmic so that it can be scaled as decibels. An electromagnetic system has been designed to move the writer logarithmically at a high recording speed. An unbalanced current in diode rectifiers causes currents to flow in one direction or the other in a coil which is free to move in a radial magnetic field. The resulting electromagnetic force moves the coil to a new position where electrical balance is established. Recording speeds of over 750 dB/second are possible with this system.

2. Oscilloscopes

The oscilloscope is a versatile, extremely useful measuring instrument. Since it can display a wide range of time-varying voltages, it has become a universal tool for all kinds of electronic investigations. The oscilloscope can present visually a variety of phenomena by using transducers which can convert pressure, acceleration, current, sound, and other physical quantities into voltage.

The oscilloscope is designed to give a visual display of one electrical quantity as a function of a second electrical quantity on a fluorescent screen at the end of a vacuum tube called a cathode ray tube (CRT). In the cathode ray tube, electrons traveling at a high velocity strike phosphorescent substances and cause the phosphors to glow and give off light. The tube consists of an electron gun, a complex combination of elements which emits, accelerates, and focuses an electron beam as a sharp point on the phosphorescent screen. The electron beam passes through a set of deflection plates mounted in the horizontal plane. When a voltage is applied to these plates, the electron beam will be deflected vertically on the screen. The beam then passes through two plates mounted perpendicularly to the first set. A voltage difference between these plates causes a horizontal deflection of the beam. The position of the electron beam and, therefore, the trace on the screen, depends on the instantaneous voltages across these two sets of plates.

Besides the cathode-ray tube, the basic components of an oscilloscope are a vertical amplifier, a horizontal amplifier, a sweep oscillator, power supplies, switching circuits, and an input attenuator. A simplified block diagram of an oscilloscope is shown in Figure 9. Frequently the voltage required to produce the necessary deflection of the electron beam falls

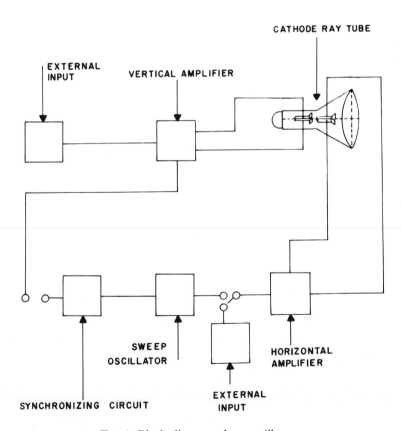

FIG. 9. Block diagram of an oscilloscope.

280   WILLIAM MELNICK

outside the limits of the signals to be measured. For this reason, amplifiers are employed if the signal is less than required. If the signal is greater, an input attenuator is employed. Calibration of the attenuator and amplifiers determines the vertical deflection factor. As a result, the signal voltage can be measured using the graticule or rectangular grid inscribed on the scope face.

When the signal is to be measured as a function of time, the most frequent application, the voltage applied between the horizontal deflection plates produces a linear trace, that is, the beam is swept across the tube at a uniform rate providing a time base. The voltage for producing this sweep comes from a sawtooth oscillator called a sweep generator.

The amplitude-time curve can be continuously displayed by the oscilloscope only if the signal to be measured is continuous and repetitive. A stationary image of the wave shape will appear on the screen if the frequency of the sweep oscillator is the same as, or some multiple of the signal frequency. The sweep generator can be synchronized to the signal frequency by feeding the signal waveform to the sweep generator.

A triggered sweep is desirable for time measurements. With this circuit the particular voltage and slope of the incoming waveform which triggers the sweep can be selected. By using the horizontal divisions of the graticule and by noting the calibrated value of time per division, time measurements of the signal such as the period of a cycle or the duration of a signal pulse can be made.

For maximum versatility, the amplifiers in an oscilloscope must have broad frequency response, low distortion, and negligible phase shift. The probes used to transfer the signal from the test circuit to the scope amplifiers should have characteristics which will not disturb the circuit or the performance of the oscilloscope. A well-designed instrument will display sawtooth waves, square waves, sine waves, triggered pulses, and complex waveforms without distortion. Frequency ranges from direct current to radio frequencies are available while time bases varying from 1 μsec cm^{-1} to several seconds per centimeter can be obtained. These ranges certainly are sufficient for measurement in a psychoacoustic laboratory.

When, instead of the sweep generator, a second input signal is connected to the horizontal amplifier, the oscilloscope becomes an X-Y plotter displaying the functional relationship between the horizontal and vertical input signals. This method of operation is useful for measuring the amplitude ratio, the frequency ratio, and especially the phase angle of two input signals. If two signals of the same frequency are connected to the horizontal and vertical inputs, the phase can be determined from patterns known as Lissajou figures on the scope face as shown in Figure

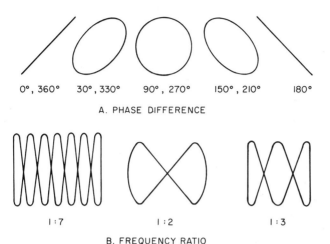

0°, 360°   30°, 330°   90°, 270°   150°, 210°   180°

A. PHASE DIFFERENCE

1 : 7   1 : 2   1 : 3

B. FREQUENCY RATIO

FIG. 10. Lissajou patterns displayed on an oscilloscope demonstrating phase (a) and frequency (b) relationships between the signals connected to the horizontal and vertical amplifier.

10a. When the two signals have a frequency ratio that can be expressed in a small whole number or a simple fraction, other Lissajou patterns (Figure 10b) are observed.

3. X-Y PLOTTERS

A graph using the Cartesian coordinates is an effective way of presenting related data. X-Y recorders have, as a result, become useful as readouts for instrument systems. Recorders are effective when precise X-Y plots are needed to obtain accurate data, or there is a need for rapid interpretation of data. An X-Y recorder automatically plots the value of a dependent variable in relation to the independent variable, if these variables can be converted to electric values.

The X-Y recorder uses servosystems to produce a pair of motions, in the vertical and the horizontal dimensions. These devices are basically two recording potentiometers, one for each variable. The recording potentiometer moves a pen across a chart according to some function of signal voltage. The circuit operates so that if the signal voltage is greater than the standard voltage in the "y" dimension, the pen moves in one direction and if the signal is less than the standard voltage, the pen moves in the other direction in the same dimension. Another servomechanism is used to move the pen in the second or "x" dimension according to the voltage of the second variable (Hewlett-Packard, 1969).

4. ELECTRONIC COUNTERS

Electronic counters provide accurate measurements of frequency and time interval. These instruments can measure frequencies from 0 to 40 GHz (billion hertz) and time intervals from 10 nanoseconds (10 nsec) (billionth of a second) to more than 100 days.

The operating principle of the counter involves comparison of an unknown frequency or time interval to a standard frequency or time. The accuracy of the measurement depends on the stability of this standard which usually is derived from an oscillator built into the counter. This oscillator frequently is a crystal kept in a controlled-temperature oven. When electrically activated, the crystal will vibrate at frequencies varying from 100,000 Hz to 10 million Hz.

All electronic counters have several common circuits as illustrated in Figure 11 (Malmstadt *et al.*, 1962). There are electronic, decade, pulse counters which register the pulses sensed and provide a visual display of the count; a circuit for providing a time base such as the crystal oscillator or the 60-Hz power line frequency; a gating circuit (usually a bistable, flip-flop multivibrator) which controls the starting

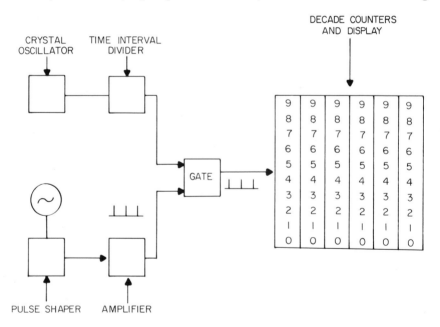

FIG. 11. Simplified block diagram of the common components for electronic counters.

and stopping of the count. There are decade-divider components which will permit a variation in gating time, scaling the output of the crystal oscillator to more manageable time units such as seconds, milliseconds, and microseconds. A Schmitt trigger is available for converting sine wave or other repetitive inputs into pulses which can be handled by the pulse-counting elements. Most counters provide variable control of the display time.

For frequency measurements, the input is first converted to pulses. The pulses are passed through the gating switch into the decade counters. The duration of the counting period is determined by the selected time base. The number of counts during the time when the gate is open is a measure of the average input frequency for the selected interval. Since the period is the inverse of frequency, period measurements are made with the input and time base connections reversed. The unknown input frequency controls the gating time and the decade counters count the pulses coming from the time-base generator.

The most versatile counters, known as "universal" counters, have separate inputs for start and stop commands and separate trigger controls which set trigger level, polarity, slope, and type of input coupling for the start and stop circuits. This type of instrument can measure the interval from one point to another on the same waveform or the time interval between two separate pulses.

Counter measurements are affected by three basic sources of error: ±1 count, time-base stability, and trigger error (Hewlett-Packard, 1969). The ±1 count ambiguity is inherent in all electronic counters because the input signal and time base are not synchronized. As a result, the counter's display may be incorrect by one count. Time-base stability is affected by crystal aging, noise generated internally in the oscillator, changes in line voltages, and temperature. The total inaccuracy in the time base is the sum of the errors from these sources. Trigger error results from noise in the gate-control signal. Because of the noise, the gate will open and close at incorrect times and will produce inaccurate counts. Trigger error is only of concern when an external signal controls the gate.

5. SOUND ANALYZERS

Sound analyzers are instruments which combine many of the components described earlier in the chapter, including a microphone and pre-amplifier, filter, or weighting networks, voltage amplifier, and a meter. The system is basically an audio, rms voltmeter calibrated to give a measurement of sound pressure.

The frequency response of the sound analyzer can be varied by using a filter system which serves a broad-band weighting function or provides band-pass filtering. Three weighting networks are incorporated in the analyzer and are called A, B, and C scales. These weighted curves approximate the inverse of the 40, 70, and 100-phon equal-loudness curves.

The broad-band weighting of these three scales permits gross comparison of the sound pressures from different sound sources. To make finer quantitative analyses, the sound must be divided into spectral components which can be measured individually and analyzed collectively. Band-pass filters must be employed.

Several filter arrangements can be used. The filters may be broad or narrow, active or passive, fixed or variable. Experience with sound level meters led to the acceptance of fixed filters with bandwidths of an octave and, even more preferable, $\frac{1}{3}$ octave.

The sweeping variable filter suffers in quality. As a constant percentage filter, the bandwidth must change continuously as it sweeps. The quality of filter function under these conditions is extremely difficult to maintain. Sweep time is also an important variable. Only the sound in a constantly shifting band can be sampled and measured at a particular time. In order to get over the entire frequency range of interest, the sweep must be rapid enough to measure all the sound components. Sweeping through $\frac{1}{3}$ octaves with a finite time constant does not provide a continuous analysis of the spectrum.

Filter quality is more readily controlled in fixed filters. A fair number of $\frac{1}{3}$ octave filters are required to cover the audible range. Automatic sound analysis can be accomplished with fixed filters and at the same time overcome the problem of slow sweep rate. Each filter is provided with a detector. The output of these detectors can be sequentially sampled electronically. The rate of sampling is independent of filter characteristics and a sweep can be completed in milliseconds, thereby providing a real-time analysis. This type of instrument is relatively expensive and, as a result, may not be available routinely.

The simplest method of frequency analysis employs manual operation of fixed, band-pass filters. This system uses a sound-level meter operating in a linear mode as the indicating system, with the filters being located in the circuit between the input amplifier and an rms detector. A continuous and periodic sound can be evaluated right in the sound field with very little difficulty. The sound is subjected to a selected filter for as long as necessary to make a measurement and then another filter is chosen with the procedure continuing until the entire frequency range is covered. When the sound field to be analyzed is interrupted and transient, the procedure becomes more complex. Usually the sound is recorded by a tape recorder in order to preserve the original waveform.

The sound can then be produced as often as required to complete the analysis.

The heterodyne wave analyzer provides a finer resolution of the spectrum. The sound to be analyzed is modulated by a variable frequency oscillator and passed through a fixed, narrow, band-pass filter usually just a few cycles wide. The frequencies of the original wave which pass through the filter depend on the frequency of the variable oscillator. The resulting effect is that of a narrow filter with a fixed bandwidth varying over the desired frequency range. The output of the filter gives the value of the power spectrum at the specified frequency. Narrow-band wave analyzers give finer resolution than thought necessary for sound-level meters (Hewlett-Packard, 1968).

The sound spectrograph (sonograph) uses a heterodyne-filter circuit and a recorded tape-loop technique. A 2.4-sec sample is recorded magnetically. The heterodyne wave analyzer performs the analysis of the sound as it is reproduced repeatedly. The frequency region is varied over the frequency range of the spectrograph as the recording is repeated. The results are displayed on a special paper moving on drum revolving in synchrony with the sound sample. The resulting display is one of frequency as a function of time. The frequency range covered in the analysis, and the bandwidth of the filter, are dictated by the design of the particular instrument.

Not all sound is continuous and repetitive. Impulsive sounds such as hammer blows, gunshots, and typewriter tapping require special circuitry to provide meaningful and predictable sound measures. The detector must have a shorter time constant (on the order of 35 msec) than other sounds analyzers. The crest factor (ratio of peak to rms) handling capabilities must be increased to ratios higher than 3. The problem of the mechanical inertia of the meter movement must be overcome. Sound level meters are available which seemingly have solved the design problems and produce usable measures of sound impulses.

6. TELEMETRY

Changes in electrophysiologic activity are often used as an indication of the effect of acoustic stimulation on the listener. The electrophysiologic action might be in the form of the galvanic skin response, electroencephalic response, myopotentials, heart rate, blood pressure, etc. Frequently the physiologic signs are influenced by artifacts of the investigative procedure. Wires connecting electrodes to measuring equipment restrict the range of activity for the subject and frequently limit the conditions under which the experiment can be conducted. The presence of the person conducting the investigation may exert an undesirable influence on the subject's behavior. Telemetry offers a possible solution to these kinds of problems.

Telemetry, or biotelemetry, is the technique for gaining and transmitting information from a living organism and its environment to a remote observer (Caceres and Cooper, 1965). While this broad definition is not specific about the method or distance of transmission, the term telemetry has traditionally meant the use of radio transmission over long distances. A biotelemetric system, however, can involve measurement over distances of a few inches or many miles from the observer. The important characteristic is that communication between the subject and the observer is made without direct physical contact.

Frequency-modulated radio transmission has become the most popular telemetry system. A simple block diagram of an FM radio system is shown in Figure 12. The signal source is the subject, human or animal. A transducer turns the signal into an electrical analog. If the signal is electrophysiologic such as an electroencephalograph, no transducer is needed. The signal is amplified and used to modulate a carrier frequency. The carrier is varied in frequency in proportion to the amplitude of the incoming signal. The modulated frequency is increased, if not already a radio frequency, by a frequency multiplier. The modulated radio frequency is delivered to the antenna where it is emitted as electromagnetic energy. The receiving antenna delivers the radio frequency to an amplifier, to a tuning circuit, to another amplifier, and then to a limiter. The limiter clips the waveform, making it a constant amplifier. The information is contained in the number of times the signal crosses its baseline or the number of zero crossings. The amplitude of the transmitted waveform has no effect on the receiver and so no information is lost. The clipped wave is delivered to a discriminating circuit where it is demodulated, changing frequency variation to amplitude variation. The resultant signal may then be filtered and finally presented to the output. This signal should be an accurate reproduction of the original, ready for storage, analysis, or whatever operation is designated by the investigator. The specifics may vary in the system but generally FM radio telemetry involves the procedure and equipment just described.

Frequency modulation has several advantages over amplitude modulation. It is less noisy than AM. It requires less power for a given transmission strength. Important to the investigator is the fact that FM is less sensitive to variations in amplitude of the transmitted signal so that it is less affected by changes in the subject's position.

The goal of a telemetry system is distortionless transmission and, as is true with other systems, this ideal is never achieved. Telemetry is affected by frequency, amplitude, phase, and noise distortion described

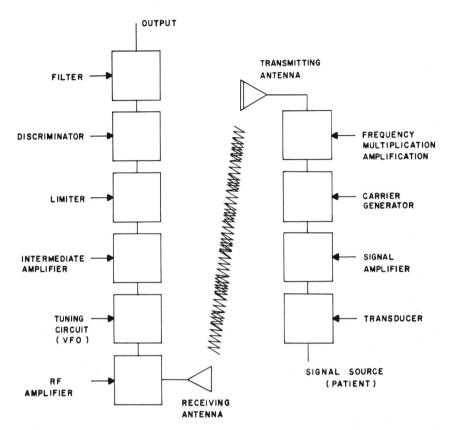

FIG. 12. A block diagram of a telemetry system which uses frequency-modulated radio transmission.

for other psychoacoustic equipment. If all of the parameters of the system are known, the effect on the input signal can be predicted, providing the input signal is known. Knowing the complete characteristics of the telemetry system will allow conversion of the distorted signal back to the original input either mathematically or electronically. With the aid of an analog computer, this conversion has been done for physiological systems where much distortion exists.

E. Tape Recorders

A basic instrument in any hearing program, research and clinical, is the tape recorder. It is a versatile, flexible device with storage of acoustic events as its primary function. The output from a tape recorder sometimes serves as a complex-signal source for subjective evaluation.

The tape recorder may be used to sample a sound environment which cannot be analyzed thoroughly under field conditions, permitting such an analysis at a more convenient place and time. The tape recorder, with appropriate modification, can serve as a programming system. It is a convenient solution for many problems in psychoacoustic investigation.

The essential components of a tape-recording system include, besides the input and output transducers, a constant-speed transport system to move the tape past the recording head (electromagnet), an amplifier to operate the recording head, a high-frequency oscillator to supply a bias current, an erase head, a reproducing head, and a playback amplifier.

The transport speeds used with $\frac{1}{4}$ inch tape vary, but several values have been accepted as standard. The speeds most frequently employed are $1\frac{7}{8}$, $3\frac{3}{4}$, $7\frac{1}{2}$, and 15 inches per second. Tape speed affects tape frequency response. Doubling the speed increases the high-frequency response by an octave. For wide frequency ranges, speeds of 30 inches per second and more may be used. For dialogue, where fidelity is not important, speeds as slow as $\frac{15}{16}$ inches per second have been used. Irregularities in speed of the tape transport produce periodic distortion in recording and reproduction of the signal known as flutter and wow. Rates of change on the order of ten per revolution are called *flutter*, while the term *wow* refers to slow rates such as once per revolution.

Recording and reproducing heads are constructed similarly. Figure 13 gives a diagrammatic sketch of head construction. The head consists of a core of laminated iron in the shape of a ring. The ring is wound with several hundred turns of wire. The magnetic ring is separated by nonmagnetic material, forming gaps.

For recording, the magnetic tape is pulled over the upper poles of the core at the gap. Audiofrequency current flowing through the wire coils causes a varying magnetic flux, similar in characteristics to the applied signal, to be generated in the gap between the pole pieces of the core. The varying flux causes a field to be introduced into the tape, aligning the molecules of the magnetic emulsion into patterns similar to the impressed waveform. The height of the gap influences the frequency response, especially at high frequencies where the height approaches the wavelength of the signal.

In the reproducing mode, the tape passes over the gap in the head and the magnetic flux of the tape causes a voltage to be generated in the head windings. These minute voltages are then amplified and reproduced in a speaker or earphones.

An erase head is constructed much the same as the record and play-

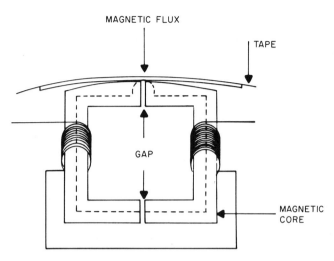

FIG. 13. Simplified operational diagram of a record or reproduce head for a tape recorder.

back head except the erase head may have one or more gaps. The gap length is generally longer than the length of the recorded sound track to assure a complete erasure. The gap height is several times the height of the recording gap. The signal is erased by passing a high-frequency current through the erase head which alters the magnetic pattern on the tape. The tape passes over the erase head before arriving at the record head. A bulk eraser using the 60-cycle line current also might be used to erase the tape. Erasures made with a bulk eraser generally result in a 4–6 dB greater signal-to-noise ratio than those made using the high-frequency bias oscillator alone.

The tape must have close and unvarying contact with the head. Poor contact might result from worn or dirty heads. A worn head will create a reduction in the inductance of the coil, resulting in a loss of sensitivity, especially at the high frequencies. Grooves worn in the head could cause dropouts or unrecorded areas on the tape, or might cause flutter, depending on whether the groove is larger or smaller than the tape. Heads should be cleaned frequently with carbon tetrachloride, acetone, or alcohol.

The record and reproduce heads may be magnetized as a consequence of surges from the motor in the tape transport system, asymmetric waveform from the bias oscillator, working around the recorder with magnetized tools, etc. A magnetized head will increase the noise 6–10 dB and will gradually erase high frequencies from tapes which are played on the recorder. The heads may be demagnetized by using a degaussing tool which consists of coil with a current running through it. Care must be exercised in the use of the degausser since it may magnetize as well as demagnetize.

The alignment of the record and reproduce heads is important for proper function. The reproduce gap must coincide with the position of the recorded track on the tape. The angle of the gap, azimuth, must be a right angle with respect to the direction of tape movement. If the tape recorder uses a common head for both recording and reproduction and the azimuth is not radically out of line, the maladjustment will have little effect. If the tape is used on other equipment, azimuth alignment problems will cause a serious loss of high frequencies, a high noise level, low output, and excessive harmonic distortion. Adjustments are made using a special lineup tape which contains a signal recorded in the proper alignment. The defective head is adjusted until the maximum signal is achieved from the reproduce head.

The tape used for recording consists of a plastic base on which a magnetic emulsion, usually iron oxide, is deposited. The tape itself can produce signal distortion. Modulation noise can be produced by irregularities in the magnetic coating. This type of noise is apparent only when a signal is present and results in a fuzzy reproduction. Dropouts can be caused by discontinuities in the magnetic coating, and if great enough, can produce noise pulses which act as a false signal. Dropouts also can be caused by clumps in the oxides which lift the tape from the recording head, causing a change of flux and a reduction in output.

Another problem with recorded tape is known as "printthrough." This problem refers to the unwanted transfer of a signal from one layer of tape on the reel to another layer by magnetic induction. Printthrough is caused by overmodulation, or recording at high levels approaching saturation. Normal printthrough will induce a signal into an adjacent layer at 50–60 dB below the maximum signal level. Printthrough levels of 20 dB below maximum level are not uncommon when the tape is saturated. This problem really becomes apparent when the investigator wishes to sequence high-intensity signals with periods of quiet.

The normal characteristic of magnetic tape is nonlinear. If recordings were to be made using this nonlinear operating characteristic, the output would be highly distorted. To correct for this nonlinearity, a high frequency current called a bias current is applied to the recording head. With the proper amount of high-frequency current, the recorded signal will be almost linear. The use of a high-frequency bias current when recording increases the signal-to-noise ratio and reduces the harmonic distortion.

The method of recording the input signal directly in its electrical analog form is inadequate for some applications, especially for signals approaching direct current as in the case of electrophysiological phenomena and where large signal-to-noise ratios are necessary. Frequency modulated (FM) recording was developed to meet these needs. In FM recording the input signal frequency modulates an oscillator and the output of the oscillator is recorded on tape. The FM carrier is applied either as a rectangular or sine wave directly to the recording head at an amplitude which will saturate the tape. The tape function is limited in this way to storing times of zero crossings of the FM signals.

The FM recording system has at least a 10–15 dB greater signal-to-noise ratio. This improvement is obtained at the expense of recorded bandwidth. Tape speeds have had to be increased considerably. For example, to obtain a bandwidth of from 0 to 10,000 Hz, the tape speed would have to be 60 inches per second. Frequency modulated recording methods which use high-frequency carriers have made strides in improving the situation but at an increase in the purchase price of the instrument.

F. Computers

The computer has come to serve an increasing role in psychological and physiological investigation. Use of the computer to analyze great quantities of data is perhaps the most familiar function. While this is still an important function, computer technology has expanded the capabilities to include uses which the investigator would find equally important. Computers can be used to develop and evaluate theoretical models of life systems including sensory processes; to analyze bioelectric potentials; for on-line monitoring, stimulating, and modifying living systems. Computers can be used in almost all phases of scientific investigation, experimental design, programming and conducting the experiment, recording responses, distilling and analyzing the data and, if properly programmed can assist in the interpretation of the experiment (Miller et al., 1965).

There are two general types of computers, digital and analog. The digital computer performs arithmetic processes. These devices are large scale, extremely fast automatic calculators capable of handling large quantities of data. The calculations performed by the digital computer could be made by hand but the amount of data and the complexity of calculation would require time expenditures which would be impractical. The digital computer, once properly programmed, can perform the myriad of operations with little or no error.

Analog computers do not deal directly with digits or numbers but with some continuous function being studied. Force, pressures, and displacements may be represented as voltages. The basis for this type of computer is that if two different physical systems can be described by a single mathematic equation, then one of the systems can be used to compute the behavior of the other. These devices are frequently used on-line or in direct connection with the experimental scheme in the laboratory.

In psychoacoustic studies the experimental design must often be complex to control all the relevant variables. As a result, an experiment may be under way for several months without the investigator having a clear idea of the tendency of the results. Computers can be used to analyze the data as the experiment progresses, appropriate revisions in the experiment can be introduced, and the collection of data could be made more efficient. A whole new class of experimental designs has become available. With a computer, it is possible to adopt experimental designs based on sequential statistics and conditional probabilities (Wald, 1947).

In many investigations a signal sequence is presented to the subject in a random order, changing from trial to trial and from subject to subject. This randomization is tedious for the experimenter but is simple for a computer. Signal sequences may have to satisfy other complex conditions. Certain probabilities of occurrence may be associated with particular signals. This task could be assigned to the computer.

Once the experimental design is set, and the equipment for presenting signals and recording responses is ready, the subject can be put into the experiment and data can be collected. It is at this stage that the computer's value is most obvious. The computer can explain the task, teach the subject to respond appropriately, present the stimuli, record responses, provide the subject with feedback, alter the experiment according to performance, repeat instructions, report subjects' performance, and when the session is over, dismiss the subject.

The wide variety of applications for the computer and the importance of this device in psychological and physiological studies of audition must be acknowledged. However, computers are expensive, not only in initial cost and maintenance, but also in programming time. Frequently the expense in time and money required for instrument programming has been underestimated, especially in the case of new applications where programs have not been developed. The investigator must be willing to sacrifice time to learn about the computer and computer programming unless adequate assistance is available. The computer is an instrument which requires expert servicing if there is malfunction. This type of support is also expensive. The potential of the computer however, is so great that these costs will be and should be paid, perhaps not by all psychoacoustic investigators but certainly by a significant number.

III. Instrument Arrangement and Problems

In the preceding sections, individual types of instruments were discussed. These instruments, in most instances, are not used by themselves but serve as essential parts of an equipment arrangement. The instruments must be combined in such a way that they do not interfere with each other or adversely affect the signal. For a good instrumentation arrangement, the characteristics of each piece of equipment must be considered and certain precautions must be taken in their assembly.

Successful, productive instrumentation arrangements depend on intelligent planning before assembly. The user must know what he wants the equipment to do, what he wants to measure, and what range of values he might expect to observe. The investigator does not have to be able to predict exactly what will happen; otherwise it would not be necessary to conduct the investigation. He can anticipate the frequencies, the intensities, and the time ranges which he will encounter. He probably will be able to estimate grossly the variation in responses by the subjects. Without this knowledge, planning will be inefficient and may result in inadequate instrumentation.

A. Interaction

When a number of instruments are combined together there is the distinct possibility of undesirable interaction. Two instruments sharing a common power supply may interact through that supply so that one may provide a positive feedback (in phase) to the other and cause the entire system to oscillate. This situation does not always occur when several instruments share a power supply, but it can. The user should be aware of any restrictions or limitations placed on the equipment.

Interaction may be produced in ways other than sharing a common element such as a power supply. Components in the equipment scheme may be coupled through a common ground, electromagnetically, and capacitively. The signal need not follow the circuit path through the obvious connections between components. Frequently the signal may enter the system by inputs which are obscure and uncontrolled. Signal leak, cross-talk, interference, and high noise levels are familiar problems.

Instruments must have compatible input and output levels. Output levels of a component higher than the rated input levels of the succeeding component may create distortion, fuse burnout, or severe instrument damage. Impedance matching problems are well known and are important enough that they merit separate consideration.

B. Impedance Matching

When two pieces of equipment are connected together in an audio system, the signal transfer will depend on their impedance relationship. Transfer of signal may involve only the transfer of voltage without concern about current, or it may involve power transfer.

In voltage transfers, the only concern is that the driven component does not load down the source and thereby create a distortion problem. When there is a power transfer the impedance problem becomes more complex. Maximum power is transferred when the input impedance is equal to that of the output impedance. If there is a reactive component in the impedance, the greatest amount of current will be transferred when the input and output impedances are conjugates, that is, are equal in magnitude and opposite in phase.

Impedance matching not only influences power transfer, but also affects frequency response, distortion, and damping. The conditions necessary for optimum power transfer may not coincide with those required by the other functions and matching is sometimes a matter of compromise. For optimum frequency response and minimal distortion, as a rule, it is better to have a source of low impedance and a load of high impedance. While some of the output power is sacrificed, risks of frequency and harmonic distortion are reduced under these conditions (Briggs, 1961).

Damping is important in loudspeaker circuits. This damping can be achieved in electromagnetic speaker systems by making the internal impedance of the amplifier lower than the nominal impedance of the loudspeaker. This is accomplished by using negative feedback in the output section of the power amplifier. The damping reduces the magnitude of resonances in the speaker frequency response and improves transient response.

The rated, working output and input impedances may not be the actual measured impedances of a device. A piece of equipment may be designed so that it would function properly with a 600-ohm device but not present 600 ohms to a source or a load.

Attenuator function is influenced by the impedance of instruments which serve as a source and as a load to the attenuator. Insertion loss depends on the ratio of the two impedances. In a decade attenuator when the attenuator is set at 0 dB attenuation, the condition of no-insertion loss indicated by the dial only exists when the impedance of the input device is equal to that of the output device. Under any other impedance condition, the first step of the attenuator will not attenuate by the amount specified by the indicator. In equipment arrangements where the attenuator does face an impedance mismatch, the nonlinearity of the first unit of attenuation must be considered.

C. Interference and Shielding

One of the most common problems in instrument systems is that of interference from external sources. The chief source of interference is that from the 60-cycle power line serving the building which houses the equipment. The current in these power lines can enter the signal circuit by capacitive and electromagnetic coupling. The power line has a varying voltage and is separated from the input lines of a circuit by a layer of air. A finite capacitance develops between these two elements as illustrated in Figure 14A.

Electromagnetic coupling results from magnetic fields being generated by the power lines. These varying magnetic fields exert an influence on the input circuits of equipment as diagrammed in Figure 14B. The phenomenon resembles that of radiowave transmission. The power line serves as an antenna and the inputs act as receivers. This type of interference is usually greater at high frequencies but can be a significant source of interference even at 60 cycles.

The result of the capacitive and electromagnetic coupling is current flow in amplifier input circuits. The voltages developed depend on the values of resistance through which the current must flow to ground. As a consequence, high-resistance circuits are much more susceptible to 60-cycle interference than those of low resistance. The magnitude of the interference depends on the gain of the amplifier stages in the circuit.

The interference from the power source is heard as hum in audio systems which has a frequency of 60 and/or 120 Hz. The power line itself is the source for 60 cycles while the source for 120 Hz is likely to be a power supply with its full-wave rectifier. Signals other than hum may be transferred from one circuit to another. This type of interference is referred to as cross-talk or signal leak.

One of the most effective methods for eliminating interference from external sources is to shield the sensitive parts of the circuit by surrounding the wire leads with a conductive material and by putting low-level amplification circuits in a conducting metal container. The shield must be grounded as shown in Figure 14C. If there is a finite resistance between the shield and the ground, a capacitive coupling will occur between the shield and the input line, thereby rendering the shield ineffective.

Noise can result electronically from the instruments themselves. The

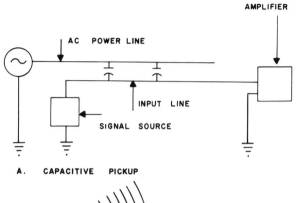

A. CAPACITIVE PICKUP

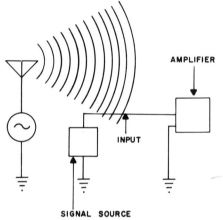

B. ELECTROMAGNETIC PICKUP

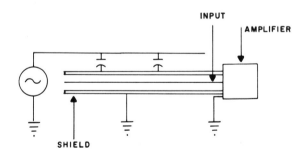

C. SHIELDING ACTION

FIG. 14. Block diagrams illustrating capacitive (a) and electromagnetic (b) coupling with external sources of interference. The action of shielding in eliminating interference is pictured in the third diagram (c).

electronic elements can develop noise by thermal agitation of electrons. If tube filaments are heated by 60-cycle alternating current, they may represent another noise source, especially in sensitive instruments. Tubes may be microphonic and, as a result, introduce ambient sounds into the circuit.

D. Grounding

Interference very frequently results from poor grounding techniques. One of the most annoying problems with instrumentation is called a ground loop. If the shielding of a circuit is grounded in more than one place, the shield itself will form a circuit with ground and may induce extraneous signals to the system as indicated in Figure 15. Ground loops are difficult to track down. The equipment arrangement should minimize the possibility for these loops to occur. All ground connections should be brought to a single, carefully grounded point.

The effectiveness of shielding and the effective operation of the components in an instrumentation scheme depend on making good electrical contact with the ground of the power lines supplying the building in which the equipment is contained. The radiators and water pipes in a laboratory are often used for grounding and are frequently not good grounds.

A good ground may be established in at least two ways. The best way is to make a direct connection with the earth. Copper rods are laid in trenches dug several feet into the ground outside the laboratory building. A large bus bar (conductor) is run to the laboratory from these rods. If the connections for the rods and the bus bar are well made, a good ground will result.

A second method for making an effective ground is to install a large bus from the ground of the fuse box supplying the laboratory. The bus must lead to the laboratory and be distributed to the equipment for convenient use. This method may not always be effective. Frequently

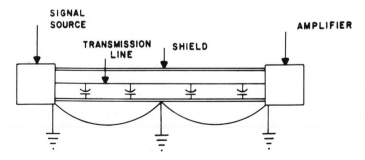

FIG. 15. Ground loops created by an unintentional ground of a bare shield.

the lines from the fuse box to the actual ground for the entire electrical system possess a finite resistance and are therefore slightly above ground or "float."

E. Calibration of the System

At any given time, an instrument or a group of instruments may stop functioning or may not function as planned for the equipment scheme. If the investigator can detect and repair the malfunction, there is no great problem. If the problem falls outside his competence, he must know how to get it corrected. Having the services of a trained electronic technician and access to an electronic workshop is extremely helpful if not indispensable.

When an instrument stops working completely, it presents no problem for detection. However, an instrument may continue to operate, but not according to plan. This condition represents a more difficult situation for detection. An instrument is functioning correctly if the output is related to the input by a set of specifications governed by the instrument design. The final indicator of proper function or malfunction is the output of the instrument. This general rule may also be applied to an instrument assembly. The functional state of the equipment should be determined at the end point and this, in most instances, is the output of the earphone or the speaker. The performance of the individual components should be established when planning and assembling the units into an instrument scheme. The final output should present the signal at appropriate levels, with minimal extraneous interference and distortion, and with a dynamic range suitable to the planned investigation. This condition must be determined before the investigation is started. The operating levels of the signal source, the amplifiers, attenuators, mixers, switches, and other signal modifiers should be noted in the initial calibration. The acoustic output of the transducer should be measured using signal levels which will actually be employed in the investigation, noting the input-output relationship. The input to the transducer may then be used as a monitor point for the entire instrumentation scheme throughout the course of the investigation.

A monitoring system consisting of an oscilloscope, a true-rms vacuum-tube voltmeter and an electronic counter connected in parallel with the input of the transducer provides an indication of the overall operation of the instrument ensemble. However, the ear of the investigator should not be neglected as a detector of malfunction. Listening to the output can reveal harmonic distortion, annoying interference, distracting transients, and inadequate signal level. The behavior, response, and reports of the subjects may also serve as clues to instrument malfunction.

Tracking down a defective instrument or instruments involves logic. If the input electrical signal shows no great change but there is a decrease in sound level produced by the transducer or an increase in distortion, the problem obviously is in the transducer. If the input signal is altered, then the problem originates at some instrument earlier in the assembly. The monitor point is moved along the instrument arrangement from output to input transducer until the deviation in performance is no longer observed. The defective instrument is isolated and, if possible, replaced. The system check then is repeated.

Once the instrument problem is found, the investigator must decide what is to be done. Some of the problems are relatively minor and can be remedied on the spot. Replacing fuses, tightening connections, resoldering contacts, replacing wires and tubes fall into the category of first-line maintenance. Other problems may require that the defective instrument be checked intensively in the electronic workshop by qualified personnel. In the shop the instrument circuit may be thoroughly checked. Defective resistors, capacitors, transformers or other electronic components are replaced. Adjustments are made in operating voltages and currents. The instrument is put into working order and calibrated to assure performance according to specification. If the electronic technician is not able to handle the problem in the workshop, the instrument may have to be returned to the manufacturer. A general rule of instrument maintenance is that required maintenance should not be attempted if it exceeds the limit of information and equipment available.

References

American Standard Method for the Coupler Calibration of Earphones, Z 24.9-1949. American Standards Association, Incorporated, New York.

American Standard Method for the Calibration of Microphones, S 1.10-1966. American Standards Association, Incorporated, New York.

Behar, M. (ed.) (1951). "Handbook of Measurement and Control." Instrument Publ. Co., Inc., Pittsburgh, Pa.

Beranek, L. L. (1949). "Acoustic Measurements." Wiley, New York.

Beranek, L. L. (1954). "Acoustics." McGraw-Hill, New York.

Bernstein, J. L. (1966). "Audio Systems." Wiley, New York.

Bogert, B. P., and Peterson, G. E. (1957). The acoustics of speech. "Handbook of Speech Pathology " (L. E. Travis, ed.). Ch. 5 pp. 109–173. Appleton, New York.

Briggs, G. A. (1961). "A to Z in Audio." Gernsback Library, Inc., New York.

Caceres, C. A., and Cooper, J. K. (1965). Radiotelemetry: A clinical perspective. In "Biomedical Telemetry " (C. A. Caceres, ed.). Ch. 5 pp. 85–105. Academic Press, New York.

Hewlett-Packard, (1968). "Acoustics Handbook." Hewlett-Packard Company, Palo Alto, California.

Hewlett-Packard, (1969). "Electronics for Measurement, Analysis, Computation."

(Ref. Cat.). p. 138 and pp. 588–592. Hewlett-Packard Company, Palo Alto, California.

Malmstadt, J. V., Enke, C. G., and Toren, E. C. Jr. (1962). "Electronics for Scientists." Benjamin, New York.

Miller, G. A., Bregman, A. S., and Norman, D. A. (1965). The computer as a general purpose device for the control of psychological experiments. *In* "Computers in Biomedical Research. Volume I" (R. W. Stacy and B. D. Waxman, eds.). Ch. 19 pp. 467–490. Academic Press, New York.

Molnar, C. E., Loeffel, R. G., and Pfeiffer, R. R. (1968). Distortion compensating condenser-earphone driver for physiological studies. *J. Acoust. Soc. Amer.* **43**, 1177–1178.

Shaw, E. A. G. (1966). Ear canal pressure generated by circumaural and supraaural earphones. *J. Acoust. Soc. Amer.* **39**, 471–479.

Stacy, R. W. (1960). "Biological and Medical Electronics." McGraw-Hill, New York.

Tremaine, H. M. (1959). "The Audio Cyclopedia." Howard W. Sams & Co., Inc., The Bobbs-Merrill Company, Inc., Indianapolis and New York.

Wald, A. (1947). "Sequential Analysis." Wiley, New York.

Zislis, T., and Fletcher, J. L. (1966). Relation of high frequency thresholds to age and sex. *J. Auditory Res.* **6**, 189–198.

Chapter 9

Adaptation and Fatigue

W. DIXON WARD

University of Minnesota

I. Early History

Temporary changes in auditory perception induced by acoustic stimulation have been studied by scientists only for the past 120 years, even though metalsmiths probably noticed millenia ago that loud noises cause a temporary loss of hearing, just as a brief flash of light produces a temporary blindness. By now, enough evidence has accumulated to show that auditory adaptation is quite a complex process or perhaps a set of complex processes. Indeed, although the title of this chapter might give the impression that *fatigue* and *adaptation* are easily separable, the terms have been used loosely and interchangeably for so long that it may be better to use a completely different classificatory scheme in approaching the topic. It appears reasonable to distinguish the phenomena commonly included under *adaptation* in two different ways: whether they are observed during or after exposure to the acoustic stimulus (concomitant or residual, respectively), and whether they require one ear (monaural) or two (binaural) for their measurement. By 1881, at least one example of each of the four categories—concomitant monaural, concomitant binaural, residual monaural, and residual binaural—had been identified. Let us take them in chronological order.

A. Concomitant Binaural: "Perstimulatory Adaptation"

To my knowledge, the first investigation of auditory adaptation of any sort was that of Dove (1859) who noted, during the course of a study of binaural beats, that if one ear were exposed for some time to a tuning fork, then binaural presentation of this same frequency would result in perception of a tone only at the unexposed ear. This is a demonstration of what has now become known as "perstimulatory adaptation"—a shift in the lateralization of a diotic tone following a period of monotic adaptation to a steady sound.

B. Residual Binaural: Loudness Reduction and Timbre Change

The next experimenter to deal with auditory adaptation was apparently J. J. Müller (1871), who did so more or less incidentally during the course of a dispute with Helmholtz over the nature of aural harmonics. Müller led the sound of a tuning fork to both of his ears by means of a stethoscope. First a fork of frequency n was presented to one ear at the highest intensity he could muster, while the tube to the other ear was squeezed shut. He then quickly substituted a fork of frequency $n/2$ and then squeezed the two tubes one after the other, so that he was able to listen with the exposed and nonexposed ears alternately. Under these conditions, he had produced a slight fatigue at what was now the second harmonic of the lower-frequency fork, and therefore noted that "im ermüdeten Ohr war der Ton stets weniger klangreich und schien etwas schwächer [p. 118]." By observing this change in timbre, Müller demonstrated (a bit indirectly) that in fatigue, the loudness of a weak but suprathreshold tone at the frequency of the adapting stimulus was diminished.

C. Residual Monaural: Temporary Threshold Shift (TTS)

However, it remained for Victor Urbantschitsch (1881) to prove that not only was loudness diminished, but that absolute sensitivity was also decreased. He used apparatus similar to Müller's, but with two completely separate tubes to the two ears. He first matched the ears of his observer by having him listen alternately with the two ears as the tone from the tuning fork gradually decayed. In case perception disappeared in one ear before the other, he reduced the sound reaching the more sensitive ear, either by constricting the tube or by moving the pickup end of the tube farther from the fork, until the tone disappeared simultaneously at both ears. Next he exposed one ear to a large (hence slowly decaying) fork for 10–15 sec. At the end of this exposure period, he damped the fork with his finger, as rapidly as possible, until the tone was just audible. As soon as it disappeared, he switched to the other ear, noting how much longer it was audible in the unfatigued ear. If we knew the rate of decay of his fork, we could calculate the magnitude of this first deliberately produced temporary threshold shift (TTS)—or at least we could if he had been more specific than saying merely that the tone was heard in the control ear for "several seconds" longer.

I call this a "residual monaural" phenomenon because although Urbantschitsch happened to use a binaural method, this was only necessitated by the primitive methods then available for study of auditory phenomena. Today, of course, electronic control of acoustic stimuli permits direct measurement of the change in absolute threshold without using the other ear as a reference.

Urbantschitsch's studies demonstrated a frequency specificity for TTS that has since been substantiated. At the intensities involved here (probably not above 80 dB sound pressure level), exposure to a low frequency did not affect the threshold of a high frequency, nor did high-frequency exposure affect low-frequency threshold, whether the exposures were given successively to the same ear or simultaneously to different ears. Finally, he showed that the loudness reduction demonstrated by Müller (1871) lasted only a few seconds: Instead of damping the fork to just *above* threshold immediately after the fatiguing exposure, he damped to just *below* threshold, and noted that it reappeared after about 1 sec (at most 5 sec); alternate comparison with the control ear revealed that from this point on, the loudness was the same in both ears.

In the same year Thompson (1881) made it clear that if one preexposes an ear to a loud tone, protecting the other ear by holding it closed, then subsequent testing at the same frequency under normal listening conditions will show errors of localization, the apparent source of the sound being shifted away from the preexposed side. This is less ambiguous an example of perstimulatory adaptation than was Dove's (1859) observation.

D. Concomitant Monaural: "Tone Decay"

About the same time, in March 1881, Lord Rayleigh (1882) was demonstrating to Helmholtz still another aspect of auditory fatigue: the phenomenon that is today called "tone decay." Lord Rayleigh produced a sustained tone by means of a "loaded gas bag" (balloon) driving a bird call whose fundamental frequency was about 10,000 Hz (10 kHz). He noted—and evidently Helmholtz agreed—that the tone soon disappeared, but that a brief interruption (merely waving the hand in front of the ear) was enough to bring it back into consciousness.

These four "classical" aspects of adaptation—tone decay, perstimulatory fatigue, temporary threshold shift, and loudness reduction—still dominate their respective categories. However, other phenomena have also since been observed, and these will be considered in the appropriate sections.

II. Concomitant Monaural

A. Tone Decay

Following Lord Rayleigh's (1882) discovery of tone decay, considerable effort was expended in an effort to find out what it meant. Jacobson (1883) observed that in some patients, a weakly struck tuning fork may actually be heard longer than one struck more vigorously. Huijsman (1884) later treated tone decay at some length, showing that it occurred much more often at high frequencies. In 1890, Corradi demonstrated that tone decay also occurs in bone conduction; if, after the tone disappears, the fork is taken off the mastoid and replaced, it can again be heard by some patients. Corradi therefore used as diagnostic measurements the duration of perception at the first application of the fork, that at the second (reapplication), and so on. In 1893, Gradenigo mentioned a procedure in which, using his "telephonic audimeter," he increased the intensity in successive steps as perception ceased. Even with a small sample of cases, he noted that tone decay was marked "in cases of neuritis (caused by trauma, compression)." However, Schäfer (1905) insisted that not everyone experiences tone decay even at high frequencies: he could hear Lord Rayleigh's bird call indefinitely. Rhese (1906) found no consistent difference in the degree of tone decay between normal ears and persons with middle-ear pathology. Bleyl (1921) tested persons with normal hearing, conductive losses, perceptive losses, and "miscellaneous," but found no consistent differences among the groups.

These results, negative except for Gradenigo's, no doubt account for the fact that tone decay as a diagnostic tool had to be rediscovered much later, under the impetus of K. Schubert's (1944) extensive monograph (even though Schubert himself was not particularly sanguine about the clinical value of the phenomenon). In 1957, Carhart proposed as a formal clinical test an adaptation of the procedure proposed by Gradenigo (1893) and studied at length by Schubert (1944). A steady tone is presented at threshold and the subject told to indicate when it disappears. If it remains audible for a minute, that ends the test at that frequency. If, however, it disappears in less than a minute, the intensity level is increased by a fixed amount—5 dB for the Carhart procedure—and the duration of perception is once again measured. If this too, disappears, then the level is raised another 5 dB, etc. The severity of the tone decay depends on the final level reached. In certain cases decay is even "complete" in that the highest intensity available on the audiometer disappears.

The underlying physiological correlate of tone decay is generally assumed to be an absence of ability of neural elements to fire continuously. They presumably will fire normally at onset of a tone or in response to a sudden change in level, but if the level is sustained, then all activity quickly ceases. A parallel can be drawn between such tone decay and the disappearance of a steadily fixated visual target; if, by means of a feedback system, one moves a visual target in order to compensate for all voluntary and involuntary movement of the eye, so that the target stimulates precisely the same area of the retina at all times, then after a few seconds the target will disappear. This general notion is consistent with observations that (1) as the percept gradually fades away, there is often a period during which it is still audible but appears noisy or even loses tonality altogether (Schubert, 1944), and that (2) the listener often reports hearing the tone being turned *off* even though it had completely disappeared (Dunlap, 1904).

A considerable body of literature has developed in the past decade bearing on the classification of degrees of tone decay into categories and on the usefulness of this test for clinical diagnosis, but the upshot seems to be merely a confirmation and extension of Gradenigo's observation that pronounced tone decay is often associated with tumors that exert pressure on nerves of the auditory system. One of the most recent studies, for example, is that of Parker *et al.* (1968) who found severe tone decay (complete in most cases) in 20 persons with confirmed pontine disease and 29 with nerve fiber lesions. Hence grossly abnormal tone

decay is highly suggestive of a retrocochlear lesion of the auditory system. However, it is far from conclusive evidence, because moderate and
even severe tone decay is sometimes observed in cochlear pathology,
and thus must be used only as one element of a battery of tests from
which a diagnosis is made (Johnson, 1968). Some rules of thumb distilled
by Stroud and Thalmann (1969) from their experience are that the
likelihood that the tone decay is a manifestation of a retrocochlear problem, rather than a cochlear one, is higher (1) the greater the total decay;
(2) the more rapid the disappearance of the tone; (3) the greater the
relative involvement of the lower frequencies (1000 Hz and below);
and (4) the lower the threshold for interrupted tones.

When tone decay is present, its influence can often be seen in tests
other than the formal tone decay test itself. The most obvious manifestation is in Békésy audiometry when the test tone is continuous. Reger
and Kos (1952) noted that when one tested at a single frequency in
a person with acoustic neuroma, the indicated threshold gradually shifted
toward a higher and higher intensity. Even when the frequency is continually shifting, the tone decay induced by the threshold-level tone
may be considerable, so that in such cases a larger separation between
Békésy audiograms gathered using continuous and using interrupted
tones emerges. Indeed, this separation provides the basis of the widely
used categorization of comparisons between continuous- and inter-
rupted-tone Békésy audiograms proposed by Jerger (1960); his Types
II, III, and IV all involve an apparently more-sensitive threshold for
interrupted than for continuous tones.

The magnitude of tone decay, as indicated by direct test or Békésy
comparison, is critically dependent on the stimulus parameters. A sudden
change in level of as little as 1 dB is generally enough to restore perception, just as Lord Rayleigh originally observed. Jerger (1960) attributes
the failure of earlier investigators to find an interrupted-continuous disparity to the fact that they used attenuators with step sizes of 1 or
2 dB. Sudden jumps of this magnitude apparently are large enough
to bring enough "unadapted elements" into play that the integrated
"on-effect" is perceptible.

Suzuki et al. (1964) actually measured the effect of amplitude modulation of an otherwise continuous tone on the standard tone decay test
(1-min duration criterion). In a group of four listeners with sensorineural
loss, the total amount of tone decay at 4000 Hz was reduced from about
20 dB with an uninterrupted tone to 16 dB with 1-dB increases and
decreases, to 10 dB with 2-dB steps, and about 3 dB with 3-dB steps;
with 4-dB steps, there was no tone decay.

Harbert and Young (1962) have shown that for an interrupted test tone, the Békésy disparity is sharply dependent on the off-time. In a patient who had suffered "accidental injury to the seventh and eighth nerves during attempts to inject the Gasserian ganglion," the Békésy tracing to a 1000-Hz tone had a midpoint of about 4 dB hearing level (HL) when the 400-msec tone bursts were separated by 400 msec of quiet, but changed to 15 dB HL when this interval was decreased to 200 msec. With 100-msec pauses, the asymptote was at 35 dB HL, 50 msec gave 50 dB HL, and 25 and 12.5 msec gave results indistinguishable from the indicated "threshold" for a continuous tone (about 62 dB HL).

This patient would be said to have a "critical off-time" (the point at which the curve relating off-time to threshold shows a break) of more than 200 msec as defined by Jerger and Jerger (1966). These authors reported similar studies on six patients; in their group, this critical off-time ranged from 200 msec down to 40 msec.

Dallos and Tillman (1966) studied the effect not only of off-time but also of frequency modulation on the Békésy disparity, finding that in their patient, a slow modulation rate (less than 10 per second) and a frequency range of at least 40 Hz was needed to prevent complete tone decay at 500 Hz as inferred from the Békésy tracing.

Various modifications of the Carhart procedure have been championed by one investigator or another, but it is still to be shown that the value of the results is enhanced by changing the criterion period from 1 min to 30 or 90 sec, by inserting a silent period between the successive steps, or by putting a weak noise in the contralateral ear.

Clinically, then, a marked tone decay, especially "accelerated tone decay" (in which the higher the intensity is raised, the shorter the duration of perception) at more than one frequency is a sufficient, but not a necessary, indicator of acoustic neuroma. Slight amounts of tone decay, and even accelerated tone decay at only a single frequency (Ward et al., 1961a) cannot as yet be regarded as diagnostically significant.

B. Change in Maskability with Time

It has long been known that the ability of a sustained stimulus to mask a test tone does not change with time. Even if the activity of neural elements stimulated by the sustained tone does decline with time, these are presumably the same elements that respond to the masked stimulus, and so the signal-to-masker ratio remains constant. Interestingly enough, however, the reverse does not hold: the *maskability* of a sustained tone by noise does increase with time. That is, a tone sustained for a minute or so can be masked by noise that is a few decibels weaker than that required immediately after onset. In normal listeners, the effect is small—only 5–10 dB (Feldmann, 1958; Thwing, 1956). Indeed, Bocca and Pestalozza (1959) indicate that they were not able to demonstrate any change in maskability with time in normal listeners. However, they give no details of procedure, and since Müller (1970) has recently published data in essential agreement with Thwing's, using a narrow-band noise masker, it seems safe to assume that the effect is real. It might well be expected that persons with marked tone decay will also show an enhanced change in maskability, and Bocca and Pestalozza did indeed find this to be true. However, the relation between tone decay and maskability change is not completely unambiguous: Müller (1970) describes a 61-year-old man with a moderate high-frequency loss who showed more than twice as great a change in maskability at 1000 Hz as normals and yet displayed no tone decay at all.

C. Change in Loudness

Under some conditions, as an exposure continues, the loudness of the adapter decreases. This is obviously the case, of course, for low-level adapters that finally disappear. In the normal ear and with exposure intensities above 70 or 80 dB SPL, however, if one asks the listener whether the fatiguing tone seems less loud after being on for a minute or two, he will generally answer "no." Because estimates of loudness changes generally involve comparison with the unstimulated ear, I will defer their discussion until later.

D. Change in Difference Limen for Intensity (SISI)

The SISI test (Jerger et al., 1959) involves the detectability of 1-dB increments superimposed on a steady tone. If a sustained stimulus did diminish steadily in loudness, it is conceivable that the SISI test might be affected, the first increments being more easily heard than later ones because the difference limen (DL) for weaker tones is, in general, larger. However, this does not seem to occur. Lüscher and Laepple (1958) found no change in the DL at 8 dB HL after 5 min of steady exposure, and although Plath (1967) has recently reported some changes of DL with time, these are not even monotonic: His DL's *decreased* during the first 30 sec and then increased. Also, his DL's were so small (0.1 to 0.2 dB) that the envelope characteristics of the increments to be detected certainly must have been quite different from those usually employed in the SISI test. Further study is indicated.

III. Residual Monaural

When the term *auditory fatigue* is used without explicit definition, what is usually meant is temporary threshold shift (TTS), a topic that has received a great deal of experimental attention since Urbantschitsch's

1881 discovery of the phenomenon. The most recent clinical interest in the topic is derived from a suggestion (Peyser, 1930; Temkin, 1933) that one might be able to predict individual differences in susceptibility to permanent damage from high-intensity sound by means of individual differences in the TTS produced by a much less intense exposure.

Figure 1 illustrates the basic scheme for the measurement of TTS. Although this paradigm is exactly as shown only for short-duration effects, it is applicable in principle to the longer-term effects as well. A TTS-arousing stimulus (the "fatiguer") is presented for a period of time T. Then the test stimulus of duration τ is presented at a time t after cessation of the TTS-arousing stimulus. If the testing is repetitive, then the duration of the total cycle—that is, from onset of one TTS-arousing stimulus to the onset of the next—will be designated by $\mathfrak{I}$. The change in detection threshold for the test stimulus, relative to the "resting" (pre-exposure) threshold, in decibels, is the threshold shift. If the threshold later returns to the original value, the threshold shift was temporary (TTS); if it does not, however, the difference between the new asymptotic threshold and the original one is a measure of permanent threshold shift (PTS), and a threshold measured before the asymptotic value is reached is defined (Miller et al., 1963) as a "compound" threshold shift (CTS).

It will be realized that the determination of TTS is nowhere near as simple as it sounds, being subject to all the problems that beset the concept of threshold in the first place. The classical meaning of the word *threshold* was a fixed and definite energy barrier: If the signal

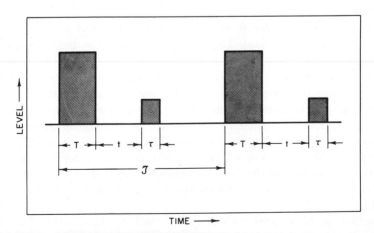

Fɪɢ. 1. Schematic temporal program for studying TTS. A fatiguing stimulus of duration T is followed, after a pause t, by a test stimulus of duration τ. In case the test is repetitive, the total cycle duration is $\mathfrak{I}$.

energy exceeded this level, it would be perceived; if the energy were less than this critical value, it would not. No one takes such a view seriously any more; it has been amply demonstrated that the signal energy necessary for detection is dependent on the shape and duration of the tone, the psychophysical method, the placement of the earphone, the instructions to the listener, and indeed, most of his past history. Even if these are held as constant as possible, there will still be considerable fluctuation of this "threshold" as indicated by the fact that at one moment a certain signal may be perceived, although at another moment a slightly stronger signal may be missed. This inherent variability of response is consistent with the notion that the task of signal detection, whether weak or strong, is always that of discriminating signal-plus-noise from noise alone. In the case of the "absolute" threshold, the noise is presumably all generated internally, but the task is still really the detection of a signal in a masker. It is well known that a person sitting in an anechoic room in "utter quiet" begins hearing his own body noises, such as breathing noise and heartbeat, superimposed upon a more steady background noise. When you are listening for a weak tone, therefore, you must distinguish the tonal signal from this physiological background—which, of course, meets the description of masking. So, in any event, if we want to study threshold shifts, either concomitant with or following exposure to some auditory stimulus, we must try to make sure that all conditions (including, hopefully, the internal noise) are as nearly the same during the determination of the shifted threshold as they were during measurement of the resting threshold.

And of course one must decide at the outset just what arbitrary definition of threshold to adopt. For example, suppose the modified method of limits is to be used, the method commonly known as the "Békésy" method (Békésy, 1947). After selecting the repetition rate and duration of the pulses (if pulses are to be used), signal shaping, rate of change of attenuation, and instructions to the subject, one still has to decide whether "threshold" should be defined as the median (or mean?) level necessary to "just hear," the level necessary to "just not hear," or the average of the two. Once all these arbitrary choices have been made, one can only hope that the threshold changes obtained will be comparable to those obtained with a different criterion (a hope that is not always fulfilled).

Another problem arises when one is running experiments involving more than one session with a given observer. Should the shifts on a given day be based on the preexposure threshold determined on that day or on the *average* resting threshold over the entire experimental period? The long-term average is intuitively more appealing, but its use assumes that the differences one observes from day to day are truly random instead of systematic. It would therefore be inappropriate if, for example, the listener were gradually shifting his response criterion, or if he had a cold that affected the transmission of sound to the inner ear on a particular day. In actual comparisons of the two alternatives, neither emerges as a clear victor (for example, Ward, 1968) : the test–retest variability is just as high when the average threshold is used as when the shifts are calculated on the basis of the threshold for that day, which means that some, but not all, of the day-to-day variability is due to conductive factors. For practical purposes, then, it is generally more efficient to base calculations on the that-day threshold, since we need then neither wait until the end of the entire experiment before calculating shifts (a foolhardy practice, because errors that could be corrected may go unnoticed until too late) nor calculate everything twice.

Obviously, anything that affects any part of the auditory chain can produce a shift in threshold. For example, all the following (at least) could conceivably be involved in TTS: residual middle-ear-muscle activity; displacement of the tectorial membrane relative to the basilar membrane; change in chemical environment of the hair cells; swelling of hair cells, making stimulation more difficult mechanically; an increase in internal noise, as for example due to increased blood flow ("pounding in the ears") or an audible tinnitus; changes in or results of efferent activity at the basilar membrane, and of course, ordinary poststimulatory decrease in nerve excitability, which could occur in the eighth nerve, cochlear nucleus, lateral lemniscus, inferior colliculus, medial geniculate, or acoustic cortex. It is no wonder, then, that there are several types of TTS. Classification is commonly made on the basis of the duration of the effect, so that convention will be followed here. However, duration of TTS is usually related monotonically to the severity (some product of intensity and duration) of the fatiguer, so that one could just as well classify types of TTS on that basis if one wished.

A. Ultra-Short-Term TTS: "Residual Masking"

In 1910, Schulze observed that if one simultaneously sounds a tuning fork and a monochord, with the latter so loud that it masks the former, then if the monochord is suddenly damped, the tuning fork is not heard immediately, but becomes audible only after a fraction of a second. The threshold, that is, has been shifted, and nowadays one determines, using the paradigm of Figure 1, just what the threshold *is* at various recovery times (t), instead of merely showing, as Schulze did, that it was first below and later above one fixed level. But for some reason,

the exact form of Schulze's demonstration has apparently influenced
what this very-short-term TTS is called. The tuning fork is masked
by the monochord; the monochord is turned off, yet the tuning fork
is still not audible—hence this is *residual masking* (Munson and Gardner, 1950)! Lately it has also been called *forward masking*, a term even
more incomprehensible unless one is aware that it was coined to be
the opposite of *backward masking*, in which a weak tone is rendered
inaudible when followed by a stronger signal. I dislike the term *residual
masking* because it implies that the shift in detectability of a weak
signal following high-level stimulation is due to an after-discharge of
neural elements ("off-fibers") that provides interference with the neural
effects of the weak signal. It seems more likely, from the evidence, that
what is involved here is not interference caused by such after-discharge,
but rather simply a manifestation of the ordinary run-of-the-mill refractory period of nerves: after it fires, a given nerve fiber cannot be fired
for a certain period (the absolute refractory period) and then, for an
additional length of time, requires greater input energy than normal
to be fired (the relative refractory period). However, no simple substitute
term suggests itself; so "residual masking" will be used to designate
that portion of TTS that disappears within a second after exposure,
even though there is probably very little masking involved.

Because in residual masking, as in TTS in general, there are so many
parameters to be studied, no one investigation has been able to cover
more than a fraction of them using enough listeners to allow much confidence in the results. Besides the various temporal parameters T, t, τ,
and $\mathfrak{J}$, the intensity and the frequency characteristics of both the fatiguer
S_f and probe tone S_p can be varied. However, a few generalizations can
be made. At levels of S_f up to 90 dB SPL or so, the shift is greatest when
S_f and S_p have the same frequency, as one would expect. The spread of
effect is asymmetric, frequencies of S_p higher than that of S_f showing
more effect than those below; however, the degree of asymmetry is
greater in some studies (for example, Zwislocki and Pirodda, 1952)
than in others (Harris and Rawnsley, 1953). The Zwislocki and Pirodda
study also indicates that the residual masking at some fixed time t is
proportional to the SPL of the fatiguer. The shift is relatively independent of the duration of S_f, from 100 msec up to a few seconds, as
long as the intensity of S_f is low enough that full recovery occurs within
half a second (that is, for levels up to 70 dB SPL) and the course of
recovery is exponential in nature, which means that if one plots the TTS
against the logarithm of the recovery time t (or against $t + \tau$, which
some authors prefer), a straight line results. These last two generalizations are illustrated by the data in Figure 2 (Bentzen, 1953). The differ-

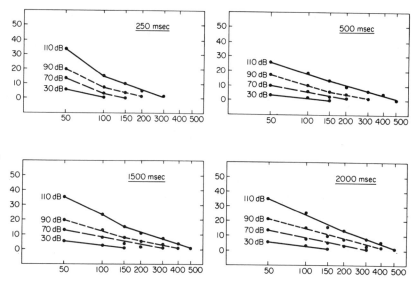

Fig. 2. Recovery of short-term TTS at 1000 Hz (ordinate) following exposure to a 1000-Hz adapting tone having durations of 250, 500, 1500, and 2000 msec. The abscissa is the delay t in milliseconds (plotted logarithmically) between the adapting tone and the 20-msec test tone. The parameter in each box is the level of the adapting tone. [From Bentzen (1953).]

ences between the residual masking from a 250- and a 2000-msec fatiguer appear to be negligible, as are most of the departures of the recovery curves from linearity.

Attempts to use residual masking as a clinical tool have not occurred in America, but in Germany the "Kietz Test" enjoys some popularity. A white noise is periodically (about twice a second) interrupted for a short time [the first descriptions of the method indicate 40 msec (Langenbeck, 1959) but apparently the standard value is now 70 msec (Langenbeck and Lehnhardt, 1970)]. The level of a pure tone that is on continuously is adjusted so that it is just audible during the pauses. With the particular parameters specified, the shifted threshold of the tone, for normal listeners, lies about halfway between the threshold in quiet and the masked threshold for masker levels that generate 60 dB or less of masking, remaining at 30 dB below the masked threshold for higher values of masker levels. If the difference is significantly smaller than 30 dB (say only 5–10 dB when the noise produces a 70-dB SPL simultaneous masked threshold), this is abnormal. It is said (Langenbeck and Lehnhardt, 1970) that such an indication is characteristic, for example, of Meniere's disease.

The Kietz test, of course, involves not only residual masking but also backward masking, so the magnitude of the total threshold shift will depend on how the effects combine. A recent study by Pollack (1964) provides information relevant to this question, and at the same time demonstrates the inappropriateness of the term *residual masking*. A 1000-Hz tone pip was sandwiched between two bursts of noise, and the effect on the tone-pip's threshold of varying the temporal distance between the pip and each of the maskers was determined.

Figure 3 is typical of the results obtained. In this case the noise bursts had a duration of 50 msec and a level of 120 dB SPL, while the tone-pip's duration was 5 msec. It can be seen that the curves are (within the experimental error) parallel, which means that the amount by which the second noise burst shifted the threshold (the backward masking) was independent of the amount of "forward masking." That is, for example, the presentation of the second noise burst 4 msec after termination

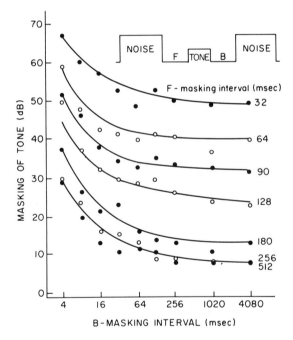

FIG. 3. Interaction of "forward" (F) and "backward" (B) masking. The ordinate represents the relative threshold of a 5-msec tone pip sandwiched between two 120-dB SPL 50-msec noise bursts. The parameter F is the pause between the end of one noise burst and the tone pip, while the ordinate (B) is the interval between tone pip and the subsequent noise burst. Three listeners. [From Pollack (1964).]

of the tone pip raised the threshold by about 20 dB more than when that particular interval was 1 sec or longer, regardless of whether "residual masking" had elevated the threshold by 4 dB (when the tone pip followed the first noise by 180 msec) or by 40 dB (when the noise-to-tone interval was 32 msec). In essence, the second noise has the same ability to override (mask) the more slowly traveling neural activity produced by the tone pip once it overtakes it, regardless of how intense the tonal signal had to be in the first place in order (1) to overcome fatigue (adaptation) processes ascribable to the first noise burst and thereby (2) to initiate neural activity along the auditory chain.

Thus a Kietz-test threshold shift represents the simple sum of the shifts in decibels produced by very-short-duration fatigue and by backward masking. So if the Kietz test does indeed have any diagnostic value, it would seem worthwhile to measure the two types of shift separately, to see whether its ability to detect certain types of malfunction is due to individual differences in very-short-term TTS or in backward masking.

B. Short-Term TTS: Low-Level Adaptation

A second type of TTS is also associated with exposure to moderate levels of pure tones. If the duration of a fatiguer below about 85 dB SPL is a minute or so, then in addition to the transitory residual masking, a more persistent TTS can be measured; it is likely that this is the type of TTS first observed by Urbantschitsch (1881). The first actual measurement of such TTS was done by Wells in 1913. In collaboration with physicist Harvey Curtis at the National Bureau of Standards, he determined the current driving a "specially constructed telephone" at the listener's threshold, for a frequency between 60 and 3000 Hz. Then the current was increased by 10, 100, or 1000 times for 1–5 min. Thus their exposures were to tones 20, 40, and 60 dB above the individual's threshold—that is, at 20, 40, and 60 dB sensation level (SL), although of course Wells could not say so because the decibel had not yet been invented. Besides confirming the frequency-specificity of TTS noted by Urbantschitsch, Wells showed that full recovery occurred within a couple of minutes, and in addition provided an illustration—perhaps the first, but certainly not the last—of the hazards of drawing generalizations on the basis of SL, when he concluded, from the fact that 60 dB SL of 60 Hz gave more TTS than 60 dB SL of 900 Hz, that low tones were more hazardous than medium-frequency ones. At 60 Hz, the typical threshold (assuming purity of signal) would be about 60 dB SPL. Hence a tone 60 dB above threshold would have a SPL of 120 dB—at least 40 dB greater than the SPL of a 60-dB SL tone at 900 Hz. Consequently,

some 10,000 times as much energy would be sent to the ear at 60 Hz
as at 900 Hz. It is hardly surprising that there was a difference in
the effect!

Subsequent experimentation on short-duration TTS established certain
facts. (1) The TTS is maximal at the exposure frequency, with a reasonably symmetrical spread to closely adjacent frequencies (Causse and
Chavasse, 1947). (2) This particular type of TTS is relatively independent of the level of the fatiguer, up to 90 dB SPL or so, being
nearly the same following an exposure at 20 dB SL as at 80 dB SL
(Flügel, 1920; Hirsh and Bilger, 1955; Lierle and Reger, 1954). (3) The
TTS increases with exposure time, but by 1 min has essentially
reached its maximum value. (4) Approximately the same magnitude
of TTS is produced by frequencies of about 800 Hz or above (the greatest
amount seldom exceeds 15 dB), but at or below 500 Hz, little TTS
of this variety can be demonstrated (Causse and Chavasse, 1947).
(5) The TTS is much diminished if an interrupted test tone is used
instead of a continuous one, and complete recovery occurs more quickly.
This result should not be surprising, however, because the continuous
test tone serves to maintain the fatigue. Thus interposition of a quiet
(rest) period between exposure and test should also reduce the TTS,
and this is indeed what happens. The longer the quiet period, the less
the TTS, so that if a full minute of quiet is provided, then no TTS
will be measured, even though if testing had been continuous, a 3- or
4-dB average TTS would still have remained after 1 min (Bell and
Fairbanks, 1963).

This last point is important if one is to avoid erroneous conclusions
about the influence of various parameters on TTS. One must, when using
a continuous test tone in a Békésy audiometer, make sure that the recording attenuator is set at precisely the same spot immediately postexposure for all conditions. Otherwise the magnitude of the indicated
TTS may be artifically inflated by the tendency of a continuous tone
to maintain this type of adaptation. For example, in an experiment
in which the effects of mental arithmetic on TTS were to be studied,
the listeners were exposed to a 40-dB SL tone for 3 min twice, once
while they were required to do mental arithmetic, and again while "in
reverie." The outcome was that more TTS was produced in the "mental
arithmetic" condition (Wernick and Tobias, 1963). However, it must
be noted that if the automatic audiometer had been turned on right
at the end of the 3-min exposure period, then while the listener was
writing down the final answer to his mental arithmetic problem (which
consisted of successive division of a large number by a smaller one),
the intensity of the test tone would have been merrily increasing; by

the time he finally got his finger over to the voting button the level would be 15–20 dB above the starting point, and so probably well above even the "true" shifted threshold, and therefore capable of maintaining the state of adaptation. This hunch (Ward, 1966) was confirmed by Price and Oatman (1967), who showed that inserting even a 5-sec post-exposure delay eliminated the difference between conditions in TTS.

Only a few attempts have been made to use this type of adaptation in a clinical test. Lierle and Reger (1955) exposed patients with various types of loss to 20-dB SL stimulation, but in many of their patients the sensorineural loss was as high as 85 dB HL, so that the exposures involved SPL's of over 100 dB; one should hardly be surprised that their threshold shifts were more persistent than those of normals!

For losses that are primarily conductive in nature, however, this criticism does not apply. In this case, "20 dB SL" probably does represent about the same energy entering the cochlea for the patient as for the normal. One would expect, therefore, that the adaptation should also be the same. However, this does not seem to be the case. Although a 3-minute exposure at 20 dB SL produces the same initial TTS in conductives as in normals, the conductives recover more slowly (Epstein *et al.*, 1962). Katz and Epstein (1962) suggest that this may be associated with the relative disuse (that is, nonexposure to sounds of high loudness) of these ears, and to support this view Katz gave the 20-dB SL test to normals after an earplug had been worn in the ear concerned for 5, 10, or 15 hours. He found a 10-dB greater TTS in the ear that had been "deprived" of stimulation for 15 hours. But any type of conductive loss will apparently produce this "disuse" phenomenon, since there was no difference between otosclerotics and nonotosclerotics (Epstein *et al.*, 1962), so there seems to be little of diagnostic value in this area.

C. Sensitization or Facilitation

Not all shifts in threshold are in the direction of decreased sensitivity. Under some conditions, an enhancement of detectability may be observed that, like low-level adaptation, also lasts only a few minutes (Josephson, 1934). Unlike it, however, sensitization seems to be best produced by exposure intensities between 70 and 100 dB SPL, and is more pronounced for exposure frequencies below 1000 Hz than above (Hughes, 1954). Although the maximum sensitization occurs at the exposure frequency itself, nearly as much is produced at adjacent frequencies. In experiments involving an increase of the intensity of the exposure tone on successive runs, an effect can be seen earlier (that is, at a lower level of exposure tone) for test frequencies below the exposure frequency than for those above it (Noffsinger and Olsen, 1970). There also appears to be greater sensitization to a continuous test tone (Hughes, 1954) than to an interrupted one (Noffsinger and Tillman, 1970), although a direct comparison does not seem to have been made. Finally, sensitization is not restricted to the ear exposed: Hughes (1954), using a special apparatus to produce an interaural attenuation of 85 dB, found nearly as much sensitization at 500 Hz after stimulation by a 500-Hz 85-dB SPL tone in the contralateral ear as after ipsilateral stimulation.

D. "Rushing Noise" Tinnitus

In 1935, Ewing and Littler reported hearing an internal noise, like rushing water, that lasted for a minute or two after cessation of a fatiguing tone. Later, Hirsh and I noticed that there was a coincidence between the appearance of sensitization and the course of this rushing noise (Hirsh and Ward, 1952). However, the effect seemed to be exactly opposite to what we would expect. Immediately after cessation of a 3-min exposure to a 500-Hz tone at 100 dB SPL, for example, this rushing noise appeared, and then, about 1 min after exposure, rather swiftly faded away, to be replaced by "dead silence" (except, of course, for the test tone). One would expect, therefore, that if this noise were providing masking of the test tone, then the least sensitive threshold would be found at the time of maximum rushing noise, and the most sensitive at its disappearance. However, the exact reverse was true. The greatest sensitivity existed during the maximum of the rushing noise, and when the noise disappeared—thus making the job of signal detection subjectively much easier for the listener—the threshold rose, often rather dramatically, by as much as 10 dB, resulting in a diphasic recovery curve. Obviously, then, this can hardly be an example of masking, and we must instead view the noise as perhaps indicating a higher rate of spontaneous discharge of neural elements, correlated with a truly enhanced sensitivity. In view of Hughes's (1954) finding that the contralateral ear also displays sensitization, these elements must include some that are fairly central—unless, of course, the noise represents a bilateral efferent discharge. Further study of this phenomenon seems to be indicated.

E. "Ordinary" TTS: Physiological Fatigue

Shifts persisting for more than 2 min may be regarded as a true "fatigue," and as early as 1930, Peyser suggested that these longer-lasting effects might be classified as either "physiological" or "pathological," the latter presumably being the precursor of permanent threshold shifts caused by chronic exposure to industrial noise. If such a concept has any validity, and if it is true that danger of permanent loss exists when a TTS caused by one day's noise exposure has not recovered before the next day's exposure begins, then perhaps a reasonable "critical value" of recovery time is 16 hours, or about 1000 min. Accordingly, *physiological fatigue* will be used to describe TTS's enduring more than 2 min but less than 16 hours. In general, this will include values of TTS_2 (TTS 2 min after cessation of exposure) up to about 30 dB, although exceptions will be cited later.

This is not to say, of course, that this type of TTS does not exist until 2 min have passed. Rather, the measured TTS following moderately severe exposures is a *combination* of adaptation, sensitization, and physiological fatigue, and only after the first two have run their course (or have become negligible in effect) can one see the third alone. Thus it is not necessary for the postexposure TTS to drop below the preexposure value for us to deduce that a sensitization process was acting; if the recovery from physiological fatigue alone is monotonic, which seems reasonable, then a short-lived improvement within the first minute or so after cessation of exposure (a "bounce") implies that sensitization was responsible. If we knew that sensitization, adaptation, and physiological fatigue all acted at different places in the auditory chain, so that one might expect simple summation of effects, then we could separate them out by inference. However, it is not at all certain that the locus of sensitization (if, indeed, there is a single locus) is actually separate from that of the others.

On the other hand, it appears, from an experiment by Selters (1964), that adaptation and physiological fatigue are independent and hence summate. First Selters determined the course of adaptation for 3000 Hz following, for instance, 30 dB SL. Then he exposed the ear to a more intense stimulus, one that required several hours for full recovery. When the persistent TTS had recovered to about 15 dB, he once again exposed the ear at 30 dB SL (which, of course, was actually 15 dB higher in intensity; however, since the adaptation in a rested ear due to a 30-dB SL tone is indistinguishable from that following a 45-dB SL tone, this is permissible). The observed TTS was now precisely the same as before, but superimposed on a 15-dB pedestal, so to speak. For example, in the unfatigued ear, the TTS at 3000 Hz 1 sec after cessation of a 10-sec 30-dB SL tone also at 3000 Hz was about 7 dB. In an ear with a 15-dB persistent TTS, the TTS 1 sec after the 10-sec tone was 22 dB. Selters concluded that because persistent TTS is probably due to fatigue at the hair cells, the adaptation process must occur somewhat more centrally.

1. Recovery

When full recovery is complete within 16 hours after exposure, the course of recovery is exponential, being rapid at first (that is, 2 min following cessation of the fatiguer, while the short-lived processes run their course), then slowing down. An exponential process is one that changes by a given fraction during any given time interval. That is, if the TTS takes 20 min to drop from 20 dB to 10 dB, then it will also take 20 min to drop from 10 to 5, from 5 to 2.5, etc. Such exponential processes are characteristic of many biological systems. Thus if one plots TTS on the ordinate using a logarithmic scale and linear time on the abscissa, the course of recovery will be a straight line. Recent discussions of several exponential processes involved in TTS have been presented by Botsford (1968) and Keeler (1968). Theoretically speaking, perhaps one should always use such a representation in presenting data on either growth or recovery of TTS in time. However, for all practical purposes, an exponential process also gives a straight line when the variable (TTS in this case) is given in linear decibels (which is already, of course, a logarithmic transform of energy) and time is scaled logarithmically. Reid (1946) seems to have been the first to plot recovery in this way.

We have found (Ward et al., 1959a) that a single set of average recovery curves does a fairly good job of fitting the course of recovery from moderate TTS's. This set of curves is shown in Figure 4. It was derived, however, from normal ears that had been given a single near-continuous exposure of up to 2 hours in duration following complete recovery from previous TTS's, and although we proceeded to use these curves as if they applied to conditions beyond those under which they were derived, this was a mistake. Recovery is not quite as rapid for TTS's produced by 8-hour exposures to noise, or when the TTS is the result of a series of exposures with time for recovery in between. Such general curves can, however, be used in the interpretation of tests designed to study individual differences in susceptibility to TTS.

2. Exposure SPL

The TTS 2 min after cessation of exposure, TTS_2, grows approximately linearly with SPL, once the level has exceeded a certain "critical" value below which only short-duration effects are produced. This critical SPL, inferred from 2-hour exposures to octave-band noise, appears to be about 70 to 75 dB (Ward et al., 1959a), for noises above 1000 Hz in center frequency. That is to say, a 75-dB SPL noise will not produce much TTS_2 no matter how long it is on; a 105-dB SPL noise will produce

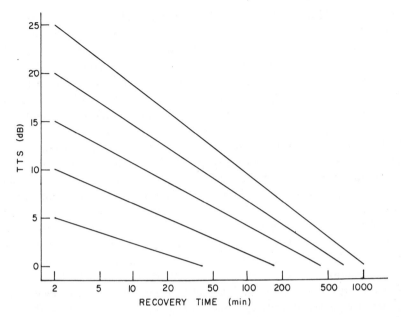

FIG. 4. Idealized average curves of recovery from TTS, for normal listeners, following 2-hour exposures to noise. [From Ward *et al.* (1959a).] A somewhat slower recovery follows 8-hour exposures, in general (Ward, 1970), while slightly faster rates are observed after exposures only a few minutes in duration (Ward, 1968).

about twice as much TTS_2 as one at 90 dB, for a given duration of exposure, and a 100-dB SPL noise will generate a value of TTS_2 halfway between those following 90 and 110 dB. For exposure frequencies below 1000 Hz, this critical level may be even greater than 70 dB SPL; the relevant general experiments have not yet been done, although the implication of a recent study by Mills *et al.* (1970) is that for their one subject, the critical level for an octave band centered at 500 Hz was 74 dB SPL. The actual rate of growth with level, of course, will depend on the exposure duration and on the exposure frequency; higher frequencies have a greater rate of growth than low frequencies, even when the critical intensity is the same.

3. DURATION

The main exception to the rule that TTS increases with intensity occurs at very high levels. In the classic Harvard study of the effects of high-intensity noise (Davis *et al.*, 1950), it was noticed that a given exposure to 130 dB SPL sometimes produces *less* TTS than the same exposure at 125 dB SPL. This observation has been confirmed by Trittipoe (1958), Miller (1958), and Ward (1962b). The most likely explanation for this reversal is that the mode of vibration of the stapes may change at very high levels, a change that is in turn produced by the maximum contraction of the middle-ear muscles (Békésy, 1949).

The middle-ear muscles may also affect the growth of TTS with intensity in a less dramatic manner. Even at intensities too low to produce the shift in mode of vibration of the stapes (80–120 dB SPL), the incoming signal produces some reflex arousal of the stapedius muscle (Møller, 1962), and this action tends to reduce the amount of signal energy reaching the inner ear, hence reducing the TTS produced. Since the degree of arousal increases with intensity, this self-limiting action does also, and therefore the observed growth of TTS with intensity will have a lower slope than it would if the middle-ear muscles were inoperative. The picture is further complicated by the fact that low frequencies are attenuated more by the action of the muscles than the high frequencies; above 2000 Hz, the transmission of sound is apparently unaffected by the contraction of the reflex. One would therefore expect that the growth of TTS with intensity should be more rapid for high-frequency than for low-frequency stimulation, and indeed this does seem to be the case. Although other factors may be involved (for example, it is conceivable that the high-frequency sensory elements are inherently more fragile than the low-frequency elements), it is clear that the auditory reflex plays an important role in limiting TTS at low frequencies.

The TTS_2 is approximately proportional to the logarithm of the exposure duration, up to 12 hours. This implies an exponential growth that reaches a maximum after about 12 hours (Mills *et al.*, 1970). Thus if a 15-min exposure produces a TTS_2 of 10 dB, and a 30-min exposure one of 15 dB, then a 1-hour exposure will result in a 20-dB TTS_2, etc. The actual rate of growth with time, again, will depend on the particular frequency and level of the fatiguer. Figure 5 illustrates the growth with time of TTS_2 at 4000 Hz for various intensities of a 1200–2400-Hz noise.

4. Test Frequency

Unlike the short-duration shifts, longer-lasting TTS's are asymmetrically distributed relative to the exposure frequency. When pure tones are used as fatiguers, the maximum TTS_2 is found at a progressively higher frequency as the intensity is raised, sometimes becoming as much as two octaves above the stimulating frequency (van Dishoeck, 1948), although it is more generally 0.5 to 1 octave above. Even at the highest intensities studied, there has been no evidence of TTS peaks at multiples of the stimulus frequency.

The above characteristics of TTS from pure tones are also true of

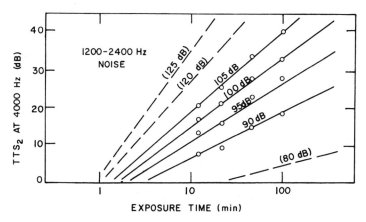

FIG. 5. Growth of TTS₂ at 4000 Hz following exposure to octave-band noise at several different intensities (parameter) as a function of exposure time; note that time is plotted logarithmically. [From Ward et al. (1959a).]

TTS produced by noise (Ward, 1962b): the maximum effect after high-level exposure is generally found one-half to one octave above the upper cutoff frequency of the noise (not one-half to one octave above the *center* frequency of the noise). Maximum TTS from impulse noise can be found at nearly any frequency in particular ears (Ward *et al.*, 1961b).

5. EXPOSURE FREQUENCY

It has already been mentioned that the higher the exposure frequency, at least up to 4000 or 6000 Hz, the greater the TTS produced. Therefore damage-risk criteria (intensity limits of noise that can be tolerated without serious risk of permanent hearing loss) generally permit exposure to higher levels in the 150–300- and 300–600-Hz octave bands than in the 600–1200- and 1200–2400-Hz bands (Kryter *et al.*, 1966).

A second characteristic of most well-known damage-risk criteria is that pure tones are assumed to be more dangerous than octave bands of noise (Anonymous, 1956). However, this was an assumption that was based on the critical-band hypothesis. The notion (Kryter, 1950) was that if a given amount of energy were concentrated within a single critical band, it would be more dangerous than if it were spread over several critical bands (for example, over an octave). However, recent research has shown that the critical-band hypothesis is no more pertinent in explaining TTS than it is in explaining the masking at high intensities. Although pure tones below 2000 Hz do indeed produce more TTS than corresponding octave bands of noise when both are at the same intensity, the effect is adequately explained by the difference in the ability of the two stimuli to produce sustained reflex arousal of the middle-ear muscles. When a pure tone is presented, the muscles, after an initial contraction, rapidly relax. However, a noise produces a more sustained reaction, presumably because of its random nature, which continuously rearouses the reflex. Therefore more energy reaches the basilar membrane under pure-tone exposure conditions. That the reflex, not the critical-band hypothesis, is the determining factor here was supported by two lines of evidence (Ward, 1962b). First, the TTS produced by a very narrow band of low-frequency noise ($\frac{1}{8}$ octave in width) was consistently less than that produced by a pure tone at the same frequency, despite the fact that both stimuli were less than a critical band in width and were equal in overall energy. The second demonstration was more involved. The TTS produced by the tone was measured, next the TTS produced by the noise. Finally, the TTS produced by the tone was again measured, but this time the noise was simultaneously presented to the other ear. Because a reflex-arousing stimulus activates both reflexes nearly equally, the middle-ear muscles of the ear receiving the tone were now as strongly contracted as when it was receiving the noise. The TTS due to the tone in this case dropped to the same value as that produced by the noise.

At low frequencies, then, pure tones are indeed more dangerous than noise, not because one is "concentrating energy in a small area," but because of the aural reflex. However, it should be clear that since the difference in degree of activation of the muscles during exposure to tone and noise respectively is a function of level (and of frequency), any single "correction factor" is at best a poor approximation. Ideally, damage-risk criteria for pure tones should simply be developed independently of criteria for octave-band noise.

TTSs produced by impulse noise differ only in minor details from those produced by tones and noise. The average maximum TTS produced by gunfire, for instance, is often at 6000 Hz instead of the 4000 Hz which is usually the maximum after broad-band noise; but this relation is not dependable enough to allow one to infer, from the fact that a particular permanent loss has a maximum at 6000 Hz, that this loss was caused by gunfire. The most striking difference between TTS's from steady noise and impulse noise is that the latter grow linearly with time instead of exponentially—as if each impulse produced the same fraction of a decibel of TTS (Ward et al., 1961b).

6. INTERMITTENT EXPOSURE

When the exposure is intermittent or varies in level with time rather than being continuous and steady, the action of the middle-ear muscles becomes even more important because even a short rest will at least partially restore their contractile strength. Let us therefore first consider the effect of intermittency at the higher frequencies, or more specifically, at 4000 Hz, where the muscles have little effect. Here the basic relation is again quite simple: If, during the total exposure time T (in this case, T is the time from the beginning of the first exposure burst to the end of the last), the exposure stimulus is only on a certain fraction R of the time, then the TTS produced will be, as a first approximation, only R times as great as that produced by a continuous exposure at that level (Ward et al., 1958). For example, if a certain noise produces a TTS of 30 dB after a 1-hour exposure, then a 1-hour exposure to a noise at the same level but one that is on for 30 sec, off for 30 sec, etc., so that $R = 0.5$, will result in only 15 dB of TTS. This relation holds for burst durations ranging from a quarter of a second or thereabouts (Rol, 1956) up to about 2 min (Selters and Ward, 1962).

When the exposure is to low frequencies, intermittency causes an even greater reduction of the resultant TTS than that produced in high-frequency exposures, presumably because of the recovery of protective action of the auditory reflex that occurs between bursts. Where an on-fraction of 0.5 produces a 50% reduction in the TTS produced by and at high frequencies, it may result in a reduction of 70% or more in the TTS from low frequencies (Ward, 1962a).

For noise bursts shorter than 0.2 sec or longer than 2–3 min, somewhat more TTS is produced than the on-fraction rule would predict (Rol, 1956; Selters and Ward, 1962). Furthermore, there is evidence that the rule also breaks down for combinations of very small on-fraction (0.1 or below) and very high intensities (above 110 dB), conditions that are found, for example, in sonar operation. Considerable research is still needed on TTS from short stimuli.

For longer burst durations, however, the cumulative final TTS can be predicted reasonably well by means of successive application of growth and recovery functions, together with what I have called the "exposure-equivalent rule" (Ward et al., 1959b). The exposure-equivalent rule is that the TTS already existing at the beginning of a particular noise exposure can be treated as additional time of exposure to the noise concerned. For example, if the TTS still existing (from an earlier exposure) at the onset of a 15-min noise burst is the value of TTS_2 that would have been produced by a 10-min exposure to the noise, then the TTS_2 at the end of the 15-min burst will be equal to the TTS_2 produced by continuous exposure for $10 + 15 = 25$ min. By successive applications of empirical equations for growth and recovery of TTS, the TTS from any complicated exposure can be predicted, although the procedure is quite tedious. The picture is further complicated by the fact that the course of recovery is somewhat slower when the TTS is the result of intermittent exposure than when it is produced by a single uninterrupted noise. In other words, it takes longer for full recovery from a TTS of 20 dB caused by an intermittent noise than from 20 dB of TTS_2 following a steady but lower-intensity exposure.

However, over a fairly large range of parameters, the TTS from an intermittent noise will be proportional to the on-fraction or smaller, so this rule of thumb can be used in calculating equinoxious exposures. Now, what about a noise that varies more irregularly in time? It appears (Ward et al., 1958) that provided that the level at all times exceeds the critical level (the level that just fails to produce TTS lasting 2 min or longer), the TTS will be a function of the *average* SPL. Thus a noise that has an intensity of 90 dB SPL half the time and 110 dB the rest of the time will produce a TTS that is equal to that produced by 100 dB acting continuously. (Again, the restrictions on burst length apply: if the periods at either level exceed 2 min, then one must calculate successively the growth of TTS during the louder periods and the partial recovery during the quieter ones.)

A final principle that applies to varying or intermittent exposures is that while the level is below the critical level, recovery proceeds just as fast as if the ear were in complete silence. After octave-band noise exposure, for example, the ear apparently recovers as fast in a noise below about 70 dB SPL as in quiet (Ward, 1960a).

All the foregoing discussion leads to the following generalization: the TTS produced is proportional to the average, over the total exposure time, of the quantity $S - S_0$, where S is the noise level and S_0 is the critical level, with negative values of $S - S_0$ excluded.

Figure 6 illustrates the point by showing four different 3-min segments of exposure to broad-band noise that will give approximately the same TTS. The critical level is indicated by the dashed line. A noise that fluctuates between $C + 20$ and C (Figure 6a) will produce no more TTS than one that goes from $C + 20$ down to $C - 15$ or even lower (Figure 6c); in both cases, the average value of $S - S_0$ over the total period is 10 dB, so the TTS will be the same as that produced by a steady noise at $C + 10$ (Figure 6b). Finally, Figure 6d shows a noise that varies irregularly over a large range; but since the average amount by which it exceeds the baseline is 10 dB, the same TTS will be produced as in the other three cases.

Notice that this does not indicate that "the ear integrates *energy* over time." Within limits, it does average *decibels* (although only decibels above the critical level), but this is not energy. The total amount of energy in the exposures pictured in Figures 6a, c, and d is much

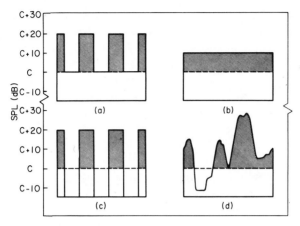

FIG. 6. Four different patterns of steady, intermittent, or interrupted exposure to broad-band noise that will produce approximately the same TTS$_2$ at 4000 Hz (see text).

greater than in Figure 6b; since halving the energy is equivalent to a 3-dB change in level, the total energy involved in Figures 6a and c is for all practical purposes the same as that produced by a continuous exposure at C + 17. However, a continuous exposure at C +17 would produce much more TTS$_2$ than any of the exposures shown. Thus much more total sound energy is required to produce a given TTS when the exposure is intermittent. Extension of this principle to permanent losses from noise may be responsible for the observation that although a continuous 8 hour per day, 5 day per week exposure to 90 dBA produces permanent damage in a few years, many persons who are exposed to noise levels well above 110 dBA do not suffer much permanent hearing loss—for example, miners (Sataloff *et al.*, 1969), chain saw operators (Kylin, 1970), and rock-and-roll musicians (Rintelmann and Borus, 1968; Speaks *et al.*, 1970). In these cases, the exposure apparently is sufficiently intermittent to keep the effective average level at a near-tolerable level.

The problem with the notion of a "critical level" at the moment is the determination of just what this level is. Our early experiments (Ward *et al.*, 1958, 1959a) implied that the critical level was 80 to 85 dB SPL for broad-band noise, about 70 dB for high-frequency octave bands. However, a direct test by several different laboratories has indicated that the true values are somewhat lower. Schwetz *et al.* (1970) found that recovery from a 20-dB TTS$_2$ was significantly retarded if the listeners were exposed to 75-dB SPL noise instead of silence during the recovery period. In addition, a series of studies at the University of Bochum reported by Klosterkötter (1970) indicate that 70 dB SPL is not equivalent to real quiet in regard to TTS from intermittent exposure, either. For example, when 10-min bursts of 105 dBA were alternated with 10-min periods of 90, 80, 70, or 30 dBA the TTS_2 after 2 hours of total exposure was significantly higher for 70 dBA intervals than for 30 dBA ones. The true values of critical levels are still to be determined, it appears, and of course it is possible that the critical level for growth of TTS may be significantly higher than the critical level for normal recovery.

7. INTERACTIVE, LATENT, AND RESIDUAL EFFECTS

A finding related to the preceding section is that even when noise *is* intense enough to produce TTS at one frequency region, it will not affect the course of recovery at frequencies outside this region (Ward, 1961). This was shown by an experiment in which a 1-hour exposure to a high-frequency noise was (1) preceded or (2) followed by a 1-hour exposure to a low-frequency noise. Although both noises produced considerable TTS at frequencies just above the corresponding noise frequency, neither had any effect on the growth or recovery of shifts produced by the other. Apparently the course of the fatigue process at one area of the basilar membrane (if that is indeed the locus of this variety of TTS) is relatively independent of conditions existing at other areas.

Just as noises that do not produce a TTS lasting 2 min or longer fail to influence the recovery from TTS from a prior exposure, so these noises do not enhance to a measurable degree the magnitude of TTS produced by a subsequent exposure (Ward, 1960a). Thus *lateral* effects of stimulation are negligible. However, a study by Harris (1955) indicates that *residual*, though subliminal, effects may sometimes be found. He repetitively restimulated his listeners with a TTS-producing stimulus just as the TTS from the previous exposure "reached zero" and found that the TTS gradually increased. The implication is therefore that the ear may still be under the influence of fatigue processes for some time after it is no longer possible to measure them by means of TTS. However, because of the difficulty of determining when the threshold has indeed recovered its preexposure value, further study is indicated in order to make sure that what is involved here is not just a cumulative effect of intermittent exposure.

8. MISCELLANEOUS FACTORS

Despite much experimentation, little direct effect on TTS by vitamins and other chemicals has been adequately demonstrated. The largest effect reported in the literature is a reduction of TTS_2 from 24 to 12 dB by the administration of hydergin, a sympathicolytic agent (Plester, 1953); however, this effect has not yet been confirmed. Doing arithmetic in one's head or other mental activity does not change the TTS produced, although Chernyak (1958) claims that some unnamed Russian investigators found less TTS to be produced by a given noise if the listener were hypnotized and told he was in silence. A recent report by Hörmann (1968), however, demands closer scrutiny. In this ingenious experiment, subjects were given a stylus tracking task whose difficulty was such that the subject was "on target" about half the time. In one group of subjects, a noise of 95 phons indicated that they were on target, in the other that they were not. The former group showed a 10-dB TTS, while the latter gave 18 dB, as if a "negative" noise were more dangerous than a "positive" one. Since there was a possibility that subjects might have been performing just a bit better in the "positive" condition (and so getting less noise), the experiment was repeated, but in this case a fixed 50%-on noise tape was used for both groups. The subjects worked without visual feedback and so had no idea that their performance was completely unrelated to the noise. Nevertheless, the same difference was found: the group for whom the noise meant "success" showed less TTS than those for whom it spelled "failure." In view of the past history of such "central" effects, however, it would be wise to wait for confirmation of this effect from other laboratories before concluding that the efferent system may play a role in this variety of TTS.

9. RESTING THRESHOLD

The foregoing material was based on normal listeners. Obviously persons with impaired hearing will show *less* TTS—but for different reasons, depending on whether the loss is conductive or perceptive. In the case of a pure conductive loss, the effective level of sound reaching the cochlea is reduced, so that, for example, if a TTS of 25 dB is produced in a normal ear by a certain exposure at 100 dB SPL, then a person with a 25-dB conductive loss will show the same 25-dB TTS only after exposure to 125 dB SPL.

Individuals with pure end-organ (recruiting) perceptive losses will also show less TTS than normal individuals, but in this case because they have less to lose, as it were. The energy entering the cochlea of such a person is no different from the normal case. But if there is already a considerable loss of sensitivity, then the *threshold shifts* produced by a given noise will be less than in normals, even though the *shifted threshold* of the impaired ear is always higher.

Figure 7 illustrates the point. This figure shows the relation between

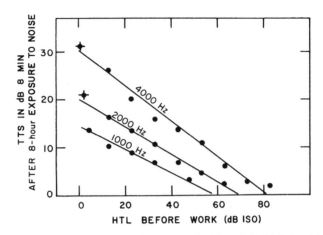

FIG. 7. Relation between TTS 8 min after a day's work in high-level broad-band noise and the resting (preexposure) threshold hearing level for a sample of 81 workers. Test frequency is the parameter.

resting threshold and the TTS produced at 1000, 2000, and 4000 Hz by an 8-hour exposure to noise in a group of 81 workers whose noise environment was unusually uniform (so that all men could be assumed to have received the same exposure). The 162 ears were categorized in terms of hearing level (HL: threshold re audiometric zero) at each frequency, and then the average TTS produced in each category of HL was determined about 8 min after leaving the noise. The two points at the extreme left represent the TTS expected, from empirical equations (Ward *et al.*, 1959a), in normal listeners (that is, men with 0 dB HL). It is clear that the TTS decreases linearly with HL. Thus where the normal ear would show a TTS at 2000 Hz of 21 dB, an ear with a 30-dB resting HL would show only 11 dB. But the shifted threshold of the latter will be 41 dB HL, compared with only 21 dB HL for the former. In other words, after exposure to a given noise, ears with end-organ deafness will still require greater signal energy for hearing than will normal ears. So the fact that he shows less TTS does *not* mean that he is "better off"—the acquisition of a permanent loss from noise does not constitute protection against further loss.

F. Long-Lasting TTS: "Pathological Fatigue"

Under some conditions, the recovery from TTS neither proceeds in the exponential manner described in Section III,E,1 nor is complete by the end of 16 hours of rest. Instead, when plotted in the ordinary way (TTS versus the logarithm of time), the curves are convex downwards.

As a first approximation, this "delayed recovery" proceeds in nearly a linear manner—that is, diminishing by a constant number of decibels each day. Delayed recovery has long been known to occur if the TTS_2 produced by a single noise exposure exceeded 40 dB or so (Reid, 1946; Ward, 1960b); however, recent evidence indicates that it may also follow intermittent exposure at high intensities (Ward, 1970) or very long exposures at low intensities (Mills *et al.*, 1970) even when the TTS_2 is moderate.

Figure 8 illustrates this delayed recovery. Shown here are the individual recovery curves at 3000 Hz of the 12 ears of 6 listeners who had been exposed for 6 hours to an intermittent 1400–2000-Hz noise at 105 dB SPL that was turned on for 3 sec and off for 7 sec. Subject B showed only an 18-dB TTS_2, yet had a residual TTS of 6 dB after 16 hours of recovery. Additional research with this 105-dB SPL noise confirmed the implication that although breaking the exposure up into separate chunks produces a drastic reduction in the TTS immediately after exposure, just as predicted by the on-fraction rule cited above (Section III,E,6), the reduction of residual TTS (after 16 hours of recovery) is probably nowhere near as great. That is, although this 6-hour

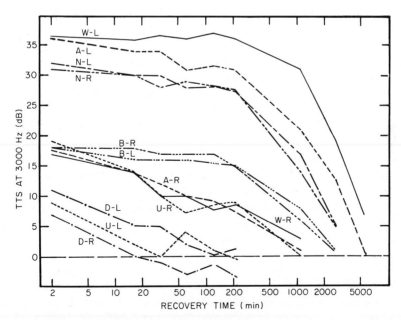

Fig. 8. Course of recovery from 6 hours of exposure to an intermittent 1400–2000-Hz noise at 105 dB SPL with an on-fraction of 0.3 (3 sec on, 7 sec off, etc.) Both normal and delayed recovery can be seen. [From Ward (1970).]

exposure with an on-fraction of 0.3 may well have produced only 30% as great a TTS_2 as a 6-hour continuous exposure, the residual TTS—the presumably dangerous component of the TTS—probably was more like 70 or 80% as great (needless to say, I did not attempt a 6-hour continuous exposure in order to check this). Thus it is apparent that if one is to use TTS at all as an index of the relative noxiousness of different noise exposures, TTS_2 is not appropriate. Instead, we should probably gauge the hazard on the basis of the TTS remaining after 16 hours of recovery.

Notice that these severe TTS's do not represent a summation of "ordinary" TTS and some more long-lasting component. The relatively rapid recovery seen in Figure 4 during the first couple of hours simply does not occur. This suggests that only one locus of damage is involved here; however, the *type* of malfunction may be different for ordinary and delayed recovery.

G. Susceptibility

About the only practical use of TTS that has been proposed is the original notion of Peyser's (1930) that perhaps individual differences in TTS might reflect individual differences in susceptibility to permanent losses caused by industrial noise exposure. However, it has become clear that if there is any merit to this scheme, one must use as a susceptibility test a sample of the noise to which the person will be exposed, because "susceptibility" seems to be relatively specific. That is, an ear that is more susceptible than another to TTS from high-frequency noise may be less susceptible to low-frequency noise, and neither of these indices of susceptibility is related to relative susceptibility to impulse noise (see Ward, 1968, for a review of the quest for a valid susceptibility test).

TTS, then, actually has as yet no proven value in audiology, although it enters into many situations as an unwanted confounding factor. Patients who ride noisy motorcycles to their appointment for an audiogram are a case in point; I once found it necessary to issue ear plugs to one of my listeners if I expected to get an accurate measurement of resting threshold on any given day.

H. Tinnitus

In addition to the rushing-noise type of tinnitus described earlier, a common result of high-intensity stimulation is a relatively high-pitched tinnitus that lasts more than 2 min. Tinnitus deliberately produced by pure tones and noise has recently been studied by Loeb and Smith (1967) and Atherley *et al.* (1968). They found that on the average, a 5-min exposure produced a tonal tinnitus when the SPL reached about 115 dB. The tinnitus tended to be higher in pitch level than the fatiguer, though not quite as high as the frequency of maximum loss (which was $\frac{1}{2}$ to 1 octave above the frequency of the fatiguer). However, variability was very large.

Zwicker (1964) has described a phenomenon he calls a "negative after-image" in hearing. If an ear is exposed to "noise with a hole" (a noise with uniform spectrum level except over a certain range in which the level is much lower), a short-duration (5–10 sec) tinnitus is heard, following cessation of the noise, whose pitch corresponds to the frequency of the suppressed band. This is a peripheral phenomenon, since if two different noises are presented to the two ears, two different aftertones are heard.

Although it has been speculated that exposures producing tinnitus are more likely to cause permanent loss than those which do not, no convincing evidence to support this notion can be found.

I. Miscellaneous Correlates of TTS

As Müller observed a century ago, suprathreshold stimuli may be altered in loudness, pitch, or timbre following stimulation. Usually the changes are so minor that a comparison with the unexposed ear is necessary to reveal them, and therefore they will be discussed under "binaural residual" effects. However, occasionally the effects are so striking that they are noticed on an absolute basis. For example, in 1947 Rosenblith et al. reported that for a few seconds after exposure to high-intensity pulses at about 100 per second, a peculiar metallic quality was added to the timbre of familiar sounds such as speech. This effect deserves further study.

In addition, an ear with a high-frequency TTS will judge most sounds containing high frequencies (for example, a watch tick) as "muffled" or "dull." Indeed, one way of inferring whether or not a worker suffers auditory fatigue from his employment is to ask him if his car sounds better on his way home from work. If he answers "yes," he probably is being given a significant daily TTS.

Musicians, particularly, also often comment on distortions of pitch correlated with TTS's. On one occasion, after I had accidentally given my left ear a 70-dB TTS at and above 2000 Hz, music sounded utterly unmusical (Ward et al., 1961b). In addition to sounding muffled, the orchestra or piano appeared completely out of tune. If I listened only with the affected ear, familiar melodies were recognizable only on the basis of rhythm. The situation was not much improved by listening with both ears, although if the affected ear were occluded, the music sounded almost normal. When the ears were occluded alternately, the affected ear heard the sound as "flatter" (lower in pitch) in a general sense. Measurements indicated that the downward shift in pitch in the affected ear was about 3 semitones at 1000 Hz, but only 1 semitone at 500 Hz. Thus, since the higher frequencies were shifted downward in pitch more than lower ones, harmonies became excruciatingly inharmonic, and consonances turned to dissonances. The effect persisted until the following morning, 19 hours after exposure, when the TTS had dropped to 40 dB (3 weeks were required for complete audiometric recovery).

Now let us turn to the problem of loudness changes, especially of the fatiguer itself.

IV. Concomitant Binaural: "Perstimulatory Adaptation"

In spite of the fact that it was the first manifestation of auditory adaptation to be described (Dove, 1859), the phenomenon commonly termed "perstimulatory adaptation" is still surrounded by controversy and confusion. However, it appears that the confusion stems from recent acceptance of a single assumption that in my opinion is quite false: the assumption that the phenomenon is based primarily on a reduction in loudness in the exposed ear. Let me eludicate.

Dove (1859), it will be recalled, simply demonstrated that if one ear were exposed to a tone for a minute or two, then introduction of the same tone simultaneously into the other ear (the control ear) resulted in perception of a tone only in the latter. Sewall, in 1907, first tried to quantify the phenomenon by reducing the intensity of the tone reaching the control ear until the percept was "normal." But just what "normal" meant, Sewall realized as he listened to the phenomenon, was not perfectly clear: were he and his subjects adjusting the intensity so that the loudness was the same in both ears, or so that the tone was judged to be in the middle of the head? That is, had the loudness of the tone in the exposed ear decreased, or had the characteristics of the ear simply shifted so that a tone in that ear no longer had the same lateralizing power as at the beginning of the exposure? In essence, is the phenomenon peripheral or central?

Three experiments more than 40 years old should, one would think, have answered the question fairly unequivocally. Flügel, in 1920, reported a series of experiments in which he systematically determined the effect of various parameters on both perstimulatory and poststimulatory adaptation, carefully done studies whose generality is limited only by the fact that tuning forks alone were used as the major source of adapter and test tones. In regard to perstimulatory adaptation, he discovered relations subsequently confirmed by modern experimenters: that the degree of final adaptation and the rate of growth are independent of frequency, and that they depend only slightly on the level (a moderate-intensity stimulus produced nearly as much effect as the loudest tone Flügel could muster). He also studied the frequency specificity of the effect: though no exact figures are given, it is claimed that exposure to, for example, 500 Hz, will shift the median-plane lateralization of 320 Hz just as much as would exposure to 320 Hz. Flügel even tried to determine the effect of "central" factors: during the adaptation period, he had his subjects (1) read, (2) look at "a series of pictures of an exciting character to be attentively contemplated," or (3) perform addition. Such activities had no effect on the adaptation. In the context of the question of losses, however, Flügel's most relevant finding was that the two ears of a given observer often displayed different degrees of asymptotic adaptation at a given frequency. Flügel argued, logically enough, that if such a difference in susceptibility existed, then when one presented the tone binaurally to begin with, the image should gradually shift to the less susceptible ear or, taking the alternate view, the loudness in the more susceptible ear should decrease. But when he subjected this hypothesis to empirical test, no such shift occurred: the image stayed right in the middle. This result implies a complicated central mechanism, not a simple peripheral comparator.

Bartlett and Mark (1922) realized this, and administered what should have been the *coup de grace* to the "loudness decrease" theory by means of an ingenious experiment. During the adaptation period, they presented the same 157-Hz tone to both ears, but shifted the phase in one ear, say the right ear, so that the tone seemed to be only in the other. At the end of the adaptation period—that is, when the phase difference between the ears was changed back to 0°—the tone was lateralized to the right side, just as if the prolonged exposure had been given only to the left ear.

Furthermore, Pattie (1927) demonstrated that if one determined the loudness of the adapter at the end of the exposure period by presenting a comparison tone in the unexposed ear successively instead of simultaneously, only a slight change in loudness was noticed. In fact, some observers indicated no change in loudness whatever. For some reason, however, the obvious conclusion—that this binaural phenomenon has virtually nothing to do with loudness in the ordinary sense—was clearly not inescapable to subsequent researchers, especially Hood (1950), who called the phenomenon "per-stimulatory fatigue" and by so doing set back understanding the phenomenon by at least 20 years. Adaptation

of sorts it may be; but fatigue it is not. Even though it must have
been apparent to each of these later investigators, as he listened to
a sustained stimulus, that the loudness of this adapter did *not* decrease
with time (except, of course, when some tone decay was present), they
all continued to talk about "perstimulatory fatigue" as a manifestation
of a "loudness decrease." I must confess I have carelessly done so myself
(Ward, 1963), even though I knew perfectly well that as one listens
to a tone at 100, 110, or 120 dB SPL, it seems, if anything, to get
louder with time (Hirsh and Ward, 1952). About the only dissenting
voices, until 5 years or so ago, were those of Bocca and Pestalozza
(1959), who concluded from their studies that perstimulatory fatigue
"has nothing to do with adaptation of cochlear receptors. In fact it
seems to be intimately bound to the effect of binaural stimulation."

Mirabella *et al.* (1967) recently studied loudness changes directly.
Their listeners' task was to keep the loudness of a sustained tone constant, on an absolute (noncomparative) basis. If indeed its loudness
tends to decrease with time, then the subject should gradually increase
the intensity to compensate for this by means of his attenuator. However,
when the tone began at 70 dB SPL, the upward drift in 10 min was
only 3–5 dB, nothing like the 20–50 dB imbalance observed in the perstimulatory adaptation paradigm. When the tone began at 90 dB, then
there was a slight average *downward* drift of the intensity, implying
that the loudness was increasing.

Perstimulatory adaptation, therefore, appearing only when both ears
are stimulated simultaneously, is a complex phenomenon involving central interaction of the auditory pathways including, perhaps, efferent
action on the nonexposed ear. The maximum effect, always reached in
5 minutes or less, seems to be obtained under the following conditions:

1. When the control ear is given a pulsed tone instead of a continuous one (this keeps the effect from diminishing during the process
   of testing for it) (Wright, 1960)
2. When the stimulus is a pure tone instead of a noise; apparently
   irregularity helps minimize the growth of perstimulatory adaptation (Carterette, 1956)
3. When the adapting stimulus is continuous; although an intermittent tone or noise shows some adaptation, it is always less than
   for a steady adapter (Sergeant and Harris, 1963)
4. When the instructions emphasize the median plane balance rather
   than "equal loudness" (Stokinger and Studebaker, 1968)
5. When the comparison stimulus has the same frequency as the
   fatiguer, although there is considerable spread of effect to both

higher and lower frequencies (Thwing, 1955) (recall that Flügel in 1920 already concluded that adaptation of one ear made *any* diotic stimulus pair appear to be shifted toward the nonadapted ear)

6. When the test subjects are adults; Kärjä (1968) found that the average perstimulatory adaptation in 7–15-year-old children was not significantly different from zero.

Just what processes underlie this fascinating phenomenon are still unknown, but no doubt the same ones are involved in (1) the shifts in lateralizing power of tones after a subject wears a hearing aid in only one ear (Elfner and Carlson, 1965); (2) the changes with time of contralateral remote masking (Ward, 1967); and (3) the decreased TTS observed after binaural exposure relative to monaural exposure, over and beyond any effects attributable to middle-ear muscle action (Ward, 1965).

Perstimulatory adaptation seems to have little clinical usefulness. So far, at least, nothing seems to correlate well with individual differences in degree of adaptation (for example, Palva, 1955). Although Tanner (1955) observed a negative correlation between perstimulatory adaptation and ordinary TTS, I have been unable to duplicate this finding (Ward, 1968). Kärjä (1968) found no change in old age. For the moment, then, perstimulatory adaptation remains a provoking enigma.

V. Residual Binaural

A. Loudness

When one determines loudness changes "correctly," that is, by alternate rather than simultaneous presentation of test stimuli, the degree of shift of the adapter itself is very small, as Pattie (1927) indicated, and as Harbert et al. (1968) and Petty et al. (1970) have recently confirmed. However, this is not true for weaker stimuli at frequencies at which an ordinary TTS exists. If an observer's resting threshold at some frequency is 10 dB SPL, and he is given a TTS of 20 dB, then a 35-dB SPL tone will be much less loud than before. This diminution of loudness of a weak tone following exposure was indeed the phenomenon demonstrated by Müller (1871) a century ago. As the level is increased, the disparity will gradually decrease; that is, recruitment is occurring. Hickling (1967) has shown that in an ear with TTS, recruitment is linear and is complete at a SPL of about 95 dB; this agrees well with the recruitment curves observed in ears with high-frequency hearing losses (Ward et al., 1961a) or Meniere's disease (Hallpike and Hood, 1959). As is true for recruiting ears in general, the difference

limen for intensity (IDL) is also reduced in the fatigued region; Elliott
et al. (1962) showed that the IDL in decibels is smaller no matter
whether the before-and-after comparison involves a standard tone of
constant SL, SPL, or loudness.

B. Pitch

Shifts in pitch probably accompany all of the different types of TTS,
although they do not seem to have yet been demonstrated for "residual
masking." Christman and Williams (1963) recently measured shifts in
pitch accompanying moderate TTS in a search for an auditory correlate
of visual figural aftereffects. In vision, if one fixates a vertical black
line on a white field for a while and then replaces the fixated line with
a pair of lines, one slightly to the right and the other slightly to the
left of the original line, these will appear to be further apart than they
really are; each has been shifted away from the "satiated" visual area.
By analogy, then, after monaural exposure to a steady tone, a 600-Hz
tone would be expected to be shifted upward in pitch (as inferred from
pitch matches with the control ear) when the fatiguer had been below
600 Hz, downward after frequencies above 600 Hz. Christman and Wil
liams report that when the SPL of both the fatiguer and test tones
were held at 85 dB SPL and the duration at 60 sec, exposure to
360, 425, or 575 Hz produced a 5-Hz upward shift in pitch of a 600-Hz
tone 2 sec after exposure, while 625, 850, and 1200 Hz give a 6-Hz
downward shift. One would expect that a larger effect might well be
shown if the test tones had been given at a much lower level. However,
the pitch seems to have been shifted symmetrically, and in this regard
this phenomenon differs sharply from pitch shifts associated with ordinary or delayed-recovery TTS. Although one can observe relatively
larger upward shifts of pitch—that is, half an octave or more—at and
above frequencies at which a relatively large TTS (40 or 50 dB) had
been produced, downward shifts are quite small (Piazza, 1966; Rüedi
and Furrer, 1946), usually being much less than a semitone. The difference is reasonable if indeed the two phenomena occur at different places,
the fatigue at the end organ, and the "satiation" at some higher center,
just as Selters's (1964) experiments implied. Only at the end organ is
a marked asymmetry to be expected, because of the pattern of motion
of the basilar membrane. If fatigue has rendered a certain area of hair
cells relatively insensitive, then, as one raises the intensity of a tone
to which this region is usually most sensitive, fibers nearer the oval
window—that is, those normally most responsive to higher frequencies—
will be stimulated before the pattern of motion involves more apical
areas.

VI. Conclusion

It is clear that there are at least three, perhaps five, completely different types of adaptation processes in the auditory system. Long-lasting postexposure phenomena (enduring more than a couple of minutes) apparently reflect fatigue processes in the cochlea. Short-lived effects (more than a second but no more than a few minutes) arise somewhere farther along the auditory pathway, but short of the final common path, since effects, except for sensitization, are specific to the ear concerned. Perstimulatory adaptation, a completely different phenomenon, reflects a change in the "potency" of stimuli in regard to lateralization following monaural stimulation; it is demonstrable only by binaural presentation of test signals, and therefore involves complex judgmental processes relatively high up the auditory chain (though the possible efferent action of monaural stimulation on the periphery of the contralateral auditory system cannot be excluded). "Residual masking"—very short-term TTS—is no doubt related most closely to refractory periods of the individual neurons, and so it probably represents a summation of such effects at all stations along the pathway. Finally, the primary locus of tone decay is simply unknown, although severe tone decay is known to be often associated with pressure on the eighth nerve produced by a pontine tumor.

Acknowledgment

Preparation of this article was supported in full by Grants NS-04403 and NS-K3-18,740 of the Public Health Service, U.S. Department of Health, Education, and Welfare.

References

Anonymous. (1956). Hazardous noise exposure. Air Force Regulation 160-3, Dept. of the Air Force, Washington, D.C.

Atherley, G. R. C., Hempstock, T. I., and Noble, W. G. (1968). Study of tinnitus induced temporarily by noise. J. Acoust. Soc. Amer. 44, 1503–1506.

Bartlett, F. C., and Mark, H. (1922). A note on local fatigue in the auditory system. Brit. J. Psychol. 13, 215–218.

von Békésy, G. (1947). A new audiometer. Acta Oto-Laryngol. 35, 411–422.

von Békésy, G. (1949). Resonance curve and the decay period at various points on the cochlear partition. J. Acoust. Soc. Amer. 21, 245–254.

Bell, D. W., and Fairbanks, G. (1963). TTS produced by low-level tones and the effects of testing on recovery. J. Acoust. Soc. Amer. 35, 1725–1731.

Bentzen, O. (1953). Investigations on short tones. Thesis; Aarhus Univ.

Bleyl, R. (1921). Die funktionelle Ermüdung des Gehörorganes. Arch. Ohren- Nasen Kehlkopfheilk. 108, 192–197.

Bocca, E., and Pestalozza, G. (1959). Auditory adaptation: Theories and facts. Acta Oto-Laryngol. 50, 349–353.

Botsford, J. H. (1968). Theory of TTS. J. Acoust. Soc. Amer. 44, 352.

Carhart, R. (1957). Clinical determination of abnormal auditory adaptation. *Arch. Otolaryngol.* **65**, 32–39.

Carterette, E. C. (1956). Loudness adaptation for bands of noise. *J. Acoust. Soc. Amer.* **28**, 865–871.

Causse, R., and Chavasse, P. (1947). Etudes sur la fatigue auditive. *Ann. Psychol.* **43-44**, 265–298.

Chernyak, R. I. (1958). Alteration in the adaptation of the hearing to silence with relation to the duration of a preliminary loud noise. *Biofizika* **3**, 75–86.

Christman, R. J., and Williams, W. E. (1963). Influence of the time interval on experimentally induced shifts of pitch. *J. Acoust. Soc. Amer.* **35**, 1030–1033.

Corradi, C. (1890). Zur Prüfung der Schallperception durch die Knochen. *Arch. Ohrenheilk.* **30**, 175–182.

Dallos, P. J., and Tillman, T. W. (1966). The effects of parameter variations in Bekesy audiometry in a patient with acoustic neurinoma. *J. Speech Hearing Res.* **9**, 557–572.

Davis, H., Morgan, C. T., Hawkins, J. E., Jr., Galambos, R., and Smith, F. W. (1950). Temporary deafness following exposure to loud tones and noise. *Acta Oto-Laryngol. Suppl.* **88**.

van Dishoeck, H. A. E. (1948). The continuous threshold or detailed audiogram for recording stimulation deafness. *Acta Oto-Laryngol. Suppl.* **78**, 183–192.

Dove, H. W. (1859). Beweis, dass die Tartinischen Töne nicht subjectiv, sondern objectiv sind. *Ann. Phys.* **107**, Ser. 2.

Dunlap, K. (1904). Some peculiarities of fluctuating and of inaudible sounds. *Psychol. Rev.* **11**, 308–318.

Elfner, L. F., and Carlson, C. (1965). Lateralization of pure tones as a function of prolonged binaural intensity mismatch. *Psychonomic Science* **2**, 27–28.

Elliott, D. N., Riach, W., and Silbiger, H. R. (1962). Effects of auditory fatigue upon intensity discrimination. *J. Acoust. Soc. Amer.* **34**, 212–217.

Epstein, A., Katz, J., and Dickinson, J. T. (1962). Low level stimulation in the differentiation of middle ear pathology. *Acta Oto-Laryngol.* **55**, 81–96.

Ewing, A. and Littler, T. S. (1935). Auditory fatigue and adaptation. *Brit. J. Psychol.* **25**, 284–307.

Feldmann, H. (1958). Eine einfache Methode zur monauralen Messung der perstimulatorisch und poststimulatorischen Adaptation oder Hörermüdung. *Arch Ohren-Nasen-Kehlkopfheilk.* **171**, 304–309.

Flügel, J. C. (1920). On local fatigue in the auditory system. *Brit. J. Psychol.* **11**, 105–134.

Gradenigo, G. (1893). On the clinical signs of the affections of the auditory nerve. *Arch. Otol.* **22**, 213–215.

Hallpike, C. S., and Hood, J. D. (1959). Observations upon the neurological mechanism of the loudness recruitment phenomenon. *Acta Oto-Laryngol.* **50**, 472–486.

Harbert, F., and Young, I. M. (1962). Threshold auditory adaptation. *J. Auditory Res.* **2**, 229–246.

Harbert, F., Weiss, B. G., and Wilpizeski, C. R. (1968). Suprathreshold auditory adaptation in normal and pathologic ears. *J. Speech Hearing Res.* **11**, 268–278.

Harris, J. D. (1955). On latent damage to the ear. *J. Acoust. Soc. Amer.* **27**, 177–179.

Harris, J. D., and Rawnsley, A. I. (1953). The locus of short duration auditory fatigue or "adaptation." *J. Exp. Psychol.* **46**, 457–461.

Hickling, S. (1967). Hearing test patterns in noise induced temporary hearing loss. *J. Auditory Res.* **7**, 63–76.

Hirsh, I. J., and Bilger, R. C. (1955). Auditory-threshold recovery after exposures to pure tones. *J. Acoust. Soc. Amer.* **27**, 1186–1194.

Hirsh, I. J., and Ward, W. D. (1952). Recovery of the auditory threshold after strong acoustic stimulation. *J. Acoust. Soc. Amer.* **24**, 131–141.

Hood, J. D. (1950). Studies in auditory fatigue and adaptation. *Acta Oto-Laryngol. Suppl.* **92**.

Hörmann, H. (1968). Lärm—psychologisch betrachtet. *Bild Wiss.* **6**, 785–794.

Hughes, J. R. (1954). Auditory sensitization. *J. Acoust. Soc. Amer.* **26**, 1064–1070.

Huijsman, A. (1884). De Afstomping der Gehoorzenuw door Geluidsindrukken. *Utrecht Rijks Univ. Physiol. Lab., Onderzoekingen, Ser.* 3, **9**, 87–142.

Jacobson, L. (1883). Bericht über die vom 1. November 1877 bis zum 1. April 1881 untersuchten und behandelden Kranken. *Arch. Ohrenheilk.* **19**, 28–54.

Jerger, J. (1960). Bekesy audiometry in analysis of auditory disorders. *J. Speech Hearing Res.* **3**, 275–287.

Jerger, J., and Jerger, S. (1966). Critical off-time in VIIIth nerve disorders. *J. Speech Hearing Res.* **9**, 573–583.

Jerger, J., Shedd, J. L., and Harford, E. (1959). On the detection of extremely small changes in sound intensity. *Arch. Otolaryngol.* **69**, 200–211.

Johnson, E. W. (1968). Auditory findings in 200 cases of acoustic neuromas. *Arch. Otolaryngol.* **88**, 598–603.

Josephson, E. M. (1934). Auditory fatigue including a new theory of hearing based on experimental findings. *Ann. Otol. Rhinol. Laryngol.* **43**, 1103–1113.

Kärjä, J. (1968). Perstimulatory suprathreshold adaptation for pure tones. *Acta Oto-Laryngol. Suppl.* **241**.

Katz, J., and Epstein, A. (1962). A hypothesis considering non-mechanical aspects of conductive hearing loss. *Acta Oto-Laryngol.* **55**, 145–150.

Keeler, J. S. (1968). Compatible exposure and recovery functions for temporary threshold shift—mechanical and electrical models. *J. Sound Vibr.* **7**, 220–235.

Klosterkötter, W. (1970). Gesundheitliche Bedeutung des Lärms. *Zbl. Bakt.* **212**, 336–353.

Kryter, K. D. (1950). The effects of noise on man. *J. Speech Hearing Dis. Monogr. Suppl.* **1**.

Kryter, K. D., Ward, W. D., Miller, J. D., and Eldredge, D. H. (1966). Hazardous exposure to intermittent and steady-state noise. *J. Acoust. Soc. Amer.* **39**, 451–464.

Kylin, B. (1970). Personal Communication.

Langenbeck, B. (1959). Messung der Hörermüdung und Adaptation am Patienten: Der "Kietz-Test" und seine klinische Bedeutung. *Z. Laryngol. Rhinol. Otol.* **38**, 202–211.

Langenbeck, B., and Lehnhardt, E. (1970). "Lehrbuch der praktischen Audiometrie." Thieme, Stuttgart.

Lierle, D. M., and Reger, S. N. (1954). Further studies of threshold shifts as measured with the Bekesy-type audiometer. *Trans. Amer. Otol. Soc.* **42**, 211–227.

Lierle, D. M., and Reger, S. N. (1955). Experimentally induced temporary threshold shifts in ears with impaired hearing. *Ann. Otol. Rhinol. Laryngol.* **64**, 263–277.

Loeb, M., and Smith, R. P. (1967). Relation of induced tinnitus to physical characteristics of the inducing stimuli. *J. Acoust. Soc. Amer.* **42**, 453–455.

Lüscher, E., and Laepple, O. (1958). Der Einfluss der Beschallung auf die Intensitätsunterschiedsschwelle des normalen und des kranken Ohres. *Arch. Ohren-Nasen-Kehlkopfheilk.* **172**, 299–309.

Miller, J. D. (1958). Temporary hearing loss at 4000 cps as a function of the intensity of a three-minute exposure to a noise of uniform spectrum level. *Laryngoscope* **68**, 660–671.

Miller, J. D., Watson, C. S., and Covell, W. E. (1963). Deafening effects of noise on the cat. *Acta Oto-Laryngol. Suppl.* **176**.

Mills, J. H., Gengel, R. W., Watson, C. S., and Miller, J. D. (1970). Temporary changes of the auditory system due to exposure to noise for one or two days. *J. Acoust. Soc. Amer.* **48**, 524–530.

Mirabella, A., Taub, H., and Teichner, W. H. (1967). Adaptation of loudness to monaural stimulation. *J. Gen. Psychol.* **76**, 251–273.

Møller, A. R. (1962). Acoustic reflex in man. *J. Acoust. Soc. Amer.* **34**, 1524–1534.

Müller, G. (1970). Änderung der Maskierungsschwelle durch Belastung. *Arch. Klin. Exp. Ohren-Nasen-Kehlkopfheilk.* **195**, 323–330.

Müller, J. J. (1871). Über die Tonempfindungen. *Akad. Wiss. Leipzig-Math.-Phys. Kl.-Berichte* **23**, 115–124.

Munson, W. A., and Gardner, M. B. (1950). Loudness patterns—a new approach. *J. Acoust. Soc. Amer.* **22**, 177–190.

Noffsinger, P. D., and Olsen, W. O. (1970). Postexposure responsiveness in the auditory system. II. Sensitization and desensitization. *J. Acoust. Soc. Amer.* **47**, 552–564.

Palva, T. (1955). Studies on per-stimulatory adaptation in various groups of deafness. *Laryngoscope* **65**, 829–847.

Parker, W. P., Decker, R. L., and Richards, N. G. (1968). Auditory function and lesions of the pons. *Arch. Otolaryngol.* **87**, 228–240.

Pattie, F. A., Jr. (1927). An experimental study of fatigue in the auditory mechanism. *Amer. J. Psychol.* **38**, 39–58.

Petty, J. W., Fraser, W. D., and Elliott, D. N. (1970). Adaptation and loudness decrement: a reconsideration. *J. Acoust. Soc. Amer.* **47**, 1074–1082.

Peyser, A. (1930). Gesundheitswesen u. Krankenfürsorge. Theoretische und experimentelle Grundlagen des persönlichen Schallschutzes. *Deut. Med. Wochenschr.* **56**, 150–151.

Piazza, R. S. (1966). The effect of the auditory fatigue upon the loudness and the pitch. *Acustica* **17**, 179–183.

Plath, P. (1967). Behaviour of the difference limen for intensity of hearing after exposure to pure tones. *Int. Audio.* **6**, 389–392.

Plester, D. (1953). Der Einfluss vegetativ wirksamer Pharmake auf die Adaptation bezw. Hörermüdung. *Arch. Ohren-Nasen-Kehlkopfheilk.* **162**, 473–487.

Pollack, I. (1964). Interaction of forward and backward masking. *J. Auditory Res.* **4**, 63–67.

Price, G. R., and Oatman, L. C. (1967). Central factor in auditory fatigue—an artifact? *J. Acoust. Soc. Amer.* **42**, 475–479.

Rayleigh, L. (1882). Acoustical observations. IV. *Phil. Mag.* **13**, Ser. 5, 340–347.

Reger, S. N., and Kos, C. M. (1952). Clinical measurements and implications of recruitment. *Ann. Otol. Rhinol. Laryngol.* **61**, 810–820.

Reid, G. (1946). Further observations on temporary deafness following exposure to gunfire. *J. Laryngol. Otol.* **61**, 609–633.

Rhese, D. (1906). Über die Beteiligung des inneren Ohres nach Kopferschütterungen mit vorzugsweiser Berücksichtigung derjenigen Fälle, bei denen die Hörfähigkeit für die Sprache garnicht oder nur in einem praktisch nicht in Betracht kommenden Grade gelitten hat. *Z. Ohrenheilk.* **52,** 320–356.

Rintelmann, W. F., and Borus, J. F. (1968). Noise-induced hearing loss and rock and roll music. *Arch. Otolaryngol.* **88,** 377–385.

Rol, C. (1956). Auditory fatigue following exposure to steady and non-steady sounds. Thesis, University of Leiden.

Rosenblith, W. A., Miller, G. A., Egan, J. P., Hirsh, I. J., and Thomas, G. J. (1947). An auditory afterimage? *Science* **106,** 333–334.

Rüedi, L., and Furrer, W. (1946). Das akustische Trauma. *Pract. Oto-Rhino-Laryngol.* **8,** 177–372.

Sataloff, J., Vassallo, L., and Menduke, H. (1969). Hearing loss from exposure to interrupted noise. *Arch. Environ. Health* **18,** 972–981.

Schäfer, K. L. (1905). Der Gehörssinn: Ermüdung. *In* "Handbuch der Physiologie des Menschen," (W. Nagel, ed.), Vol. 3, pp. 509–512. Braunschweig.

Schubert, K. (1944). Hörermüdung und Hördauer. *Z. Hals-Nasen-Ohrenheilk.* **51,** 19–74.

Schulze, F. A. (1910). Ermüdung des Ohres. Ges. z. Beförderung d. ges. Naturwiss. zu Marburg, *Sitzungber.* **45,** 76–77.

Schwetz, F., Donner, R., Langer, G., and Haider, M. (1970) Experimentelle Hörermüdung und ihre Rückbildung unter Ruhe- und Lärmbedingungen. *Mschr. Ohrenheilk.* **104,** 162–167.

Selters, W. (1964). Adaptation and fatigue. *J. Acoust. Soc. Amer.* **36,** 2202–2209.

Selters, W., and Ward, W. D. (1962). Temporary threshold shift with changing duty cycle. *J. Acoust. Soc. Amer.* **34,** 122–123.

Sergeant, R. L., and Harris, J. D. (1963). The relation of perstimulatory adaptation to other short-term threshold-shifting mechanisms. *J. Speech Hearing Res.* **6,** 27–39.

Sewall, E. (1907). Beitrag zur Lehre von der Ermüdung des Gehörorgans. *Z. Sinnesphys.* **42,** 115–123.

Speaks, C., Nelson, D., and Ward, W. D. (1970). Hearing loss in rock-and-roll musicians. *J. Occup. Med.* **12,** 216–219.

Stokinger, T. E., and Studebaker, G. A. (1968). Measurement of perstimulatory loudness adaptation. *J. Acoust. Soc. Amer.* **44,** 250–256.

Stroud, M. D., and Thalmann, R. (1969). Unusual audiological and vestibular problems in the diagnosis of cerebellopontine angle lesions. *Laryngoscope* **79,** 171–200.

Suzuki, T., Yoshie, N., Sakabe, N., and Igarashi, E. (1964). Abnormal auditory adaptation with use of amplitude modulated tones. *J. Auditory Res.* **4,** 213–226.

Tanner, K. (1955). Über Hörermüdung und Akustisches Trauma und deren Beeinflussung durch Vegetativ wirksame Pharmaka. *Acta Oto-Laryngol.* **45,** 65–81.

Temkin, J. (1933). Die Schädigung des Ohres durch Lärm und Erschütterung. *Mschr. Ohrenheilk. Laryngol-Rhinol.* **67,** 257–299, 450–479, 527–553, 705–736, 823–834.

Thompson, S. P. (1881). Phenomena of binaural addition. *Phil. Mag.* **12,** Ser. 5, 351–355.

Thwing, E. J. (1955). Spread of perstimulatory fatigue of a pure tone to neighboring frequencies. *J. Acoust. Soc. Amer.* **27,** 741–748.

Thwing, E. J. (1956). Masked threshold and its relation to the duration of the masked stimulus. *J. Acoust. Soc. Amer.* **28,** 606–610.

Trittipoe, W. J. (1958). Temporary threshold shift as a function of noise exposure level. *J. Acoust. Soc. Amer.* **30,** 250–253.

Urbantschitsch, V. (1881). Zur Lehre von der Schallempfindung. *Arch. Gesamte Physiol. Menschen Tiere* **24**, 574–595.

Ward, W. D. (1960a). Latent and residual effects in temporary threshold shift. *J. Acoust. Soc. Amer.* **32**, 135–137.

Ward, W. D. (1960b). Recovery from high values of temporary threshold shift. *J. Acoust. Soc. Amer.* **32**, 497–500.

Ward, W. D. (1961). Noninteraction of temporary threshold shifts. *J. Acoust. Soc. Amer.* **33**, 512–513.

Ward, W. D. (1962a). Studies on the aural reflex. II. Reduction of temporary threshold shift from intermittent noise by reflex activity; implications for damage-risk criteria. *J. Acoust. Soc. Amer.* **34**, 234–241.

Ward, W. D. (1962b). Damage-risk criteria for line spectra. *J. Acoust. Soc. Amer.* **34**, 1610–1619.

Ward, W. D. (1963). Auditory fatigue and masking. *In* "Modern Developments in Audiology," (J. Jerger, ed.), pp. 240–286. Academic Press, New York.

Ward, W. D. (1965). Temporary threshold shifts following monaural and binaural exposure. *J. Acoust. Soc. Amer.* **38**, 121–125.

Ward, W. D. (1966). Audition. *In* "Annual Review of Psychology," (P. R. Farnsworth, ed.), Vol. 17, pp. 273–308. Annual Reviews, Palo Alto.

Ward, W. D. (1967). Further observations on contralateral remote masking and related phenomena. *J. Acoust. Soc. Amer.* **42**, 593–600.

Ward, W. D. (1968). Susceptibility to auditory fatigue. *In* "Contributions to Sensory Physiology" (W. D. Neff, Ed.), Vol. 3, pp. 191–226. Academic Press, New York.

Ward, W. D. (1970). Temporary threshold shift and damage-risk criteria for intermittent noise exposures. *J. Acoust. Soc. Amer.* **48**, 561–574.

Ward, W. D., Glorig, A., and Sklar, D. L. (1958). Dependence of temporary threshold shift at 4 kc on intensity and time. *J. Acoust. Soc. Amer.* **30**, 944–954.

Ward, W. D., Glorig, A., and Sklar, D. L. (1959a). Temporary threshold shift from octave-band noise: Applications to damage-risk criteria. *J. Acoust. Soc. Amer.* **31**, 522–528.

Ward, W. D., Glorig, A., and Sklar, D. L. (1959b). Temporary threshold shift produced by intermittent exposure to noise. *J. Acoust. Soc. Amer.* **31**, 791–794.

Ward, W. D., Fleer, R. E., and Glorig, A. (1961a). Characteristics of hearing losses produced by gunfire and by steady noise. *J. Auditory Res.* **1**, 325–356.

Ward, W. D., Selters, W., and Glorig, A. (1961b). Exploratory studies on temporary threshold shift from impulses. *J. Acoust. Soc. Amer.* **33**, 781–793.

Wells, W. A. (1913). The influence of sounds of different pitch, duration and intensity in the production of auditory fatigue. *Laryngoscope* **23**, 989–998.

Wernick, J. S., and Tobias, J. V. (1963). Central factor in pure-tone auditory fatigue. *J. Acoust. Soc. Amer.* **35**, 1967–1971.

Wright, H. N. (1960). Measurement of perstimulatory auditory adaptation. *J. Acoust. Soc. Amer.* **32**, 1558–1567.

Zwicker, E. (1964). "Negative afterimage" in hearing. *J. Acoust. Soc. Amer.* **36**, 2413–2415.

Zwislocki, J., and Pirodda, E. (1952). On the adaptation, fatigue and acoustic trauma of the ear. *Experientia* **8**, 279–284.

Chapter 10

Measurement of Acoustic Impedance at the Tympanic Membrane

DAVID J. LILLY

University of Iowa

I. Introduction

Although the concept of acoustic impedance was introduced in 1914 (Webster, 1919), its application to clinical audiology did not become evident until Metz (1946) published his classic monograph. Measurement of acoustic impedance at the lateral surface of the tympanic membrane is "not just another audiological test," it constitutes "a whole new field of investigation with an inherent new-methodology." (Zwislocki, 1965, p. 19). This new clinical technique involves concepts, terminology, and mathematical procedures that traditionally have not been emphasized in audiology training programs. The basic concepts are well developed; the terminology has been standardized (ASA S1.1-1960); and the mathematical operations require only elementary trigonometry and the algebra of complex numbers. Still, a systematic introduction to acoustic impedance is not available in existing audiology textbooks. Accordingly, a primary goal of this chapter is to provide the audiologist with the information needed to understand basic literature in the area of acoustic impedance.

It is difficult for the student or the busy clinician to concentrate upon the fundamentals of a new technique if he does not have an overview of its clinical utility. Consequently, a secondary goal of this chapter is to provide a source of references and a summary of clinical applications for acoustic-impedance measurements.

A. Basic Acoustic-Impedance Measurements

In simplest terms, acoustic-impedance measurements tell us something about the "opposition" encountered by an acoustic wave. Acoustic-impedance techniques are used clinically to measure the "opposition" that exists at the lateral surface of the tympanic membrane or at some plane ·within the external auditory meatus. These clinical acoustic-impedance measurements may be classified as either *static or dynamic*.

1. STATIC ACOUSTIC-IMPEDANCE MEASUREMENTS

Static acoustic-impedance measurements are made with ambient (atmospheric) air pressure in the external auditory meatus and with the middle-ear muscles in a state of "normal" tonus. The words static (Dallos, 1964; Lilly, 1964, 1966; Lilly and Shepherd, 1964; Pinto and Dallos, 1968) and quiescent (Hecker and Kryter, 1965) have been used to distinguish these measurements from measurements of *dynamic* changes in acoustic impedance at the tympanic membrane.

Static acoustic-impedance measurements usually are reported in absolute physical units. As a result, some investigators (Bicknell and Morgan, 1968; Feldman, 1963, 1964, 1969; Lamb and Norris, 1969; Neergaard *et al.*, 1965; Priede, 1970; Robertson *et al.*, 1968; Simmons, 1964; Wilber *et al.*, 1969; Zwislocki, 1963b, 1964; Zwislocki and Feldman, 1970) have used the word *absolute* as a synonym for the word *static*, and have used the word *relative* as a synonym for the word *dynamic*. This terminology creates an artificial dichotomy since it suggests that dynamic changes in acoustic impedance can be measured only in relative terms. In general, nearly any measurement of dynamic change in the transmission characteristics of the middle ear is more valuable when it is reported in absolute physical units than when it is reported in units that are relative only to a specific instrument or to a specific patient.

2. DYNAMIC ACOUSTIC-IMPEDANCE MEASUREMENTS

Acoustic impedance at the lateral surface of a normal tympanic membrane will change when the middle-ear muscles contract, when the Eustachian tube opens, or when air pressure in the external auditory canal is made higher or lower than ambient pressure. These dynamic changes in acoustic impedance must be measured in absolute physical units if the audiologist wishes to compare the magnitude of a given change with corresponding data from other patients or from subjects with normal ears.

When the audiologist does not plan to compare a measured change in acoustic impedance with data from other individuals, calibration of the instrumentation may be simplified, and dynamic changes may be reported in relative terms. Measurements of relative dynamic changes in acoustic impedance have been used to determine: (1) the existence of an acoustic reflex, (2) the "threshold" of the acoustic reflex, (3) "adaptation" of the acoustic reflex, (4) opening of the Eustachian tube, (5) contraction of the stapedius muscle, (6) contraction of the tensor tympani muscle, and (7) the general effects of air pressure upon the middle-ear transmission system.

B. Application of Basic Measurements to Clinical Problems

It would be impossible in this chapter to review and evaluate the hundreds of articles that deal with clinical applications of acoustic-impedance measurements. The summary that follows indicates the scope of these applications, and provides a source of selected references. This summary has four major headings. The first three headings reflect general test procedures that currently are used clinically: (1) measurement of static acoustic impedance, (2) determination of reflexive contraction of the middle-ear muscles, and (3) tympanometry. Each of these procedures has been used to evaluate Eustachian-tube function, and therefore this clinical application is considered separately under a fourth heading.

1. STATIC ACOUSTIC-IMPEDANCE MEASUREMENTS

Measurements of static acoustic impedance at the tympanic membrane are of primary value in differential diagnosis of conductive lesions. These measurements reflect directly the transmission characteristics of the middle-ear system. In general, acoustic impedance at the tympanic membrane is (1) lower than normal with ossicular discontinuity, (2) higher than normal with clinical otosclerosis, and (3) very much higher than normal with acute inflammatory and chronic diseases of the middle ear. An historical review of static acoustic-impedance measurements, a classification of measurement techniques, and a summary of clinical findings are provided with references in Section V.

2. REFLEX MEASUREMENTS

In a normal middle ear, contraction of the stapedius muscle or contraction of the tensor tympani muscle produces a measurable, time-locked change in acoustic impedance at the lateral surface of the tympanic membrane. In the first edition of *Modern Developments in Audiology*, Jepsen (1963) devotes a chapter to the "middle-ear muscle reflexes in man." The reader is referred to this chapter for a comprehensive discussion of anatomy and physiology of the reflex arcs, and methods for recording contraction of the middle-ear muscles.

The normal relation between changes in acoustic impedance and reflexive contraction of the middle-ear muscles is modified by middle-ear disease, by cochlear disease, and by lesions that affect the trigeminal nerve (Nerve V), the facial nerve (Nerve VII), and the statoacoustic nerve (Nerve VIII). Auditory, electrical, pneumatic, and tactile stimuli are used clinically to activate one or both of the middle-ear muscles. These activation methods have been classified as either "acoustic" or "nonacoustic" in this section. For convenience, clinical measurements of dynamic changes in acoustic impedance (with contraction of the middle-ear muscles) have been grouped under five application headings.

a. Acoustic-Impedance Audiometry. The relation between threshold of audibility and threshold of the acoustic reflex for pure tones has been used: (1) as an objective measure of hearing sensitivity for neonates and for young children (Jerger, 1970; Robertson *et al.*, 1968; Terkildsen, 1960a; Wedenberg, 1963) ; (2) to determine the existence and magnitude of nonorganic hearing impairment (Harper, 1961; Jepsen, 1953, 1963; Lamb and Peterson, 1967; Lamb *et al.*, 1968; Terkildsen, 1964; Thomsen, 1955a,b; Wilmot, 1969).

b. Conductive Hearing Impairment. Acoustic and nonacoustic activation methods have been used: (1) to discriminate between clinical otosclerosis and ossicular discontinuity (Anderson and Barr, 1971; Djupesland, 1964a,b, 1965, 1967, 1969b; Floberg *et al.*, 1969; Flottorp and Djupesland, 1970; Jepsen, 1963; Jerger, 1970; Klockhoff, 1960, 1961, 1963;

Klockhoff and Anderson, 1959, 1960; Lidén, 1969a; Lidén *et al.*, 1970c; McPherson, 1971; Terkildsen, 1964; Wilmot, 1969); and (2) to determine the existence of a conductive lesion (Anderson and Barr, 1966; Brooks, 1968, 1969, 1970; Farrant and Skurr, 1966; Hecker and Kryter, 1965; Holst *et al.*, 1963; Jerger, 1970; Klockhoff, 1961, 1963; Klockhoff and Anderson, 1959; Lidén, 1969b; Metz, 1946; Onchi, 1963; Terkildsen, 1960a; Thomsen, 1955b).

c. Sensorineural Hearing Impairment. Acoustic and nonacoustic activation methods have been used: (1) to provide an "objective" measure for recruitment of loudness (Alberti and Kristensen, 1970; Anderson and Barr, 1966; Beedle and Harford, 1970; Djupesland, 1964a; Djupesland and Flottorp, 1970; Ewertsen *et al.*, 1958; Franzen and Lilly, 1970; Harper, 1961; Jepsen, 1963; Jerger, 1970; Klockhoff, 1961; Klockhoff and Anderson, 1959; Kristensen and Jepsen, 1952; Lamb *et al.*, 1968; Lidén, 1969b, 1970; Metz, 1952; Terkildsen, 1960a, 1964; Thomsen, 1955b,d; Wilmot, 1969); (2) as an "objective" measure of abnormal auditory adaptation for patients with pressure lesions or demyelinating lesions of Nerve VIII (Alberti and Kristensen, 1970; Anderson *et al.*, 1969, 1970a,b); and (3) to rule out the existence of conductive lesions for patients with severe sensorineural hearing losses (Farrant and Skurr, 1966; Favors and Lilly, 1971; Klockhoff, 1961; Klockhoff and Anderson, 1959; Lamb *et al.*, 1968; Robertson *et al.*, 1968).

d. Neurotology. Again, both acoustic and nonacoustic activation methods have been used: (1) for topographic localization of lesions to Nerve VII (Cawthorne, 1963; Djupesland, 1969a; Feldman, 1967; Harper, 1961; Holst *et al.*, 1963; Jepsen, 1963; Jerger, 1970; Klockhoff, 1961; Kristensen and Zilstorff, 1967; Lidén *et al.*, 1970c; Metz, 1946; Terkildsen, 1964; Thomsen, 1955b); (2) in differential diagnosis for patients with brainstem lesions (Greisen and Rasmussen, 1970; Jepsen, 1963); (3) as an indirect measure of changes in intracranial pressure (Klockhoff *et al.*, 1965); and (4) as a test for motor function of Nerve V, or as a test for contraction of the tensor tympani muscle (Djupesland, 1964b, 1965, 1967, 1969a,b; Klockhoff, 1961, 1963; Klockhoff and Anderson, 1960; Lidén, 1969a,b; Lidén *et al.*, 1970c; Lindström and Lidén, 1964).

e. Miscellaneous Applications. Measurement of the acoustic reflex has been: (1) considered as a possible index of susceptibility to noise exposure (Hecker and Kryter, 1965; Johansson *et al.*, 1967; Lilly *et al.*, 1969; Ward, 1962); (2) used to aid in the identification of normal-hearing "carriers of genes for recessive deafness" (Anderson and Wedenberg, 1968); and (3) used to provide an "objective" estimate of temporal summation within the auditory system for pure tones (Djupesland and Zwislocki, 1971).

3. Tympanometry Measurements

Acoustic impedance at the tympanic membrane of a normal middle ear will *increase* if air pressure in the external auditory meatus is made higher or lower than ambient (atmospheric) air pressure. This predictable relation between changes in air pressure and changes in acoustic impedance is modified by middle-ear disease, by perforations of the tympanic membrane, by abnormal air pressures in the middle ear, or by scars on the tympanic membrane. The general term *tympanometry* refers to methods and techniques for measuring, for recording, and for evaluating changes in acoustic impedance with systematic changes in air pressure. In this section, clinical tympanometry measurements have been grouped under six application headings.

a. Middle-Ear Fluid. Tympanometry has been used to detect or to confirm the presence of effusion within the middle-ear cavity (Alberti and Kristensen, 1970; Brooks, 1968, 1969, 1970; Hood and Lamb, 1969; Jerger, 1970, 1971; Lamb and Norris, 1969; Lamb et al., 1969; Lidén, 1969b; Lidén et al., 1970a,b; Lilly, 1970; McPherson, 1971; Terkildsen, 1964; Terkildsen and Thomsen, 1959; Thomsen, 1961; Wilber et al., 1970).

b. Perforations of the Tympanic Membrane. Tympanometry has been used to determine the integrity of the tympanic membrane, or to determine the patency of pressure-equalization tubes (Alberti and Kristensen, 1970; Lidén et al., 1970a,b; Lilly, 1970; Terkildsen, 1964; Terkildsen and Thomsen, 1959).

c. Air Pressure within the Tympanum. Tympanometry has been used to estimate the air pressure in the middle-ear cavity (Alberti and Kristensen, 1970; Brooks, 1968, 1969, 1970; Holmquist, 1969; Hood and Lamb, 1969; Jepsen, 1963; Jerger, 1970; Lamb and Norris, 1969; Lamb et al., 1969; Lidén et al., 1970a,b; Lilly, 1970; McPherson, 1971; Terkildsen, 1964; Terkildsen and Thomsen, 1959; Thomsen, 1961; Wilber et al., 1970).

d. Cicatricial Lesions of the Tympanic Membrane. Tympanometry has been used to evaluate the effects of atrophic scars on the tympanic membrane (Lidén et al., 1970a,b; Lilly, 1970; Terkildsen and Thomsen, 1959; Terkildsen, 1964; Wilber et al., 1970).

e. Acoustic and Nonacoustic Reflexes. Contraction of the middle-ear muscles will produce maximum impedance change at the tympanic membrane when the air pressure in the external auditory meatus is identical to the air pressure within the middle-ear cavity. The tympanometry system provides a method for equalizing these air pressures *before* measuring changes in acoustic impedance (Jepsen, 1963; Klockhoff, 1961; Lilly, 1970; Robertson *et al.*, 1967; Terkildsen, 1960b, 1964; Thomsen, 1958b).

f. Static Acoustic Impedance. Tympanometry has been used to estimate the magnitude of static acoustic impedance at the tympanic membrane (Alberti and Kristensen, 1970; Hood and Lamb, 1969; Jerger, 1970, 1971; Lamb *et al.*, 1969; Lilly, 1970; Terkildsen, 1964; Terkildsen and Thomsen, 1959; Thomsen, 1961; Wilber *et al.*, 1970).

4. MEASUREMENT OF EUSTACHIAN-TUBE FUNCTION

Each of the three basic measurement techniques (static acoustic-impedance measurement, reflex measurement, and tympanometry) has been used to evaluate Eustachian-tube function. In this section, clinical measurements of Eustachian-tube function have been grouped under five headings.

a. Patulous Eustachian Tube. Static acoustic impedance at the tympanic membrane is lower than normal and changes in synchrony with respiration if the Eustachian tube is open continuously. Acoustic-impedance measurements have been used to provide quantitative diagnosis, and evaluation of treatment for patients with patulous Eustachian tubes (Harper, 1961; Metz, 1953; Thomsen, 1955c).

b. Static Acoustic-Impedance Measurements. Static acoustic-impedance techniques have been used in conjunction with "inflation," "aspiration," and "pressure-chamber" procedures to provide quantitative measurements of Eustachian-tube function (Harper, 1961; Thomsen, 1955c, 1957, 1958a,b).

c. Reflex Measurements. Absence of the "nonacoustic stapedial reflex" provides support for a diagnosis of subnormal air pressure within the tympanic cavity. This reflex returns with normal ventilation of the middle ear (Djupesland, 1969b).

d. Tympanometry. Tympanometry also has been used in conjunction with "inflation" and "aspiration" procedures to provide a quantitative recording of Eustachian-tube function (Alberti and Kristensen, 1970; Holmquist, 1969; Terkildsen and Thomsen, 1959; Thomsen, 1961).

e. "Aspiration and Deflation Measurements." All tympanometry instruments contain a subsystem for producing and for measuring air-pressure changes within the external auditory meatus. This pneumatic subsystem may be used, in isolation, to evaluate Eustachian-tube function for patients with perforations of the tympanic membrane (Flisberg, 1964; Flisberg *et al.*, 1963; Holborow, 1962; Holmquist, 1970; Miller, 1965; Silverstein *et al.*, 1966; van Dishoeck, 1970).

C. The Need for Understanding Basic Concepts

The foregoing summary has focused upon a wide range of potential diagnostic applications for clinical acoustic-impedance measurements. Unfortunately, relevant research cannot be evaluated critically without a broad understanding of: (1) the general concept of impedance; (2) impedances that exist within the peripheral, human auditory system; (3) standard methods for reporting acoustic-impedance data; and (4) average, static acoustic-impedance results for subjects with normal hearing and for patients with middle-ear disease. These topics are covered, in order, in the following sections.

II. The Concept of Impedance

The study of impedance involves an analysis of the "opposition" offered by a system to the "flow" of energy. In audiology we are concerned with the performance of electrical, mechanical, and acoustical systems. The concept of impedance may be applied to each of these systems.

Heaviside (1886) first used the term *impedance* in an analysis of an alternating-current (ac) network. The utility of this concept was enhanced when Steinmetz (1893) formulated a complex-notation method for use with ac circuits.[1] Webster (1919) probably was the first to suggest that complex notation and the concept of impedance could be used to simplify the analysis of mechanical and acoustical circuits. He suggested that "Whenever we have permanent vibrations of a single given frequency . . . the notion of impedance is valuable in replacing all the quantities involved in the reactions of the system by a single complex number."

The term *impedance* may be defined generically as the complex ratio of a force-like quantity (force, voltage, or sound pressure) to a related velocity-like quantity (velocity, current, or volume velocity). This operational definition tells us that the concept of impedance involves *vector quantities*. Vector quantities always are "complex" quantities. This means that, in a two-dimensional plane, two numbers are required to specify completely a vector quantity such as force. One number denotes the magnitude of the force and the second number denotes the direction in which the force is acting.[2] Moreover, the definition states that imped-

---

[1] In this chapter, the word complex always will mean "composed of two or more related parts." It will not mean "involved, complicated, or difficult."

[2] A vector quantity in physics is distinguished from a scalar quantity (such as mass, time, density, distance, or speed) that can be specified completely with a single number (Davis, 1967).

ance is a complex ratio of two vector quantities. This means that impedance also is a vector quantity, and therefore, two numbers are required to specify completely the electrical impedance (Z), the mechanical impedance (Z_M) or the acoustic impedance (Z_A) of a system.

Unfortunately, our operational definition does not explicate the relation between impedance and the transmission of electric current, mechanical vibrations, or sound. In the sections that follow, we shall consider the impedance at the input of several systems. Therefore, to simplify discussion, we shall define the *input impedance* of a given system or network as the "total opposition" offered by that system to the flow of energy. This intuitive definition suggests that less energy will flow into a system with a high input impedance than into one with a low input impedance. Stated differently, knowledge of the input impedance of a system can tell us how much energy will flow *into* the system; it cannot tell us, however, how much energy will be transmitted *through* the system unless we know the amount of energy that will be dissipated or stored *within* the system.

III. Impedances at the Input of the Auditory System

A. Electrical, Acoustical, and Mechanical Impedance

The labels along the top of Figure 1 identify the four interrelated systems that usually are involved during measurement of acoustic impedance at the tympanic membrane. At the left-hand side of the figure, a sinusoidal electrical signal from the output of an audiofrequency generator (or a pure-tone audiometer) is delivered to the input terminals of a magnetic hearing-aid earphone. This signal usually is referred to as a "carrier signal" (Dallos, 1964; Klockhoff, 1961; Klockhoff *et al.*, 1965; Lilly, 1964; Onchi, 1963). Most audiologists recognize that it is not difficult to measure the "total opposition" provided by a hearing-aid transducer to the flow of electric current. We call the result of such a measurement the input or driving-point impedance, we symbolize it with an uppercase Z, and we report its value as a complex number, with units ohms (Ω). The input impedance of an earphone is related directly to the acoustic load that exists at its output. It is interesting to note that some of the earliest methods for measurement of acoustic impedance involved an analysis of the electrical impedance at the input of transducers (Fay and Hall, 1933; Fay and White, 1948; Kennelly, 1925; Kennelly and Kurokawa, 1921; Kosten and Zwikker, 1941).

The hearing-aid transducer in Figure 1 constitutes an electromagnetic system. Its diaphragm is driven into vibration by the applied electrical

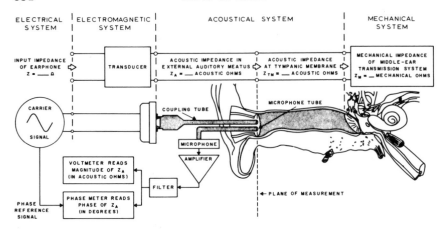

FIG. 1. Four physical systems involved during measurement of acoustic impedance at tympanic membrane. Under clinical conditions, impedance can be measured at input of the electromagnetic system (Z in ohms), at a plane of measurement through the external auditory meatus (Z_A in acoustic ohms), and at the surface of the tympanic membrane (Z_{TM} in acoustic ohms). Instrumentation blocked out in lower left-hand corner comprises a simple electroacoustic system for direct measurement of Z_A.

signal, and the frequency and amplitude of diaphragm vibration are related directly to the frequency and amplitude of the carrier signal. Since the vibrating diaphragm is in contact with air (an elastic, gaseous medium), and since this quantity of air exists at some static (barometric) pressure, periodic changes in air pressure at the face of the diaphragm are considered as "excess pressures"[3] above and below the pressure of the atmosphere. These alternating deviations in atmospheric pressure are propagated outward from the diaphragm as a longitudinal acoustic wave.

The shading in Figure 1 represents a compression of the air particles[4] that are trapped between the diaphragm of the earphone and the tympanic membrane (TM). No attempt has been made to depict a series of alternating compressions and rarefactions of air particles in the external auditory meatus (EAM). Under clinical conditions, this type of wave motion does not occur because the column of air enclosed is too

---

[3] The term excess pressure commonly is used in acoustics texts to describe the sound pressure produced by a vibrating body (Beranek, 1960; Morse, 1948; Randall, 1951; Rettinger, 1968; Stewart, 1932).

[4] For many problems in acoustics it is common to ignore molecular composition and molecular activity of the gases that compose our atmosphere. Accordingly, the term particle of air is used to describe a small quantity of the atmospheric medium (Stewart, 1932, p. 10).

short. To be specific, carrier frequencies used for acoustic-impedance measurements usually are lower than 1000 Hz. At 34°C the wavelength of a 1000-Hz signal is approximately 35.2 cm/cycle.[5] When the earmold or ear tip of the acoustic-impedance probe is sealed in place, however, the effective length of the EAM does not exceed 2 cm. This means that, for clinical acoustic-impedance measurements, it is not necessary to consider the incident and reflected waves separately.

The coupling tube shown in Figure 1 is a hypodermic needle with a small lumen. This type of tube has been used by many investigators (Lilly, 1964; Møller, 1960, 1961a,b, 1962, 1964; Onchi, 1961, 1963; Pinto and Dallos, 1968; Söhoel and Arnesen, 1962; Terkildsen and Scott Nielsen, 1960; Zwislocki, 1957a,b) to prevent impedance changes within the EAM from affecting the transfer characteristics of the transducer. The earphone with its coupling tube is the source of energy for the middle (acoustical) section of the complete system. Since we now are concerned with acoustic energy, in an acoustic system, the impedance at the tip of the coupling tube will be an acoustic impedance. In this chapter we shall use the term *acoustic impedance* and the symbol Z_A to refer to the "total opposition" encountered by a longitudinal acoustic wave.[6] The standard unit for this quantity is the mks (meter-kilogram-second) acoustic ohm or the cgs (centimeter-gram-second) acoustic ohm. If a system of units is not specified we assume that the cgs system was used.

The cgs system of units was used for most of the early work in acoustics. The mks system of units, however, is more satisfactory for systems that contain electrical, mechanical, and acoustical components (Beranek, 1954, p. 8; Randall, 1951, p. 7). Consequently, within the past 20 years

---

[5] Auricular acoustic-impedance measurements usually are made with a coupling tube sealed hermetically into the EAM. Temperature of the air in this tube depends upon how long it has been sealed in the EAM, upon its volume, and upon the ambient room temperature. In our laboratory, average air temperatures range from about 31°C in the coupling tube to almost 37°C at the surface of the tympanic membrane. Consequently, on the basis of these preliminary measurements and the data of Becker (1930), Benzinger (1959), and Scevola (1938), we have elected to use 34 ± 3°C for computations that involve the air trapped within the EAM during clinical acoustic-impedance measurements.

[6] A standard definition for acoustic impedance (Z_A) is given in the American standard for acoustical terminology (ASA S1.1-1960, p. 22): "The acoustic impedance of a fluid medium on a given surface lying in a wave front is the complex ratio of the sound pressure (force per unit area) on that surface to the flux (volume velocity, or particle velocity multiplied by the area) through the surface." The term *analogous acoustic impedance* also is used to describe the quantity we have labelled acoustic impedance (Z_A) (Morse, 1948, p. 243; Randall, 1951, p. 106).

there has been a trend toward adoption of the rationalized[7] mks system of units for acoustical computations. This trend has been supported in published American standards (ASA Z24.11, 1954, pp. 9–10; ASA S3.3, 1960) and was given international sanction at the Eleventh General Conference on Weights and Measures (Anon., 1960). For acoustic-impedance measurements, the same numerical values may be reported in either system, if the notation (10^5 mks acoustic ohms) is used interchangeably with the unit (acoustic ohm) [500 acoustic ohms (cgs) = 500 (10^5 mks acoustic ohms)].

There is no standard symbol for the acoustic ohm. It is incorrect and confusing to use an uppercase omega or the word ohms (without the adjective acoustic) when referring to acoustic-impedance measurements.

The input acoustic impedance of the human auditory system (Z_A) usually is measured at the point in the EAM where the coupling tube terminates. The tip of the tube defines a cross-sectional plane (through the canal) that often is called the *plane of measurement*. The acoustic signal in the plane of measurement will depend upon the acoustic impedance that exists in this plane. It is common practice to speak of the acoustic impedance that is *seen* in the plane of measurement.

The coupling tube in Figure 1 does not contact the tympanic membrane. This situation exists in every clinical system that is used for acoustic-impedance measurements. It is an important consideration because the acoustic impedance measured within the external auditory canal (Z_A) is a combination of the acoustic impedance seen at the distal surface of the tympanic membrane (Z_{TM}) and the acoustic impedance of the volume of air that is interposed between the tip of the coupling tube and the tympanic membrane (Z_C). This means that if we wish to know the acoustic impedance at the tympanic membrane (Z_{TM}), we must make an electrical, a mathematical, or an acoustical correction for the acoustic impedance of the volume of air within the external auditory canal (Z_C).

For clinical measurements, it usually is assumed that Z_A is equal to Z_C *in parallel with* Z_{TM}. The phrase "in parallel with" and the concept of impedances in parallel have been borrowed from electrical network theory to provide a method for computing Z_{TM} when Z_A and Z_C are known.[8] In

---

[7] Varner (Chapter III, 1947) reviews the basic differences between the two mks systems of units. He suggests that the adjective "rationalized," although in common use, is not mathematically accurate.

[8] This simple concept of impedances in parallel may produce excessive computational errors for carrier frequencies above 500 Hz when earmolds are used or when the patient has a long external auditory meatus. Acoustic transmission-line theory (Beranek, 1949; Morse, 1948) provides a computational approach that is

general, if two acoustic impedances (such as Z_C and Z_{TM}) are in parallel, the total acoustic impedance (Z_A) will be lower than either acoustic impedance in the parallel combination.

In Figure 1, the coupling tube and the EAM serve as waveguides for the acoustic carrier signal. When the incident wavefront reaches the tympanic membrane: (1) some of the available acoustic energy is used to set the membrane into vibration; (2) some is absorbed at the surface of the membrane; and (3) the remaining acoustic energy is propagated back toward the source as a reflected wave. The magnitude and the relative phase angle of the reflected signal will depend upon the mechanical impedance (Z_M) of the middle-ear transmission system. In acoustical terms we would say that the "total" instantaneous air particle velocity (u_i) at the surface of the TM is the vector sum of u_i for the incident wave and u_i for the reflected wave. Moreover, the "total" instantaneous sound pressure (p_i) at the surface of the TM is the vector sum of p_i for the incident wave and p_i for the reflected wave.

For clinical acoustic-impedance measurements, the magnitude and the relative phase angle of the "total" sound pressure in the plane of measurement: (1) is nearly the same as the magnitude and relative phase angle of the "total" sound pressure at the lateral surface of the TM; (2) is dependent upon boundary conditions at the TM; (3) is dependent upon the acoustic impedance of the column of air within the EAM; and (4) is proportional to Z_A in the plane of measurement.

The microphone tube in Figure 1 samples the "total" sound pressure in the plane of measurement. The electrical output of the microphone is amplified, filtered, and then delivered to a voltmeter and to a phase meter. The complete electroacoustic system then is calibrated so that the voltmeter reads the magnitude of Z_A (in acoustic ohms) and the phase meter reads the phase angle of Z_A (relative to the phase of the carrier signal). This simple, direct-reading electroacoustic impedance system does not require a bridge or comparison circuit. A system of this type first was used for clinical acoustic-impedance measurements by Lilly (1964). The design of his system was based upon the work of Mawardi (1949), Møller (1958, 1960), and Zwislocki (1957a).

B. Relations between Input Impedances and Anatomical Structures

Figure 2 shows the peripheral auditory system and a block diagram of the air cavities and the middle-ear structures that contribute to the

---

more precise for these special problems. Olson (1947, p. 459) and Pinto and Dallos (1968) discuss the application of acoustic transmission-line theory to the external auditory meatus.

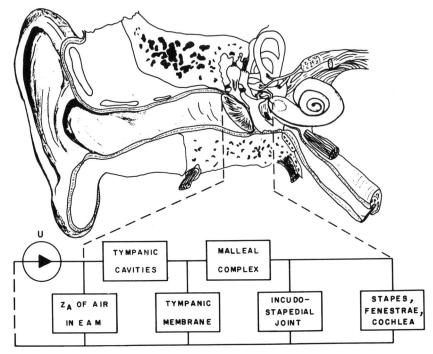

Fig. 2. Peripheral auditory system and block diagram of air cavities and middle-ear structures that contribute to acoustic impedance (Z_A) at plane of measurement in external auditory meatus.

acoustic impedance at the input of the system (Z_A). This composite model has been assembled from the work of Bauer *et al.* (1968), Møller (1961c, 1963, 1965), Onchi (1949, 1961), and Zwislocki (1957b, 1962, 1963a,b). The source of acoustic energy for the model is a constant volume–velocity generator. This generator is designated by an arrow within a circle (Beranek, 1954, p. 51). A sinusoidal acoustic wave produces an alternating flow of air particles perpendicularly through a specified surface area or plane (S). The rate of flow of these air particles is called volume-velocity (U), with units cubic meters per second.[9] In simplest terms, the rate of flow of air particles through the generator in this model will remain constant regardless of the acoustic load con-

---

[9] Volume velocity is analogous to current in electrical systems. The quantity volume velocity (U) also has been called "volume current" (ASA Y10.11-1953; Olson, 1943, 1947; Randall, 1951; Stewart and Lindsay, 1930), "rate of volume displacement" (Stewart and Lindsay, 1930; West, 1928), "analogous current" (Morse, 1948), and "flux" (ASA S1.1-1960; Beranek, 1949).

nected to its terminals. In general, a constant volume-velocity source is analogous to a constant-current source in electric-circuit theory.

The first block (from the left) in Figure 2 represents the acoustic impedance of the volume of air within the external auditory canal (Z_C). The human EAM is a warm, moist, skin-lined cul-de-sac (McLaurin, 1954) that varies in length from about 2 cm in neonates (Perry, 1957) to almost 3 cm in adults (Wever and Lawrence, 1954, p. 416). The volume of the EAM during acoustic-impedance measurements depends upon the insertion depth of the earmold or ear tip. If the dimensions of the EAM are small compared to the wavelength (λ) of the carrier signal, the volume of air enclosed usually is regarded as a pure acoustic compliance (C_A), with units m^5 per newton.[10] Since an elastic medium can be compressed by an acoustic force, we may think of an acoustic compliance as the acoustical analog of a mechanical spring. Acoustic compliance (C_A) is the reciprocal of acoustic stiffness. In general, as a volume of air becomes smaller, it becomes less compliant (more stiff), and its acoustic impedance (Z_A) becomes higher. Although it takes acoustic energy to compress a closed volume of air, this energy is not dissipated (converted to heat) or lost. An enclosed volume of air opposes the applied acoustic force or "reacts" against this force. Accordingly, we say that an acoustic compliance provides a "reactance" to the propagation of acoustic energy. In the words of Kennelly and Kurakawa (1921, p. 4), an "acoustic reactance cyclically stores and releases, without dissipation, the energy of acoustic vibration." In this chapter we shall use the term *compliant reactance* and the symbol $-X_A$ to denote the acoustic reactance provided by an acoustic compliance or produced at the surface of a diaphragm (such as the TM) that is loaded by a mechanical spring.[11]

It is appropriate at this point to consider an acoustic element that provides a second basic type of acoustic reactance. A column of air within an *open* tube is considered an acoustic mass (M_A) with units kg per m^4. Since the end of the tube is not sealed, this column or "slug" of air can be displaced by an acoustic force.[12] A comparison of M_A with C_A shows that a "pure" acoustic mass M_A involves acceleration of a column of air *without compression* whereas a "pure" acoustic compliance involves com-

---

[10] Acoustic compliance (C_A) is analogous to capacitance (C) in electrical systems. Acoustic compliance also has been called "acoustical capacitance" (Olson, 1943, 1947).

[11] Compliant reactance ($-X_A$) also has been called "elastic reactance" (West, 1928).

[12] Acoustic mass (M_A) is analogous to inductance (L) in electrical systems. Acoustic mass also has been called "acoustic inertance" (Zwislocki, 1962).

pression of a volume of air *without acceleration* (Beranek, 1954, pp. 63–65).

Acoustic energy is required to displace an acoustic mass, but again, this energy is not dissipated or lost. An acoustic mass, like a mechanical mass, opposes or "reacts" against positional changes. Accordingly, we say that an acoustic mass provides a second type of acoustic reactance. In this chapter we shall use the term *mass reactance* and the symbol X_A to denote the acoustic reactance provided by an acoustic mass or produced at the surface of a diaphragm (such as the TM) that is loaded with a mechanical mass. The mass reactance (X_A) of the air in the EAM is not an important factor during acoustic-impedance measurements unless we use an earmold with a long, small-diameter drill hole.

Mass reactance (X_A) and compliant reactance ($-X_A$) both may contribute to the complex acoustic impedance (Z_A) in a given plane (S). Consequently, the unit for either type of acoustic reactance is the acoustic ohm.

A small fraction of the acoustic energy within the EAM will be dissipated or absorbed. "Sound absorption is the change of sound energy into some other form, usually heat, in passing through a medium or on striking a surface." (ASA S1.1-1960) It has been shown experimentally (Knudsen, 1933; Neklepajev, 1911; Pielemeier, 1945) and mathematically (Kneser, 1933; Rayleigh, 1896, Volume II, Chapter XVII; Stokes, 1868) that acoustic energy is dissipated as a result of friction within the medium. Sound absorption in this small sample of air would depend upon its viscosity, its heat conductivity, and upon collisions between gas molecules within the EAM. An acoustic element or surface that dissipates or absorbs acoustic energy is called an acoustic resistance (R_A). Acoustic resistance is another component that may contribute to the complex acoustic impedance in a given plane. The "opposition" provided by an acoustic resistance also is reported in acoustic ohms.

The walls of the EAM are lined with stratified squamous epithelium that contains sebaceous glands, ceruminous glands, and vellus hair. The canal also contains varying amounts of cerumen, macerated epithelium, dust, and debris. Although most investigators have ignored acoustic absorption at the cutaneous surface of the EAM, Ithell (1963a) observed a steady increase in acoustic resistance (R_A) for some subjects during a 20-minute test session. He attributed this increase in R_A to "variations of the moisture content of the sealed ear." Ithell (1963a) concluded that, "The change of relative humidity is not significant in its effect upon the impedance of the medium but the presence of drops of perspiration may alter the absorption of the cavity walls [pp. 142–143]." This hypothesis may explain why Lilly and Shepherd (1964) observed a similar increase in R_A during 50-min acoustic-impedance experiments.

The function of each remaining block in Figure 2 has been analyzed in detail by Zwislocki (1962). In general: (1) some of the energy "transmitted" to the middle ear is used to produce alternating compression and rarefaction of the air within the tympanic cavities; (2) some energy is dissipated in frictional resistance within the transmission system; and (3) some energy is used to produce proportional displacement of the ossicular chain (which in turn, produces displacement of the cochlear fluids and the basilar membrane). Every block in Figure 2 is composed of mechanical or acoustic elements, and nearly every block contains a mass (inertial) component, a compliance (elastic) component, and a resistance (dissipative) component. The transmission and impedance characteristics of some blocks in the model will be affected by congenital malformations of the transmission system. The characteristics of others will change with ear disease and with contraction of the middle-ear muscles.

The complicated interaction of mass, resistance, and compliance elements within the middle ear produces a complex mechanical impedance (Z_M) at the lateral surface of the TM. The "total opposition" presented by this mechanical impedance to an acoustic wave will determine the acoustic impedance that we measure at the tympanic membrane (Z_{TM}).

IV. Standard Methods for Presenting Acoustic-Impedance Data

The concept of acoustic impedance allows us to consider simultaneously the combined effect of mass, compliance, and resistance: (1) with one word, (2) with one complex number, and (3) with one type of unit—the acoustic ohm.

We noted in our original definition that any impedance involves a complex ratio of two vector quantities. Accordingly, acoustic impedance at the TM: (1) will be a vector quantity, and (2) will require two numbers for complete specification. The form used for writing these two numbers will differ with the type of notation. In this section we shall examine some common numerical and graphical methods for presenting acoustic-impedance data in *polar notation, rectangular notation, trigonometric notation,* and *exponential notation.*

A. Polar Notation

It is important for the audiologist to understand polar notation because most electroacoustic-impedance instruments provide measurement data in polar form. When a complex number is reported in polar form we are given a *magnitude* and a *phase angle*. For example, the input or driving-point impedance of a (ISC/Telephonics Corp.) TDH-39 earphone might be written

$$Z_i = 9.9\angle 6° \; \Omega.$$

We would read this statement: "Input impedance equals 9.9 ohms at an angle of 6 degrees." Sometimes we are concerned only with the magnitude of an impedance. If this had been the case for our TDH-39 earphone, we would have written

$$|Z_i| = 9.9 \; \Omega.$$

When the impedance symbol is enclosed within two vertical lines we must read: "The *magnitude* (or the absolute value) of the input impedance equals 9.9 ohms." In polar notation the phase angle tells us how the phase of the force-like quantity (force, voltage, or sound pressure) differs from the phase of the related velocity-like quantity (velocity, current, or volume velocity).

When the polar form is used to report acoustic impedance at the tympanic membrane (Z_{TM}), we usually indicate the carrier frequency as well as the magnitude and phase angle. For example, we might write

$$Z_{TM} \bigg|_{500 \; Hz} = 610\angle -55° \quad \text{acoustic ohms.}$$

We would read this statement: "At 500 hertz, acoustic impedance at the tympanic membrane equals 610 acoustic ohms at an angle of negative 55 degrees." Dallos (1964) used a Zwislocki acoustic bridge to measure acoustic impedance at the right tympanic membrane of six subjects with normal hearing. His data are plotted in terms of magnitude $|Z_{TM}|$ and the phase angle $\angle \theta$ of Z_{TM}. The second and third columns of Table I show his individual measurements for each subject, plus the mean magnitude and phase angle for Z_{TM} when his carrier frequency was 500 Hz. Dallos' data are written in standard polar notation in the fourth column of Table I. The negative phase angles in Column 4 were obtained by subtracting each phase angle in Column 3 from 360°.

A special configuration of the Cartesian system of rectangular coordinates is used to plot complex numbers in polar form. This graphical representation is called a "polar plot," a "polar diagram," or a "phasor diagram." In Figure 3, two coordinate axes are drawn perpendicular to each other with zero at the origin. This two-dimensional plane is labeled the "Z_A plane" when it is used for acoustic-impedance data. When a separate polar diagram is used for each carrier signal, the carrier frequency can be stated below the notation "Z_A plane." The fixed refer-

TABLE I

ACOUSTIC IMPEDANCE AT TYMPANIC MEMBRANE
(Z_{TM}) FOR SIX SUBJECTS WITH NORMAL
HEARING WHEN CARRIER FREQUENCY
WAS 500 Hz[a]

Subject	Plotted values (acoustic ohms)		Standard polar notation (acoustic ohms)
	$|Z_{TM}|$	θ	
1	775	312°	$775\angle -48°$
2	437	323°	$437\angle -37°$
3	488	297°	$488\angle -63°$
4	438	304°	$438\angle -56°$
5	438	311°	$438\angle -49°$
6	388	301°	$388\angle -59°$
Mean	494	308°	$494\angle -52°$

[a] Based on data from Dallos (1964).

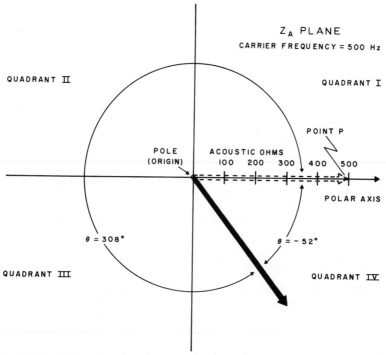

FIG. 3. Polar diagram for complex acoustic-impedance data. Phasor plotted in quadrant IV represents mean Z_{TM} data reported by Dallos (1964) for normal ears at 500 Hz.

ence point at the origin (0) of a polar diagram is called the *pole*. The horizontal axis extending to the right of this pole is called the *polar axis*.

The mean Z_{TM} for Dallos's six subjects is shown in Table I as 494∠308° acoustic ohms. To plot this complex number on our polar diagram we could (1) scale the polar axis in acoustic ohms; (2) mark a point P at 494 acoustic ohms; (3) draw a line segment from the pole (origin) to point P (in Figure 3 this initial line segment is shown as a dashed line tipped with an arrowhead); and then (4) rotate the line segment 308° counterclockwise from the polar axis. A mathematician would call this directed line segment a *radius vector*. Many operations (in formal vector analysis) that apply to a general vector in the plane, however, do not apply to a radius vector (Davis, 1967). Other mathematical operations that are applicable to radius vectors have been developed specifically for network analysis. Consequently: "In an attempt to differentiate between vectors in formal vector analysis and the type of vector of concern here, the term 'phasor' has been rather widely adopted" (Stewart, 1960.)[13] In this chapter we shall follow the trend in electrical engineering and refer to our radius vector as a *phasor*.

The length of the directed line segment in Figure 3 ($|Z_{TM}| = 494$ acoustic ohms) is called the *magnitude*, the *absolute value*, the *modulus*, or the *radius* of the phasor. The phase angle ($∠θ = 308°$) is called the *argument* or the *amplitude* of the phasor. The coordinate axes in Figure 3 divide the plane into four parts or *quadrants* that conventionally are numbered I, II, III, and IV. Phasors representing clinical acoustic-impedance measurements always fall in quadrant I, on the polar axis, or in quadrant IV. When a phasor lies in quadrant IV, electrical engineers usually measure its argument clockwise from the polar axis and report an angle of 0° to −90° rather than an angle of 360° to 270°. This procedure simplifies algebraic and trigonometric computations, and therefore, we shall use it for acoustic-impedance measurements.

The tip of the phasor in Figure 3 describes one point, and only one point in the Z_A plane. This same point also can be described uniquely using rectangular notation.

B. Rectangular Notation

Although most electroacoustic-impedance instruments provide measurement data in polar form, acoustic-impedance bridges provide equivalent data in rectangular form. It will be easier to understand the rectan-

---

[13] Stewart (1960, pp. 1–28) presents an evaluation of the applications and limitations of vectors, phasors, and sinors for systems analysis.

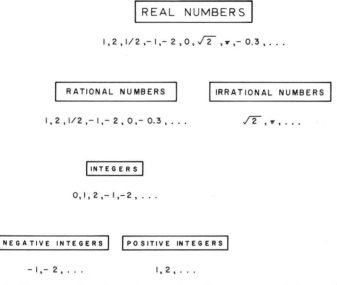

FIG. 4. Hierarchy of real number system with some numerical examples.

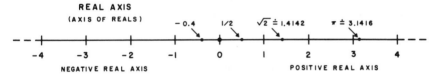

FIG. 5. Real axis. All real numbers could be plotted as points on this horizontal line.

gular form of a complex number if we review first the nature of complex numbers. By definition, a complex number is composed of a "real component" and an "imaginary component." In this section, we shall plot each of these components on the rectangular coordinate axes of a special graph that is called an "argand diagram."

We recall from our study of algebra that *real numbers* can be rational or irrational. The positive integers, the negative integers, and zero are rational numbers. Figure 4 depicts the hierarchy of the real number system with some numerical examples. Any of the real numbers in this hierarchy can be represented as points on a line. Conceivably, the numbers on the horizontal line in Figure 5 could extend from $-\infty$ on the left, through zero, to $+\infty$ on the right.[14] Real numbers always are plotted

---

[14] The phrase "extended real number system" often is used when the system under consideration includes the real number system together with the symbols $+\infty$ and $-\infty$ (James and James, 1959, p. 152).

on the horizontal axis of an argand diagram. Consequently, the axis of abscissas is called the "real axis" or the "axis of reals." The positive real axis begins at zero and extends indefinitely to the right, whereas the negative real axis begins at zero and extends indefinitely to the left.

Most algebraic operations on real numbers yield results that are real numbers. The exception to this statement becomes apparent when we attempt to take the square root of a negative number. For example: find x if

$$x^2 = -4. \tag{1}$$

taking the square root of both sides gives

$$x = \sqrt{-4}, \tag{2}$$

but our definition for multiplication states that either $(+2)^2$ or $(-2)^2$ equals $+4$. Since no real number multiplied by itself will give a negative number, the square root of a negative number does not fit in the real number system. To solve problems like the example in Eq. (1), we must define a new kind of number whose square is a negative number. This number is called an *imaginary number*. Just as the integer 1 is the unit of the real number system, the symbol

$$j \equiv \sqrt{-1} \tag{3}$$

is the unit of the imaginary number system.[15] This means that every imaginary number is a multiple of the "imaginary unit" j. Thus, imaginary numbers (such as $j2$, $-j470$, and $j0.5$) are easy to identify because they always are preceded by j.

Our new number system may be used to solve Eq. (2) if we rewrite the square root of -4 as the square root of 4 times the square root of -1. Thus

$$x = \sqrt{-4} = \sqrt{(-1)(4)} = \sqrt{-1}\sqrt{4},$$

but since $\sqrt{-1} = j$,

$$x = j\sqrt{4} = \pm j2. \tag{4}$$

Imaginary numbers always are plotted on the vertical axis of an argand diagram. Consequently, the axis of ordinates is called the "imaginary axis" or the "axis of imaginaries." In Figure 6, the positive imaginary

---

[15] Mathematicians use the symbol $i = \sqrt{-1}$ as the imaginary unit. Electrical engineers and investigators working in electroacoustics have adopted the symbol j to avoid confusion between the imaginary unit and the conventional symbol for instantaneous electric current (i).

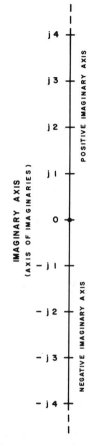

Fig. 6. Imaginary axis. All imaginary numbers could be plotted as points on this vertical line.

axis begins at zero and extends upward indefinitely, whereas the negative imaginary axis begins at zero and extends downward indefinitely.

If two real numbers are added, the sum is another real number. We know that

$$2 + 3 = 5. \tag{5}$$

If two imaginary numbers are added, the sum is an imaginary number. Thus

$$j4 + j2 = j6. \tag{6}$$

If the real number 5 is added to the imaginary number $j6$, the result

$$5 + j6 \tag{7}$$

is called a *complex number*. When a complex number is given in the form of Eq. (7), we say that it is written in "rectangular" or "algebraic" form. The rationale for the phrase "rectangular form" becomes clear when this complex number is plotted.

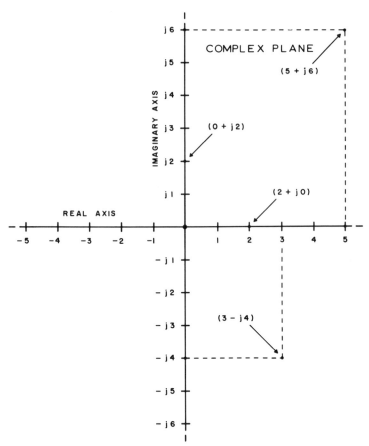

FIG. 7. Argand diagram constructed from real axis of Figure 5 and imaginary axis of Figure 6. Four complex numbers (expressed in rectangular form) are plotted in this complex plane.

If we draw the real axis of Figure 5 perpendicular to the imaginary axis of Figure 6; and if we set zero at the intersection (origin) of these two coordinate axes, we obtain the complex plane of Figure 7. To plot the complex number $5 + j6$ in this plane: (1) We plot the real number 5 as a point on the real axis and draw a dashed line parallel to the imaginary axis through this point. (2) We plot the imaginary number $j6$ on the positive imaginary axis and draw a dashed line parallel to the real axis through this point. (3) We plot a point at the intersection of the two dashed lines. This procedure shows that the complex number $5 + j6$ describes uniquely a point in the complex plane that lies at one corner of a *rectangle* formed by the two dashed lines and the coordinate axes. A similar procedure has been used to plot $3—j4$ in the complex plane of Figure 7.

To summarize, all of the numbers we have discussed may be plotted in the complex plane. In practical terms, we note that: (1) A real number has only one component, and therefore, it can be represented as a point on a line (the real axis). (2) A pure imaginary number also has only one component, and it too can be represented as point on a line (the imaginary axis). (3) A complex number has two components, and therefore, it must be represented as a point in the complex plane. In analytical terms, however, we recognize that the real and the imaginary number systems are subsystems of the complex number system. To illustrate, the real number 2 is a complex number with zero as its imaginary component. This number $(2 = 2 + j0)$ is plotted on the real axis of Figure 7. Likewise, the pure imaginary number $j2$ is a complex

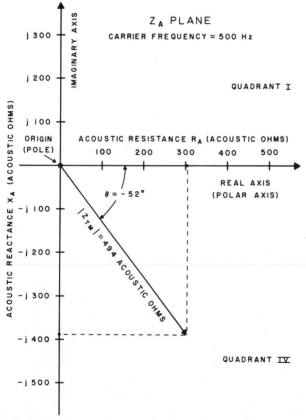

Fig. 8. Complex acoustic-impedance plane combines characteristics of polar diagram (Figure 3) with axes and notation of argand diagram (Figure 7). Phasor plotted in quadrant IV represents mean Z_{TM} data reported by Dallos (1964) for normal ears at 500 Hz. Auricular acoustic-impedance values always lie in quadrant I, on positive real (polar) axis, or in quadrant IV.

number with zero as its real component. This number $(j2 = 0 + j2)$ is plotted on the imaginary axis of Figure 7.

The relation between the rectangular form and the polar form of a complex number can be shown best when we combine the basic characteristics of a polar diagram (Figure 3) with the axes and notation of an argand diagram (Figure 7). This has been done in Figure 8. Seven characteristics of this complex Z_A plane should be emphasized: (1) An arrowhead on an axis identifies it as the positive (real or imaginary) segment of the axis. (2) Acoustic-resistance (R_A) data are plotted on the positive real (polar) axis. Since negative acoustic resistance does not exist, the negative real axis is neither scaled nor labeled. This situation was suggested earlier when we noted that, "Phasors representing acoustic-impedance measurements always fall in quadrant I, on the polar (*positive real*) axis, or in quadrant IV." (3) Mass-reactance data $(X_A \equiv jX_A)$ are plotted on the positive imaginary axis. (4) Compliantreactance data $(-X_A \equiv -jX_A)$ are plotted on the negative imaginary axis. (5) Both the imaginary axis and the real axis are scaled and labeled in acoustic ohms. (6) Scale divisions on the real axis are *identical* to those on the imaginary axis. (7) The origin (pole) represents an acoustic impedance of zero acoustic ohms.

It should be emphasized at this point that j or $-j$ normally will precede an acoustic-reactance (X_A) value *only* when it is written as a complex number [together with an acoustic-resistance (R_A) value]. Throughout the remainder of this chapter, however, the imaginary unit (j) will be used with all X_A and $-X_A$ values to remind the reader where these values would be plotted in the complex Z_A plane.

For a carrier frequency of 500 Hz, the mean Z_{TM} for Dallos' six subjects was $494\angle-52°$ acoustic ohms (Table I). A phasor representing this complex number has been plotted in quadrant IV of Figure 8. The tip of this phasor occupies a unique point in the complex plane. To describe this point in rectangular form: (1) We draw from the tip of the phasor a vertical (dashed) line that intersects the real axis at an angle of 90°. (2) We draw from the tip of the phasor a horizontal (dashed) line that intersects the imaginary axis at an angle of 90°. (3) We read the rectangular coordinates of the complex number from the intersection point on each axis. In Figure 8, the vertical dashed line intersects the real axis at $R_A = 304$ acoustic ohms, and the horizontal dashed line intersects the imaginary axis at $X_A = -j389$ acoustic ohms. Dallos's mean data now may be expressed in polar form and in equivalent rectangular form as

$$Z_{TM}\Big|_{500\ Hz} = 494\angle-52° \equiv 304 - j389 \quad \text{acoustic ohms.} \quad (8)$$

The rectangular coordinates of the phasor in Figure 8 show that Z_{TM} is composed of a resistive component (R_A), and a negative reactive (stiffness) component $(-jX_A)$. We did not determine a point for the positive reactive (mass) component (jX_A). This does not mean that the mass of the middle-ear transmission system was absent for Dallos' subjects. Rather, it means that the average stiffness component was larger than the average mass component at 500 Hz. Had we been able to measure the two reactive components separately, we might have seen the following:

$$\text{Compliant reactance} = -j560 \quad \text{acoustic ohms}$$

$$\text{Mass reactance} = \underline{\quad j171} \quad \text{acoustic ohms}$$

$$\text{Total acoustic reactance} = -j389 \quad \text{acoustic ohms}$$

The values in this example are hypothetical. They illustrate, however, that total acoustic reactance always is the algebraic sum of the mass reactance and the compliant reactance at the lateral surface of the TM. The relative size of the mass, stiffness, and resistive components (in a given middle-ear transmission system) will vary with the frequency of the carrier signal. For frequencies below 500 Hz: (1) the stiffness component $(-jX_A)$ usually is larger than the mass component (jX_A); (2) the phasor for Z_{TM} lies in quadrant IV; and (3) we say that the middle-ear transmission system is "stiffness-controlled." For frequencies between 500 and 1000 Hz, we may find that: (1) jX_A is larger than $-jX_A$; (2) the phasor for Z_{TM} lies in quadrant I; and (3) the transmission system is said to be "mass-controlled." Mass-controlled middle-ear transmission systems are most common (in the frequency range from 500 to 1000 Hz) for adult males with large ears, for patients with interrupted ossicular chains, and for patients who have had stapes surgery or other middle-ear surgery. At any frequency where $jX_A \equiv -jX_A$, the two reactive components cancel each other and we are left with only a resistive component. For this condition, the phasor for Z_{TM} lies on the positive real (polar) axis and we say that the transmission system is in resonance.

C. Trigonometric Notation

It is not necessary to plot an impedance phasor each time we wish to convert a polar quantity to rectangular form. A phasor in quadrant I or in quadrant IV of the Z_A plane constitutes the hypotenuse of a right triangle. In Figure 8, the length of this hypotenuse $= |Z_{TM}| = 494$ acoustic ohms. To convert Dallos's mean data from polar to rectangular form we must determine the length of each of the remaining sides of the right triangle. The positive real (polar) axis is the side of the triangle adjacent to the angle θ. We recall from trigonometry that

$$\cos \theta = \frac{\text{side adjacent}}{\text{hypotenuse}} = \frac{R_A}{|Z_{TM}|}, \tag{9}$$

but since $|Z_{TM}|$ and θ are known, we can multiply both sides of the equation by $|Z_{TM}|$ to obtain

$$R_A = |Z_{TM}| \cos \theta \quad \text{acoustic ohms.} \tag{10}$$

Ii we substitute into this equation the mean Z_{TM} for Dallos's six subjects, we find that

$$R_A = 494 \cos -52° \tag{11}$$
$$= 494(0.61566) \tag{12}$$
$$= 304 \quad \text{acoustic ohms.} \tag{13}$$

This value for R_A is identical to the one we obtained graphically.[16]

In Figure 8 the dashed line from the tip of the phasor to the real axis forms the side of the triangle opposite θ. The length of this line is the reactive component of Z_{TM} since it has the same length as the segment of the imaginary axis that lies between the origin and the horizontal projection from the tip of the phasor. Again, we recall from trigonometry that

$$\sin \theta = \frac{\text{side opposite}}{\text{hypotenuse}} = \frac{X_A}{|Z_{TM}|}, \tag{14}$$

but since $|Z_{TM}|$ and θ are known, we multiply both sides of the equation by $|Z_{TM}|$ to obtain

$$X_A = |Z_{TM}| \sin \theta \quad \text{acoustic ohms.} \tag{15}$$

When we substitute into this equation the mean Z_{TM} for Dallos's six subjects, we find that

$$X_A = 494 \sin -52° \tag{16}$$
$$= (494)(-0.78801) \tag{17}$$
$$= -389 \text{ acoustic ohms.} \tag{18}$$

This negative reactance value is identical to the one we obtained graphically. When we write the value of this reactive component together with the value computed for the resistive component, we multiply -389 by the "imaginary unit" j to obtain a complex number in rectangular form [as in Eq. (8)].

Although we have computed R_A and X_A separately for the Dallos data, Eq. (10) and Eq. (15) usually are combined to provide a general computational formula that may be used with any Z_A data in polar form. An

---

[16] The negative sign preceding $52°$ in Eq. (11) does not appear in Eq. (12) because the cosine function is an "even" function. This means that $\cos(-\theta) = \cos \theta$. We shall see in Eq. (16) and in Eq. (17) that the sine function is an "odd" function of θ. Consequently, $\sin(-\theta) = -\sin \theta$.

equation of the form

$$|Z_A|\angle\theta = |Z_A|(\cos\theta + j\sin\theta) \qquad (19)$$

is called Euler's formula.[17] When a value for $|Z_A|$ and a value for θ are substituted into the right-hand side of Eq. (19), we say that the data are presented in "trigonometric form." For example, the mean Z_{TM} for Dallos's subjects (Table I) could be written in trigonometric form as

$$Z_{TM}\Big|_{500\ Hz} = 494(\cos -52° + j\sin -52°) \quad \text{acoustic ohms.} \qquad (20)$$

In our examples, we have used Dallos's (1964) data because they were published in polar form. Since his measurements were made with a Zwislocki acoustic bridge, we know that Dallos converted the data from rectangular to polar form before analysis. This type of conversion is the converse of the one developed in the preceding section, and it too can be accomplished graphically or mathematically. To illustrate, suppose we had been given $Z_{TM} = 304 - j389$ acoustic ohms as the mean value for Dallos' six subjects. Referring back to Figure 8 we see that the horizontal side of the right triangle has a length of $R_A = 304$ acoustic ohms, whereas the vertical (orthogonal) side has a length of $X_A = -389$ acoustic ohms. We must determine from these two sides the hypotenuse of the triangle and the angle θ. The theorem of Pythagoras states that the sum of the squares of the sides of a right triangle is equal to the square of the hypotenuse of the triangle. We may use this theorem to compute the length of the phasor in Figure 8, if we write

$$(|Z_{TM}|)^2 = (R_A)^2 + (X_A)^2. \qquad (21)$$

Taking the square root of both sides of this equation gives

$$|Z_{TM}| = \sqrt{(R_A)^2 + (X_A)^2} \quad \text{acoustic ohms.} \qquad (22)$$

When we substitute into this equation the mean rectangular coordinates for Dallos' six subjects we find that

$$
\begin{aligned}
|Z_{TM}| &= \sqrt{(304)^2 + (-389)^2} \\
&= \sqrt{(92{,}416) + (151{,}321)} \\
&= \sqrt{243{,}737} \\
&= 493.7 \quad \text{acoustic ohms.} \qquad (23)
\end{aligned}
$$

---

[17] The Swiss mathematician Leonhard Euler (1707–1783) first proposed the basic formula for converting polar data to rectangular form (James and James, 1959, p. 149).

This value for $|Z_{TM}|$ rounds to the mean value (494 acoustic ohms) we computed in Table I.

We must use another trigonometric definition to solve for the polar angle θ. Recall that

$$\tan \theta = \frac{\text{side opposite}}{\text{side adjacent}} = \frac{X_A}{R_A}. \tag{24}$$

When an impedance value is given in rectangular form both X_A and R_A are known, and the function tangent θ can be determined by division. Since we wish to know the angle θ rather than the function tangent θ, we write

$$\theta = \angle\tan^{-1} \frac{X_A}{R_A}. \tag{25}$$

We would read this equation: "The argument theta equals the angle whose tangent is X_A/R_A."[18] For Eq. (12) and Eq. (17) we entered a table of natural trigonometric functions to find the cosine function and the sine function of an angle. For Eq. (25), we reverse the process, and enter the table with the computed function (tan θ) to find the angle. If we substitute into Eq. (25) the mean rectangular coordinates for Dallos's six subjects we find that

$$\theta = \angle\tan^{-1} \frac{-389}{304}$$

$$= \angle\tan^{-1} -1.2796$$

$$= \angle -52°. \tag{26}$$

This value for θ is identical to the mean value that we computed in Table I. Although we have determined $|Z_{TM}|$ and θ separately for the Dallos data, Eq. (22) and Eq. (25) usually are combined to provide a general computational formula that may be used with any Z_A data in rectangular form. Thus,

$$|Z_A|\angle\theta = \sqrt{(R_A)^2 + (X_A)^2} \;\angle\tan^{-1} \frac{X_A}{R_A} \quad \text{acoustic ohms.} \tag{27}$$

D. Exponential Notation

In Section IV, A we introduced the angle notation $\angle\theta$ for complex numbers in polar form. This particular notation is cumbersome to manipulate mathematically. Consequently, polar quantities often are written in an equivalent *exponential form* for computational work and for publica-

---

[18] The arc tangent of a number x usually is written $\tan^{-1} x$ or arc tan x. The function may be called the inverse tangent function or the antitangent function.

tion. In general, an exponential function may be written

$$y = a^u, \tag{28}$$

where a is a constant and u is a variable. The base of the Napierian system of logarithms e usually is the constant in exponential functions that represent polar quantities, and the definition

$$\angle\theta = e^{j\theta} \tag{29}$$

frequently is applied to acoustic-impedance data. We would read this definition as: "The polar argument theta equals e to the j theta." As an example, we can use either the angle notation $\angle\theta$ or the exponential notation $e^{j\theta}$ to report the mean Z_{TM} for Dallos's six subjects (Table I):

$$Z_{\text{TM}} \Big|_{500 \text{ Hz}} = 494\angle-52° \equiv 494e^{-j52°} \quad \text{acoustic ohms.} \tag{30}$$

Equation (30) shows that the notation e^j may be regarded as an alternative method for writing the angle symbol $\angle$.[19] A negative sign preceding the exponent j means that the impedance phasor will lie in quadrant IV of the Z_A plane. The polar argument θ normally is reported in sexagesimal measure (with units degrees) for the angle notation, and in circular measure (with units radians) for the exponential notation. Accordingly, the relation shown in Eq. (30) ordinarily would be written

$$Z_{\text{TM}} \Big|_{500 \text{ Hz}} = 494\angle-52° \equiv 494e^{-j0.9757} \quad \text{acoustic ohms,} \tag{31}$$

since

$$1 \text{ degree} = \frac{\pi}{180} \doteq 0.01745 \quad \text{radians.} \tag{32}$$

If the argument of an exponential function is complicated, it may be

---

[19] Rigorous proof of Eq. (29) involves mathematical assumptions and operations that normally are not emphasized in audiology training programs. The derivation below is presented in outline form for the reader who has studied analytic functions of a complex variable: (1) For any real number θ, the expression $e^{j\theta}$ can be expanded in an infinite series according to Maclaurin's theorem. (2) When we separate the real and imaginary terms that result from such an expansion, we see that the collection of real terms is identical to the Maclaurin expansion for cosine θ, whereas the collection of imaginary terms constitutes the Maclaurin expansion for sine θ. (3) Recognition of these two relations allows us to write

$$e^{j\theta} = \cos\theta + j\sin\theta,$$

and

$$\cos\theta + j\sin\theta = 1\angle\theta$$

was derived trigonometrically for Eq. (19). Euler's formula usually is written in the form of the first equation shown above.

confusing to write the function in the form e^u. For example, the expression

$$4e^{j628}\left(t - \frac{\pi}{2}\right),$$ (33)

is easier to understand (and is easier for the typesetter to set) if we substitute the *exponential operator* (exp) for the symbol e and write

$$4 \exp\left[j628\left(t - \frac{\pi}{2}\right)\right].$$ (34)

The exponential operator exp or the symbol e, normally is used in place of the angle symbol when polar quantities are reported in scientific journals.

E. Rationale and Applications for Alternative Presentation Methods

Although the mathematical exposition in this section is not difficult, it involves number systems and operations that traditionally are not stressed in audiology training programs. At this point it is appropriate for the audiologist to ask: "Why are there four interrelated methods for presenting acoustic-impedance data?" There is a mathematical answer and a physical answer to this question. When we consider the usual algebraic operations that are performed on acoustic-impedance data, we discover that: (1) *Addition* and *subtraction* may be done graphically, but usually are accomplished with the complex number in rectangular form. (2) *Multiplication* and *division* may be performed with the complex number in any form, but these operations are simpler in polar or in exponential form. (3) *Raising to a power* and *extracting a root* must be performed with the complex number in polar or in exponential form. (4) *Taking a logarithm* must be performed with the complex number in exponential form and with the polar angle in radians. An example of each of these operations is provided by Cassell (1964, pp. 589–593).

The "physical" answer to our question relates to the measurement values we obtain in the laboratory and in the clinic. We have noted already that acoustic measurement systems normally provide impedance data in rectangular form, whereas electroacoustic measurement systems normally provide impedance data in polar form. Unfortunately, it is not possible to compare acoustic-impedance measurements (obtained from several sources or from different instruments) without first converting all data to the same form.

V. Static Acoustic-Impedance Measurements

In this section we shall consider *static* impedance characteristics at the input of the human auditory system. We have noted already that static acoustic-impedance measurements are made with ambient (atmospheric) air pressure in the EAM, and with the middle-ear muscles in a state of "normal" tonus.

Beranek (1949, pp. 302–361) has reviewed 12 basic methods for measuring Z_A. At least eight of these methods have been adapted for the measurement of complex acoustic impedance: (1) in a plane through the cavum conchae, (2) within the EAM, or (3) at the lateral surface of the TM. In this section we shall use a simple dichotomy to classify all measurement systems as either "acoustic" or "electroacoustic." If one is interested only in static measurements of Z_{TM}, valid and reliable data can be obtained with nearly any acoustic or electroacoustic impedance method. Zwislocki (1957a) summarized this point concisely when he wrote: "Considering the difficulties arising from the anatomy of the ear, the theoretical precision of the acoustical method itself becomes of secondary importance." In this paper, Zwislocki discusses three problems that still plague accurate measurements of Z_{TM}. These problems emanate from difficulties with: (1) precise determination of Z_C (the acoustic impedance of the air trapped between the tip of the probe device and the TM); (2) an hermetic seal between the probe device and the EAM; and (3) methods for holding the distance and the azimuth of the probe device constant relative to the TM.

A. Electroacoustic Systems

Electroacoustic impedance systems have been used for a majority of the basic studies of static Z_A at the input of the *normal*, human auditory system. The earliest auricular Z_A measurements were made by telephone engineers (Fay and Hall, 1933; Inglis *et al.* 1932; Kennelly, 1925; Kennelly and Kurokawa, 1921; West, 1928). These investigators were concerned primarily with the acoustic load provided by human ears to telephone transducers. Data from their experiments and from subsequent investigations (Ithell, 1963a,b; Ithell *et al.*, 1965; Kosten and Zwikker, 1941; Morton and Jones, 1956) have been valuable in the development of acoustic couplers that are used for calibration of audiometric earphones and hearing-aid transducers.

The work of Tröger (1930) usually is regarded as the first systematic investigation of complex acoustic impedance at the tympanic membrane Z_{TM}.[20] Subsequent studies (Geffcken, 1934; Keibs, 1936; Kurtz, 1938; Lilly, 1964; Møller, 1960, 1961c, 1963, 1964, 1965; Pinto and Dallos,

---

[20] Wegel (1932) compared Tröger's average acoustic-reactance data (for low frequencies) with similar, unpublished measurements that had been made earlier (at the Bell Telephone Laboratories) by Wegel and Lane (1923) and Thuras (1925). The Thuras data subsequently were tabulated by Sivian and White, (1933, p. 316), and plotted by Zwislocki (1957a).

1968; von Békésy, 1932; Waetzmann, 1936; Waetzmann and Keibs, 1936; Zwislocki, 1957a,b, 1961, 1962, 1963a,b, 1964) have reflected technological advancements in electroacoustics and in electronics. The procedures and results reported in these investigations have produced: (1) improvements in measurement and calibration techniques, and (2) a body of normative data for Z_{TM}.

Although electroacoustic impedance systems have been used for some clinical studies (Lilly, 1964; Waetzmann, 1936; West, 1928; Zwislocki, 1957b, 1961, 1962, 1963b), acoustic measurement systems have been used for most static Z_{TM} measurements on patients with hearing impairments.

B. Acoustic Systems

The acoustic-impedance bridge has been the primary *acoustic* system for static measurements of Z_{TM}. The first practical acoustic-impedance bridge probably was constructed by Stewart (1926). An acoustic-impedance bridge developed by Schuster (1934, 1936) was improved and modified by Robinson (1937), by Waetzmann (1938), and by Schuster and Stöhr (1939). These basic instruments served as prototypes for most modern acoustic-impedance bridges. All "Schuster-type" bridges are balanced by adjusting sequentially an acoustic control for R_A and an acoustic control for X_A.

Waetzmann (1938) used a Schuster-type bridge (Schusterschen Brücke) to measure Z_{TM} in normal ears, and Menzel (1940) used a similar instrument for Z_{TM} measurements with three patients. In 1939, Metz constructed a Schuster-type bridge (similar to the one used by Waetzmann in 1938) and began a systematic study of acoustic impedance at the human tympanic membrane. A complete report of this investigation was published as a monograph in 1946. One section of the Metz (1946) monograph focused upon the relation between changes in Z_{TM} and contractions of the middle-ear muscles. In another section, Metz showed that measurement of changes in Z_{TM} might provide a quantitative test for Eustachian-tube function. Both of these applications stimulated additional research, and subsequently were developed as clinical techniques.

The primary emphasis in the Metz (1946) study, however, was on the measurement of static Z_{TM}. Metz demonstrated that these measurements could be used to diagnose accurately the presence of middle-ear disease. Still, evaluation of static Z_{TM} did not develop as a clinical test for several reasons: (1) Accurate measurements of Z_{TM}, and meaningful presentation of the data involved procedures, concepts, terminology, and quantitative methods that were not familiar to audiologists and to otolaryngologists. (2) Measurement of Z_{TM} with *any* acoustic-impedance bridge is time consuming. With the Metz bridge, additional time was required to convert the raw data to standard notation. (3) Static Z_{TM} measurements are especially valuable in differential diagnosis of (clinical) otosclerosis from interruption of the ossicular chain. In 1946, however, this type of diagnosis was of minor importance since the otologist did not have access to many of the operative techniques that currently are used in stapes surgery and in reconstructive surgery of the middle ear. (4) An acoustic-impedance instrument designed and calibrated to read static Z_A or static Z_{TM} (in absolute physical units) is more difficult to construct and to maintain than an instrument that reads only relative changes in Z_A. (5) Finally, as a corollary, an instrument for static Z_{TM} measurements was not available commercially. This final problem was not solved until Zwislocki (1963b) developed a stable acoustic-impedance bridge for clinical use.[21]

A thorough discussion of the theory and operation of the Zwislocki acoustic bridge is provided in the literature (Bicknell and Morgan, 1968; Feldman, 1963; Lamb and Norris, 1969; Zwislocki, 1963b, 1968; Zwislocki and Feldman, 1963, 1970) and in the manual that accompanies the instrument. The Zwislocki acoustic bridge is a Schuster-type bridge that incorporates several features that were not available on its predecessors. This instrument (1) is small and portable; (2) is constructed with all calibrated parts made of stainless steel; (3) contains an extremely stable, variable acoustic-resistance element; and (4) has a variable compensation cavity on the comparison side of the bridge. When the variable compensation cavity is preset to the volume of the patient's EAM, and when the bridge is sealed in the EAM and balanced, the two readings that produce this balance are approximately proportional to the rectangular coordinates of Z_{TM} (R_A and $-jX_A$).

To simplify calibration, the scales engraved on the Zwislocki acoustic bridge do not read directly in acoustic ohms. The variable acoustic-resistance control is scaled in equally spaced arbitrary units. The relation between these arbitrary units and R_A (in acoustic ohms): (1) is nonlinear and inverse; (2) is different for every Zwislocki acoustic bridge; but (3) may be determined from a calibration chart provided with each instrument. It follows, therefore, that presentation of "arbitrary resistance" (R_{ARB}) values is meaningless without calibration data for the specific model and serial number of the instrument that was used. Clinically, the most efficient approach is to convert every R_{ARB} value to R_A (in acoustic ohms) before plotting. This conversion is recommended

---

[21] The basic patent that covers the Zwislocki acoustic bridge (U.S. Patent No. 3,295,513) was issued to Paul W. Dippolito on January 3, 1967 and assigned to the Grason-Stadler Co. Inc. (Dippolito, 1967).

by Feldman (1967, p. 172) and may be done quickly if a table of values is prepared in advance from the calibration curve (Nilges *et al.*, 1969, p. 729).

The variable acoustic-reactance control on the Zwislocki acoustic bridge is calibrated relative to the acoustic compliance (C_A) of an equivalent volume of air (V_e), with units of cubic centimeters (cm^3). The relation between a reading on this control (in cubic centimeters). and $-jX_A$ (in acoustic ohms) is: (1) frequency dependent; (2) non-linear and inverse; and (3) contingent upon the temperature, the atmospheric pressure, and the relative humidity at the location of measurement (Lilly, 1970, 1971). Consequently, every scale reading from the bridge (in cubic centimeters) must be converted to an acoustic-reactance value ($-jX_A$, in acoustic ohms) if data are to be comparable from one clinic to another. This conversion should not create a clinical problem since it can be done in less than a minute (for all carrier frequencies and for both ears) if a table of values is prepared in advance. A discussion of the "acoustic impedance of an equivalent volume of air," and a description of the basic equation for this conversion are available (Lilly, 1971).[22]

C. Static Z_{TM} Data for Normal Ears

Many electroacoustic and acoustic systems have been used to measure static Z_{TM} at normal tympanic membranes. When published measurements are converted to the same form (polar or rectangular), systematic differences appear between data collected with the various systems. The experimental populations in most studies have been too small to permit detailed analysis of these differences. In general, Z_{TM} values obtained with the Zwislocki acoustic bridge appear to be higher than those obtained with electroacoustic systems. Consequently, to avoid intersystem differences, the data presented in the remainder of this section all have been gathered with Zwislocki instruments. This emphasis on a single system is appropriate, however, because the Zwislocki acoustic bridge is the only commercial instrument that currently can be used to measure complex acoustic impedance at the TM.

---

[22] A formula for converting scale readings (in cubic centimeters) to $-jX_A$ (in acoustic ohms) is given in the manual supplied with the Zwislocki acoustic bridge. Unfortunately, this equation contains no correction for the atmospheric pressure in the clinic or laboratory. Our computations show that this formula will provide precise conversion values (on a standard day, at 22°C, and with 0% relative humidity) only in a laboratory that is approximately 55 meters (55 m) below sea level. The use of this equation will produce a conversion error that is directly proportional to the altitude of the clinic or laboratory. The magnitude of the error is about 3% in Iowa City, Iowa (224 m above sea level) and about 23% in Denver, Colorado (1613 m above sea level).

Evidently, all models of the Zwislocki instrument contain a residual volume of air in the comparison arm of the bridge (Feldman, 1963, p. 317; 1964, 1967, p. 160; Feldman and Zwislocki, 1965). After "careful calibration," Feldman and Zwislocki (1965, p. 217) elected to correct for the residual volume in their instrument by adding a constant of 0.1 cm³ to each measured V_e (cm³) value. This correction apparently was used from 1965 to 1967. Following a second "careful analysis" of the instrument, Feldman (1967, p. 167) discovered that the calibration error was frequency dependent. As a result, he decided to add an average correction constant of 0.05 cm³ to every published V_e (cm³) value. The most recent median V_e (cm³) values for normal ears (Zwislocki and Feldman, 1970, p. 18) are almost identical to the medians that Feldman (1967) computed *before* adding his correction term. Apparently, Zwislocki and Feldman have made another calibration of their instrument and now find that a V_e correction is unnecessary.

A constant V_e correction of 0.1 or 0.05 cm³ seems like a trivial matter until we recognize that the magnitude of these corrections varies inversely with frequency and directly with $-jX_A$ at the patient's TM. Table II shows the approximate corrections (in acoustic ohms) that Feldman and Zwislocki have *subtracted* from average $-jX_A$ data for normal ears. It is not clear whether these corrections ever have been applied to data from patients.

Field calibration of the Zwislocki acoustic bridge is difficult because an adequate calibration standard and procedure are not provided with each instrument. Since only Zwislocki and Feldman have published evidence of field calibration, we have relied upon their normative data whenever possible. Table III provides a summary of Z_{TM} data in rectangular form and in polar form (in acoustic ohms) for normal ears, at the five most common (audiometric) carrier frequencies. These data have been computed (for each frequency) from the median and the

TABLE II

APPROXIMATE CORRECTIONS (ACOUSTIC OHMS) SUBTRACTED FROM
NORMAL $-jX_A$ DATA PUBLISHED BY FELDMAN AND
ZWISLOCKI SINCE 1965

Approximate correction subtracted (acoustic ohms)	Carrier frequency (Hz)				
	125	250	500	750	1000
1965–1967	396	221	84	36	21
1967–1970	267	134	57	22	13
1970	0	0	0	0	0

TABLE III

Summary of Z_{TM} Data in Rectangular Form and in Polar Form (Acoustic Ohms) for Normal Ears at Five Audiometric Carrier Frequencies[a]

Carrier frequency (Hz)	Z_{TM} (acoustic ohms)		Statistic
	Rectangular form $R_A - jX_A$	Polar form $Z_{TM}\angle\theta$	
125	$800 - j3922$	$4003\angle -78.5°$	90th centile
125	$510 - j2941$	$2985\angle -80.2°$	Median
125	$280 - j2076$	$2095\angle -82.3°$	10th centile
250	$630 - j1961$	$2060\angle -72.2°$	90th centile
250	$420 - j1471$	$1530\angle -74.1°$	Median
250	$280 - j1038$	$1075\angle -74.9°$	10th centile
500	$510 - j882$	$1019\angle -60.0°$	90th centile
500	$330 - j679$	$755\angle -64.1°$	Median
500	$230 - j441$	$497\angle -62.5°$	10th centile
750	$630 - j490$	$798\angle -37.9°$	90th centile
750	$390 - j346$	$521\angle -41.6°$	Median
750	$230 - j235$	$329\angle -45.6°$	10th centile
1000	$630 - j368$	$730\angle -30.3°$	90th centile
1000	$410 - j232$	$471\angle -29.5°$	Median
1000	$250 - j63$	$258\angle -14.1°$	10th centile

[a] Computed from data of Zwislocki and Feldman (1970).

"80% range" of normal Z_{TM} values provided by Zwislocki and Feldman (1970, p. 18).[23] If we define the median point as the *50th centile* of their frequency distribution, the "lower bound" of their "80% range" may be called the *10th centile* and the "upper bound" of this range many be called the *90th centile* (Guilford, 1950, p. 124). These labels have been used in Tables III, IV, V, and VII.

We have compared our measurements of static Z_{TM} for normal ears with corresponding data reported in the major studies since 1930. In

[23] Zwislocki and Feldman (1970) present R_A values in acoustic ohms, and therefore, no conversion is necessary. Their acoustic-reactance values, however, are presented in terms of the acoustic compliance (C_A) of an equivalent volume of air (V_e, in cm^3). We have converted all such values to $-jX_A$ values (in acoustic ohms), since V_e values are precisely correct only for atmospheric conditions that existed at the original location of measurement.

The following constants have been used for the Laboratory of Sensory Communication in Syracuse, New York: (1) Altitude, $h = 182$ m above sea level; (2) latitude $= 43°$ 2′ N; (3) barometric pressure on a "standard day," $P_0 = 741.1$ mm Hg; (4) laboratory temperature, $t = 22°$C; and (5) relative humidity, $f = 50\%$.

general, if the number of measurements is sufficiently large, Z_{TM} values appear to be distributed normally about the arithmetic mean of the frequency distribution. Moreover, the arithmetic mean of a large sample of Z_{TM} values does not differ significantly from the median point. The trend toward a normal distribution is evident in Table III.

Assumptions regarding a normal sampling distribution are tenable, however, only when Z_{TM} measurements are expressed in acoustic ohms, and in one of the standard forms (polar, rectangular, or exponential). As an example, consider a sample of Z_{TM} values that are distributed normally about an arithmetic mean. If a nonlinear transformation is applied to each complex number in this sample, and if each new value then is plotted in a histogram, the resulting frequency polygon will have a skewed distribution. Unfortunately, the conversion of a negative acoustic-reactance value ($-jX_A$, in acoustic ohms) to the acoustic compliance (C_A) of an equivalent volume of air (V_e, in cubic centimeters) requires a nonlinear transformation (Lilly, 1971). Table IV illustrates this point for a 500-Hz carrier signal. The data in the second column are V_e values at the 10th, the 50th, and the 90th centile for a sample of 33 subjects with normal hearing. Zwislocki and Feldman (1970, p. 18) present this "normal 80% range" and note that: "The compliance [V_e] values defining the upper boundary are about twice the compliance [V_e] values of the lower boundary." Clearly, the V_e value at the 10th centile (1.0 cm³) in Table IV is twice as large as the V_e value at the 90th centile (0.5 cm³). Since the V_e value at the median point (0.65 cm³) is closer to 0.5 cm³ than it is to 1.0 cm³, the distribution is positively skewed (Bicknell and Morgan, 1968; Feldman, 1963, 1964, 1967; Zwislocki and Feldman, 1970). This skewed distribution becomes symmetrical, however, when each V_e value is converted to a $-jX_A$ value (in acoustic ohms); or when the entire complex number is converted to polar form (Lilly et al., 1968, p. 307; Lilly, 1971).

TABLE IV

ACOUSTIC COMPLIANCE OF AN EQUIVALENT VOLUME OF AIR V_e (CM³), ACOUSTIC REACTANCE X_A (ACOUSTIC OHMS), AND MAGNITUDE OF ACOUSTIC IMPEDANCE $|Z_{TM}|$ (ACOUSTIC OHMS) AT NORMAL TYMPANIC MEMBRANES WHEN CARRIER FREQUENCY IS 500 Hz[a]

Statistic	V_e (cm³)	X_A (acoustic ohms)	$|Z_{TM}|$ (acoustic ohms)
90th centile	0.50	$-j882$	1019
Median	0.65	$-j679$	755
10th centile	1.00	$-j441$	497

[a] Based on data from Zwislocki and Feldman (1970).

The X_A values in the third column of Table IV were computed from the V_e values in the second column. These X_A values also appear in Table III as reactive components for Z_{TM} at 500 Hz. The $|Z_{TM}|$ values in the fourth column of Table IV were computed from the R_A values provided by Zwislocki and Feldman (1970, p. 18), and from the associated V_e values in the second column of Table IV. A test proposed by Kelley (1923, p. 77) may be used to determine the "skewness" of a frequency distribution when the 10th, the 50th, and the 90th centiles are known. A second test (Garrett, 1953, p. 241) then may be used to determine whether the computed measure of "skewness" deviates significantly from zero (the skewness of a normal distribution). When these two statistical tests are applied to the centile points in each column of Table IV: (1) we must reject the hypothesis that the three (V_e) values in Column 2 were drawn from a normal distribution; but (2) the probability of obtaining the centile points in Column 3 $(-jX_A$ values) and in Column 4 $(|Z_{TM}|$ values) from a skewed distribution is less than 1 in 100. Indeed, the entries in Column 4 emphasize the symmetry of the distribution. Stated differently, when Zwislocki and Feldman's (1970) "skewed" R_A and V_e data (for normal ears) are converted to polar form, the median $|Z_{TM}|$ value for 500 Hz lies within 3 acoustic ohms of the distribution midpoint.

Our experience with descriptive statistics suggests that the arithmetic mean is the most *efficient* measure of central tendency, and that the standard deviation is the most appropriate measure of variability for Z_{TM} data. This generalization will hold, however, only when the data are reported as complex numbers (in acoustic ohms). Furthermore, since each raw measurement reading from a Zwislocki acoustic bridge consists of an R_{arb} value (arbitrary units) and a V_e value, and since these quantities represent nonlinear transformations of R_A and $-jX_A$ at the TM, R_{arb} and V_e values must be converted to R_A and $-jX_A$ (in acoustic ohms) *before* means and standard deviations may be computed. More specifically, the arithmetic mean of a sample of $-jX_A$ values will be a different number than the mean obtained when the same measurements are summed as V_e values, averaged, and then converted to acoustic reactance (Burke *et al.*, 1967; Lilly, 1971; Lilly *et al.*, 1968). An analogous problem occurs if R_{arb} values are not converted to R_A values before a mean is computed.

D. Static Z_{TM} Data for Otosclerotic Ears

The localized bone disease of otosclerosis is present in its (asymptomatic) histologic form in about 10% of the adult, white population. It produces hearing impairment, however, for only about 1% of this population (Guild, 1944). Although otosclerotic lesions may originate in many regions of the otic capsule (Nager, 1969; Nylén, 1949; Rüedi and Spoendlin, 1957), the occurrence of otosclerotic bone is most common in the region of the fissula ante fenestram (Anson and Martin, 1935; Anson and Wilson, 1933; Bast, 1929, 1933, 1936; Wilson, 1935). This "area of predilection" (Bast and Anson, 1949; Beickert, 1965; Nager, 1969) lies just anterior to the oval window. Nager (1969, p. 362) points out that the otosclerotic exostosis will begin to affect hearing sensitivity:

> when a lesion near the oval window involves the annular ligament, grows across it, and causes fixation of the stapes, or when the otosclerotic process distorts the contours of the oval window and produces a jamming, subluxation, or fibrous immobilization of the footplate. . . . Each mechanism may occur independently, the former being probably the more frequent; more often the two occur jointly.
>
> Increasing stiffness in the stapedio-vestibular articulation leads to an impairment of hearing which is, in general, of the conductive type.

Since clinical otosclerosis usually produces increased "stiffness in the stapedio-vestibular articulation," and since increases in the mechanical stiffness of the middle ear produce proportionate increases in negative acoustic reactance at the TM, we should expect $-jX_A$ values to be higher for patients with clinical otosclerosis than for subjects with normal hearing. This correspondence between abnormally high $-jX_A$ values and stapes fixation has been predicted from analog models of the middle ear (Møller, 1961c; Zwislocki, 1957b, 1962, 1963a,b), and has been observed experimentally (Bicknell and Morgan, 1968; Feldman, 1963, 1964, 1969; Feldman and Zwislocki, 1965; Lilly, 1964, 1970; Lilly and Shepherd, 1964; Metz, 1946; Nilges et al., 1969; Zwislocki, 1957b, 1961, 1962, 1963a,b, 1968; Zwislocki and Feldman, 1970).

When the stapes becomes immobilized by an otosclerotic lesion, the mechanical impedance of the cochlea is replaced by a much higher impedance; and as a result, acoustic resistance (R_A) at the lateral surface of the TM is controlled by the frictional resistance of the incudostapedial joint. Analog models of the middle ear may be used to predict R_A values for patients with complete stapes fixation. Sepcifically, Zwislocki's (1957b, 1962, 1963a) models suggest that measured R_A should: (1) be higher than normal for carrier frequencies below 500 Hz; (2) approximate normal values between 500 Hz and 750 Hz; and (3) be lower than normal for 750 Hz and 1000 Hz. This abnormal, inverse relation between carrier frequency and R_A has been observed experimentally (Feldman and Zwislocki, 1965; Lilly, 1970; Metz, 1946; Nilges et al., 1969; Zwislocki, 1957b, 1961, 1962, 1963a, 1968; Zwislocki and Feldman, 1970).

Table V provides a summary of Z_{TM} data in rectangular form and in

TABLE V

Summary of Z_{TM} Data in Rectangular Form and in Polar
Form (Acoustic Ohms) for Ears with Clinical Otosclerosis
at Five Audiometric Carrier Frequencies[a]

| | Z_{TM} (acoustic ohms) | | |
Frequency (Hz)	Rectangular form $R_A - jX_A$	Polar form $Z_{TM}\angle\theta$	Statistic
125	$1550 - j11766$	$11868\angle -82.5°$	90th centile
125	$725 - j6471$	$6512\angle -83.6°$	Median
125	$520 - j5042$	$5069\angle -84.1°$	10th centile
250	$1190 - j5883$	$6002\angle -78.6°$	90th centile
250	$520 - j3530$	$3568\angle -81.6°$	Median
250	$322 - j2332$	$2354\angle -82.1°$	10th centile
500	$622 - j2647$	$2719\angle -76.8°$	90th centile
500	$380 - j1471$	$1519\angle -75.5°$	Median
500	$230 - j1103$	$1127\angle -78.2°$	10th centile
750	$646 - j1471$	$1607\angle -66.3°$	90th centile
750	$295 - j980$	$1023\angle -73.2°$	Median
750	$218 - j614$	$652\angle -70.4°$	10th centile
1000	$556 - j735$	$922\angle -52.9°$	90th centile
1000	$280 - j421$	$506\angle -56.4°$	Median
1000	$209 - j250$	$326\angle -50.1°$	10th centile

[a] Computed from data of Feldman (1971).

polar form (in acoustic ohms), at the five most common (audiometric)
carrier frequencies, for ears with clinical otosclerosis. These data have
been computed (for each frequency) from the median and the "80%
range" of Z_{TM} values for 24 patients with surgically confirmed stapedial
ankylosis (Feldman, 1971). Computational constants used for the con-
versions in Table III also were used for these data.

Comparison of the data in Table V with corresponding entries in
Table III shows that differential diagnosis (between normal middle ears
and ears with stapes fixation) is facilitated if Z_{TM} measurements are
available for several carrier frequencies. To expand this point:

Middle-ear disease usually modifies the transmission characteristics
of the middle ear.

If a (mechanical, electrical, or acoustical) transmission system
possesses one or more resonance frequencies, changes in its transmission characteristics can be determined most easily (from input-im-

pedance measurements) when the carrier frequency approximates a resonance frequency of the system.

Although the principle resonance frequency of the normal middle-ear transmission system lies near 1200 Hz, a smaller resonance peak consistently has been observed between 750 Hz and 900 Hz (Geffcken, 1934; Møller, 1961a,c, 1964; Tröger, 1930; Waetzmann, 1936; Waetzmann and Keibs, 1936; Zwislocki, 1957b, 1962, 1963a).

This first resonance peak (between 750 Hz and 900 Hz) disappears with stapes fixation (Zwislocki, 1962, 1963a), and with vigorous contraction of the stapedius muscle (Møller, 1961c).

The audiometric carrier frequencies that have been used by Zwislocki and Feldman provide measurement data at frequencies below the first resonance peak (125, 250, and 500 Hz), near this peak (750 Hz), and above the first resonance peak (1000 Hz).

Comparison of static Z_{TM} measurements for low frequencies with those obtained near the first resonance peak provides more diagnostic information than data obtained at only one frequency.

The effects of stapes fixation upon Z_{TM} are especially clear when data are presented in polar form. As the carrier frequency is increased from 125 Hz to 750 Hz, the data in Table III and Table V show that: (1) median $|Z_{TM}|$ changes only 2464 acoustic ohms for normal ears, but 5489 acoustic ohms for ears with stapes fixation; (2) median phase angle $\angle\theta$ changes 38.6° for normal ears, but only 10.4° for ears with stapes fixation.

The data in Table III and in Table V also can be used to emphasize the necessity for converting every V_e value (in cm³) to a $-jX_A$ value (in acoustic ohms). As an example, consider a patient for whom $-jX_A = 880$ acoustic ohms at 500 Hz. This value falls within the "normal 80% range" proposed by Zwislocki and Feldman (1970), and therefore, below the 90th centile point in Table III. Most models of the middle-ear transmission system (Møller, 1961c, 1963, 1965; Onchi, 1949, 1961; Zwislocki, 1957b, 1962, 1963a,b) suggest that Z_{TM} for this patient would not change significanty from Astrakhan, U.S.S.R. (altitude $h = 20$ m below sea level) to Bogota, Colombia (altitude $h = 2645$ m above sea level). Zwislocki (1968, p. 95) summarized this point when he noted that: "The middle ear cavities have little effect on the acoustic properties of the human middle ear at low sound frequencies. This is in contradistinction to conditions in the middle ear of small mammals where the acoustic properties at low frequencies are almost completely determined by the

TABLE VI

ACOUSTIC-REACTANCE DATA FOR A HYPOTHETICAL PATIENT AT
EIGHT LOCATIONS IN THE UNITED STATES[a]

Location of clinic	Altitude (meters)	Data for hypothetical patient	
		X_A (acoustic ohms)	Equivalent volume of air (cm^3)
Miami, Florida	6	$-j880$	0.513
Syracuse, New York	182	$-j880$	0.501
Iowa City, Iowa	224	$-j880$	0.499
Wichita, Kansas	414	$-j880$	0.488
Boise, Idaho	835	$-j880$	0.463
El Paso, Texas	1152	$-j880$	0.445
Denver, Colorado	1613	$-j880$	0.420
Santa Fe, New Mexico	2138	$-j880$	0.393

[a] Carrier frequency is 500 Hz. Anticipated X_A values (in acoustic ohms) are identical at all locations, whereas associated "equivalent volume" values (in cm^3) are related inversely to the altitude of the clinic.

air volume of the bulla." Unfortunately, the acoustic impedance of an equivalent volume of air (V_e) is about 31% higher in Astrakhan than in Bogota on a "standard day."

Table VI shows the acoustic-reactance ($-jX_A$) measurements that we might obtain for our hypothetical patient at eight different locations in the United States. If we use $-j882$ acoustic ohms (from Table III) as the upper limit for the "normal 80% range," we can conclude that this patient's middle-ear transmission system is on the stiff side of the normal range at all eight clinics. If we follow the convention of Zwislocki and Feldman (1970), and use 0.5 cm^3 as the "lower" limit for the "normal 80% range" and 0.4 cm^3 as the "upper" limit of the "otosclerotic 80% range," the middle ear of our hypothetical patient falls within the normal range in Miami and in Syracuse, and within the otosclerotic range in Sante Fe.

The disease process in otosclerosis may involve: (1) a relatively small lesion that is isolated to the annular ligament and to the footplate of the stapes (Guild, 1944; Rüedi and Spoendlin, 1957); (2) two or more independent lesions developing from different regions of the otic capsule (Nager, 1969); (3) three or more independent lesions (Beickert, 1965); (4) a diffuse disease process that covers large areas of the otic capsule (Nager, 1938; Nylén and Nylén, 1952); and that often obliterates the oval window, the round window, or both windows (Nager and Fraser, 1938); (5) the carotid canal, the tegmen tympani, the cochleariform process, the walls of the epitympanum, the malleus, and the incus (Altmann, 1951, 1965; Anderson *et al.*, 1962; Covell, 1940; Covell and Feinmesser, 1959; Goodhill, 1966; Guild, 1944; Guilford, 1963; House, 1956; Kelemen, 1943; Lempert and Wolff, 1945; Nager, 1941; Nylén, 1949; Sleeckx *et al.*, 1967; Wustrow, 1956). Analog models of the middle ear suggest that a close relation should exist between the structures affected by the otosclerotic process and static Z_{TM}. This relation has not been investigated systematically. It is conceivable, however, that the variability in locus and magnitude of the otosclerotic lesion may contribute to the variability that is observed in Z_{TM} measurements from patients with clinical otosclerosis.

E. Static Z_{TM} Data for Ears with Ossicular Discontinuity

Advances in otologic microsurgery have been paralleled by an increase in exploratory tympanotomy for patients with conductive hearing losses of obscure origin. Findings at tympanotomy suggest that ossicular discontinuity occurs more frequently than the early literature (prior to 1950) would indicate. Interruption of the ossicular chain in man may be partial or complete. It may involve a small, focal discontinuity or total destruction of the ossicles. In general, ossicular separation is produced by: (1) surgical (iatrogenic) trauma, (2) external (exogenic) trauma, (3) chronic middle-ear disease, or (4) congenital malformations.

Elimination of infection is the primary objective in surgery for chronic middle-ear disease. Accordingly, when the surgeon encounters advanced mastoid disease and cholesteatoma, he may dislocate the ossicular chain or remove completely the incus and the head of the malleus during surgical eradication of pathologic tissue (Davison, 1957; Guilford, 1969; Palva and Pulkkinen, 1960a, 1960b; Proctor, 1960; Rambo, 1969; Turner, 1969; Wullstein, 1956; Zöllner, 1957). Occasionally, unintentional dislocation of the ossicular chain has occurred during paracentesis, myringotomy, simple mastoidectomy, stapes mobilization, section of the chorda tympani nerve, or resection of the mastoid process (Alberti and Dawes, 1961; Andersen *et al.*, 1962; Anklesaria, 1963; Bauer, 1958; Brünner *et al.*, 1962; Donaldson and Selters, 1961; Flisberg and Floberg, 1960; Freeman, 1959; Goodhill, 1960; Hall and Rytzner, 1957; House, 1960; Hough, 1958; Kos, 1959; Plester, 1959; Rosen, 1958; Schuknecht and Davison, 1956; Schuknecht and Trupiano, 1957).

In the normal middle ear, the manubrium and the lateral process of the malleus are embedded in the TM. The malleus also is supported by the superior, the anterior, and the lateral malleolar ligaments. The footplate of the stapes is bound by the annular ligament to the cartilage-covered rim of the oval window. By comparison, the incus lacks the secure anchorage of the other two ossicles, and thus, is more susceptible to traumatic dislocation (Anklesaria, 1963; Does and Bottema, 1965; Sadé, 1965). Many investigators have observed dislocation of the incus following traumatic head injury (Anklesaria, 1963; Ballantyne, 1962; Bicknell, 1966; Does and Bottema, 1965; Farrior, 1969; Flisberg and Floberg, 1960; Gisselsson, 1958; Kelemen, 1944; Kelly, 1961; Seltzer, 1962; Thorburn, 1957; Ulrich, 1926). Although traumatic injury to the stapes is not as common as dislocation of the incus, the literature contains case studies involving: (1) fracture of the head or neck of the stapes (Sadé, 1965; Williams, 1958); (2) fracture of both crura of the stapes (Does and Bottema, 1965; Donaldson and Selters, 1961; Farrior, 1960; Hammond, 1964; Sadé, 1964); (3) fracture of the footplate of the stapes (Sadé, 1964); (4) fragmentation of the stapes and loss of the lenticular process of the incus (Scott, 1964); (5) avulsion of the intact stapes from the oval window (Hammond, 1962; Hough, 1959; Sadé, 1965); or (6) a forcing of the stapes into the vestibule (Sadé, 1964). Bicknell (1966) noted the incidence of fractured crura in ears with stapes fixation, and suggested that "an otosclerotic stapes is more liable to fracture than a normal one which, subjected to a similar force, might remain intact allowing the incudo-stapedial joint to dislocate."

The incus, "from an embryological and from nutritional and static points of view, is the weakest link of the ossicular chain" (Andersen et al., 1962). In general, the long process (long crus) of the incus and the incudostapedial joint are most susceptible to inflammatory and cholesteatomatous disease processes, and to trophic deficiencies (Alberti and Dawes, 1961; Andersen et al., 1962; Hough, 1958; Nager and Nager, 1953; Sadé, 1965). The literature contains reports of: (1) erosion of the incus in ears with chronic discharge from the middle ear (Davison, 1957; McGuckin, 1960; Sadé, 1965; Tabor, 1970); (2) necrosis of the long process or of the lenticular process of the incus (Alberti and Dawes, 1961; Andersen et al., 1962; Goodhill, 1960; Kos, 1959; Sadé, 1965; Sheehy, 1962; Sooy, 1960); (3) cholesteatomatous erosion of the lenticular process or of the long process of the incus (Farrior, 1969; House et al., 1964; Sadé, 1965); (4) atrophy of one or more of the incudal processes (Alberti and Dawes, 1961; Gisselsson, 1958; Goodhill, 1960); (5) erosion of the lenticular process of the incus "in a simple atelectatic ear where the drum, or squamous epithelium, contacts the incus and erodes its terminal portion" (Farrior, 1969); and (6) ischemic necrosis of the lenticular process of the incus following barotrauma (Donaldson and Selters, 1961).

Congenital malformation, interruption, or absence of the ossicular chain frequently is accompanied by visible evidence of disturbed embryologic development. These external signs usually appear as facial anomalies involving: (1) the malar bone, the zygomatic arch, and the lower eyelid; (2) the auricle and the external auditory meatus; (3) the mandible; and (4) the lips and mouth. The general term "mandibulofacial dysostosis" (Franceschetti and Zwahlen, 1944) has been used to describe this complex of facial symptoms. Other investigators have used the terms "Treacher-Collins syndrome" (Berry, 1888; Collins, 1900); "syndrome of Franceschetti" (Brégeat and Naud, 1949); "Treacher Collins-Franceschetti syndrome" (Harrison, 1957); or "congenital atresia of the ear" (Livingstone, 1959) to label the complete syndrome or a particular aspect of the complex. Congenital ossicular discontinuity also has been observed without concomitant anomalies of the face, the external ear, or the tympanic membrane (Andersen et al., 1962; Elbrønd, 1970; Goodhill, 1957, 1960; Hajek, 1961; Hough, 1958; House et al., 1964; Noguera and Haase, 1964; Sooy, 1960).

Nearly any interruption of the ossicular chain will produce a decrease in the stiffness of the total middle-ear transmission system. Since decreases in the mechanical stiffness of the middle ear produce proportionate decreases in negative acoustic reactance at the TM, we should expect $-jX_A$ values to be lower for patients with ossicular discontinuity than for subjects with normal hearing. Analog models of the middle ear (Møller, 1961c; Zwislocki, 1957b, 1962) have been used to predict that ossicular separation will produce abnormally low $-jX_A$ values for frequencies below 500 Hz. These models suggest that (for many lesions) the effective stiffness of the system may be less than the effective mass for frequencies above 500 Hz. Under these conditions: (1) positive (mass) reactance (jX_A) is greater than negative (compliant) reactance $(-jX_A)$; (2) the middle-ear transmission system is mass-controlled; (3) it will be impossible to balance a standard Zwislocki acoustic bridge.

Acoustic resistance (R_A) values for patients with ossicular separation also can be predicted from analog models. With complete interruption of the ossicular chain, the mechanical resistance contributed by the cochlea and the incudostapedial joint does not appear at the TM. Therefore, we should expect R_A values also to be lower than normal for most cases of ossicular discontinuity.

Clinical reports provide good support for the results predicted from analog models. Abnormally low Z_{TM} values have been observed consistently for patients with ossicular discontinuity (Bicknell and Morgan, 1968; Feldman, 1963; Nilges et al., 1969; Priede, 1970; Zwislocki, 1957b; Zwislocki and Feldman, 1970). Unfortunately, statistical analysis of Z_{TM} data is not available for this class of patients. Therefore, for the purposes of this chapter, experimental data from two sources have been combined

TABLE VII

Summary of Z_{TM} Data in Rectangular Form and in Polar
Form (Acoustic Ohms) at Five Audiometric Carrier
Frequencies for Ears with Ossicular Discontinuity[a]

	Z_{TM} (acoustic ohms)		
Frequency (Hz)	Rectangular form $R_A - jX_A$	Polar form $Z_{TM}\angle\theta$	Statistic
125	$230 - j1790$	$1805\angle-82.7°$	90th centile
125	$120 - j1261$	$1267\angle-84.6°$	Median
125	$79 - j872$	$876\angle-84.8°$	10th centile
250	$229 - j950$	$977\angle-76.4°$	90th centile
250	$120 - j609$	$621\angle-78.8°$	Median
250	$63 - j369$	$374\angle-80.3°$	10th centile
500	$175 - j323$	$367\angle-61.6°$	90th centile
500	$90 - j188$	$208\angle-64.4°$	Median
500	CNB[b]	CNB	10th centile
750	CNB	CNB	90th centile
750	CNB	CNB	Median
750	CNB	CNB	10th centile
1000	CNB	CNB	90th centile
1000	CNB	CNB	Median
1000	CNB	CNB	10th centile

[a] Tabled values were computed from raw data provided by
Feldman (1971) and from data obtained at the University of Iowa
(see text).

[b] Indicates Zwislocki acoustic bridge could not be balanced.

to provide a preliminary estimate of expected Z_{TM} values for patients with
complete ossicular separation.

Table VII presents a summary of Z_{TM} data in rectangular form and in
polar form (in acoustic ohms), at the five most common (audiometric)
carrier frequencies, for ears with ossicular discontinuity. These data have
been computed (for each frequency) from the median and the "80%
range" of Z_{TM} values for 13 patients with surgically confirmed separation
of the ossicular chain. Raw data for seven patients in this series were
provided by Feldman (1971). Data for the other five patients were
obtained in our laboratory at the University of Iowa.

We have noted, for frequencies above 500 Hz, that mass reactance
(jX_A) often is larger than compliant reactance ($-jX_A$) for patients with
ossicular discontinuity. A standard Zwislocki acoustic bridge, however,
has an adjustable control for R_A, and adjustable control for $-jX_A$, but

no method for adjusting jX_A. Thus, it is not possible to balance the instrument when the patient has a "mass-controlled" middle-ear transmission system. This result is coded CNB (could not balance) in Table VII.

Comparison of the data in Table VII with corresponding entries in Table III and in Table V shows again that diagnosis of middle-ear disease is facilitated if Z_{TM} measurements are available for several carrier frequencies.

F. Summary of Static Z_{TM} Data

Figure 9 provides a graphic summary of the static acoustic-impedance data presented in this section. Median Z_{TM} values for the otosclerosis group (coded "0") and for the ossicular-separation group (coded "S") are plotted on a form that is used for clinical Z_{TM} measurements at the University of Iowa. On the right side of the form, acoustic-resistance values (R_A in acoustic ohms) and negative acoustic-reactance values ($-jX_A$ in acoustic ohms) are plotted against frequency (in hertz) on two graphs that share a common axis of abscissas. The shaded area on each graph contains the "80% normal range" as defined in Table III. On the left side of the form, blocks are provided for recording "arbitrary-resistance" values (R_{ARB}) and "equivalent-volume" values (V_e) from the Zwislocki acoustic bridge. Below each of these entry blocks, space is provided for converting bridge readings to R_A and $-jX_A$. Space also is provided for noting the volume of the EAM and the type of speculum that was used.

Although the form in Figure 9 is convenient for acoustic-bridge measurements, the graphic format may be used to plot nearly any Z_{TM} data that: (1) fall in quadrant IV of the complex Z_A plane (Figure 8), and (2) are available in rectangular notation. In our experience, a summary form (like Figure 9) provides a valuable reference for otolaryngologists and others who must interpret the results of our acoustic-impedance studies.

VI. The Future for Acoustic-Impedance Measurements

The introduction to this chapter focused upon clinical applications for acoustic-impedance measurements. The future of these measurements will be shaped by careful, systematic research in each application area. This research cannot proceed efficiently until the audiologist becomes familiar with: (1) the concept of acoustic impedance, (2) standard terminology, (3) appropriate computational methods, and (4) the relation between acoustic-impedance measurements and the middle-ear transmission system. Accordingly, the emphasis of this chapter has been on basic information rather than on procedures that apply to current

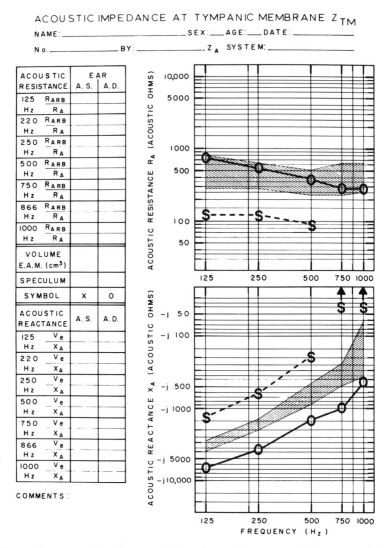

FIG. 9. Summary of static acoustic-impedance data presented in chapter. Median Z_{TM} values for otosclerosis group, (coded "O") and for ossicular-separation group (coded "S") are plotted in rectangular notation on clinical form used at the University of Iowa. Shaded area on each graph contains the "80% normal range" defined in Table III.

instrumentation. All static Z_{TM} data have been presented in absolute physical units (acoustic ohms). These data should be of value to any audiologist (working at any altitude above sea level) long after the Zwislocki acoustic bridge has been superseded by a single instrument that can be used for all of the clinical applications outlined in Section I,B. Commercial instruments available in 1971 will be obsolete in 5 years. The basic concepts, and the application of these concepts to clinical needs, will remain.

References

Alberti, P. W. R. M., and Dawes, J. D. K. (1961). Necrosis of the lenticular process of the incus after stapes surgery and its treatment. *J. Laryngol. Otol.* **75**, 821–825.

Alberti, P. W. R. M., and Kristensen, R. (1970). The clinical application of impedance audiometry. *Laryngoscope* **80**, 735–746.

Altmann, F. (1951). Malformations of the eustachian tube, the middle ear and its appendages. *Arch. Otolaryngol.* **54**, 241–266.

Altmann, F. (1965). The finer structure of the auditory ossicles in otosclerosis. *Arch. Otolaryngol.* **82**, 569–574.

Andersen, H. C., Jepsen, O., and Ratjen, E. (1962). Ossicular-chain defects. *Acta Oto-Laryngol.* **54**, 393–402.

Anderson, H., and Barr, B. (1966). Conductive recruitment. *Acta Oto-Laryngol.* **62**, 171–184.

Anderson, H., and Barr, B. (1971). Conductive high-tone hearing loss. *Arch. Otolaryngol.* **93**, 599–605.

Anderson, H., and Wedenberg, E. (1968). Audiometric identification of normal hearing carriers of genes for deafness. *Acta Oto-Laryngol.* **65**, 535–554.

Anderson, H., Barr, B., and Wedenberg, E. (1969). Intra-aural reflexes in retrocochlear lesions. *In* "Disorders of the Skull Base Region", (C.-A. Hamberger, and J. Wersäll, eds.), pp. 49–55. Nobel Symposium, 10th. Almqvist and Wiksell, Stockholm.

Anderson, H., Barr, B., and Wedenberg, E. (1970a). Early diagnosis of VIIIth-nerve tumours by acoustic reflex tests. *Acta Oto-Laryngol. Suppl.* **263**, 232–237.

Anderson, H., Barr, B., and Wedenberg, E. (1970b). The early detection of acoustic tumours by the stapedius reflex test. *In* "Sensorineural Hearing Loss" (G. E. W. Wolstenholme, and J. Knight, eds.). Churchill, London.

Anklesaria, D. M. (1963). The dislocated incus. *J. Laryngol. Otol.* **77**, 528–532.

Anon. (1960). "Comptes rendus des séances de la onzième conférence générale des poids et mesures." Gauthier-Villars & Cie, Paris. [A complete translation of the proceedings of this conference now is available as: National Aeronautics and Space Administration, *Trans. Meet. 11th Gen. Conf. Wts. Measures,* NASA TT F-217, Washington: Off. Tech. Serv., Dept. Commerce (1964).]

Anson, B. J., and Martin, J. Jr. (1935). Fissula ante fenestram: Its form and contents in early life. *Arch. Otolaryngol.* **21**, 303–323.

Anson, B. J., and Wilson, J. G. (1933). The fissula ante fenestram in an adult human ear. *Anat. Rec.* **56**, 383–393.

ASA Y10.11 (1953). American standard letter symbols for acoustics. American National Standards Institute, New York.

ASA Z24.11 (1954). American standard method for the free-field secondary calibration of microphones. American National Standards Institute, New York.

ASA S1.1 (1960). American standard acoustical terminology. American National Standards Institute, New York.

ASA S3.3 (1960). American standard methods for measurement of electroacoustical characteristics of hearing aids. American National Standards Institute, New York.

Ballantyne, J. C. (1962). A case of traumatic disruption of the incudo-stapedial joint. *J. Laryngol. Otol.* **76**, 661–664.

Bast, T. H. (1929). Osteogenesis of the human periotic capsule. *Arch. Otolaryngol.* **10**, 459–471.

Bast, T. H. (1933). Development of the otic capsule: II. The origin, development and significance of the fissula ante fenestram. *Arch. Otolaryngol.* **18**, 1–20.

Bast, T. H. (1936). Development of the optic capsule: III. Fetal and infantile changes in the fissular region and their probable relationship to the formation of otosclerotic foci. *Arch. Otolaryngol.* **23**, 509–525.

Bast, T. H., and Anson, B. J. (1949). "The Temporal Bone and the Ear." Thomas, Springfield, Illinois.

Bauer, B. B., Rosenheck, A. J., and Abbagnaro, L. A. (1968). External-ear replica for acoustical testing. *J. Int. Audiol.* **7**, 77–84.

Bauer, F. (1958). Dislocation of the incus due to head injury. *J. Laryngol. Otol.* **72**, 676–682.

Becker, B. M. (1930). Aural thermometry as a diagnostic aid in otology. *Arch. Otolaryngol.* **11**, 205–209.

Beedle, R. K., and Harford, E. R. (1970). An investigation of the relationship between the acoustic reflex growth and loudness growth in normal and pathological ears. *ASHA* **12**, 435.

Beickert, P. (1965). Otoklerose. *In* "Handb. d. Hals-Nasen-Ohrenheilk" (J. Berendes, R. Link, and F. Zöllner, eds.), Band III, Teil 1. Thieme, Stuttgart.

von Békésy, G. (1932). Zur Theorie des Hörens bei der Schallaufnahme durch Knochenleitung. *Ann. Phys.* **13**, 5, 111–136.

Benzinger T. H. (1959). On physical heat regulation and the sense of temperature in man. *Proc. Nat. Acad. Sci.* **45**, 645–659.

Beranek, L. L. (1949). "Acoustic Measurements." Wiley, New York.

Beranek, L. L. (1954). "Acoustics." McGraw-Hill, New York.

Beranek, L. L. (ed.) (1960). "Noise Reduction." McGraw-Hill, New York.

Berry, G. A. (1888). Note on a congenital defect (?coloboma) of the lower lid. *Roy. London Ophthal. Hosp. Rep.* **12**, 255–257.

Bicknell, M. R. (1966). Bilateral traumatic interruption of the ossicular chain. *J. Laryngol. Otol.* **80**, 748–752.

Bicknell, M. R., and Morgan, N. V. (1968). A clinical evaluation of the Zwislocki acoustic bridge. *J. Laryngol. Otol.* **82**, 673–692.

Brégeat, P., and Naud, G. (1949). Un nouveau cas de dysostose mandibulo-faciale (syndrome de Franceschetti). *Arch. Ophtalmol.* New Ser. **9**, 427–440.

Brooks, D. N. (1968). An objective method of detecting fluid in the middle ear. *J. Int. Audiol.* **7**, 280–286.

Brooks, D. N. (1969). The use of the electro-acoustic impedance bridge in the assessment of middle ear function. *J. Int. Audiol.* **8**, 563–569.

Brooks, D. N. (1970). Secretive otitis media in school-children. *J. Int. Audiol.* **9**, 141.

Brünner, S., Petersen, O., and Stoksted, P. (1962). Roentgenologic description of the auditory ossicles. *Ann. Otol.* **71**, 882–890.

Burke, K. S., Shutts, R. E., and Milo, A. P. (1967). On the Zwislocki acoustic bridge. *J. Acoust. Soc. Amer.* **41**, 1364.

Cassell, W. L. (1964). "Linear Electric Circuits." Wiley, New York.

Cawthorne, T. (1963). Bell's palsies. *Trans. Amer. Otol. Soc.* **51**, 290-297.

Collins, E. T. (1900). Congenital abnormalities: 8 and 9, Case with symmetrical congenital notches in the outer part of each lower lid and defective development of the malar bones. *Trans. Ophthal. Soc. U.K.* **20**, 190-192.

Covell, W. P. (1940). The ossicles in otosclerosis. *Acta Oto-Laryng.* **28**, 263-276.

Covell, W. P., and Feinmesser, M. (1959). Further studies on pathology of ossicles in otosclerosis. *Laryngoscope* **69**, 164-173.

Dallos, P. J. (1964). Dynamics of the acoustic reflex: phenomenological aspects. *J. Acoust. Soc. Amer.* **36**, 2175-2183.

Davis, H. F. (1967). "Introduction to vector analysis." Allyn and Bacon, Rockleigh, New Jersey.

Davison, F. W. (1957). Atticomastoidectomy. *Laryngoscope* **67**, 191-199.

Dippolito, P. W. (1967). Acoustic bridge for impedance measurements of the ear. *J. Acoust. Soc. Amer.* **42**, 1127.

van Dishoeck, H. A. E. (1970). Tubal resistance measuring in perforated eardrums by means of the pneumophone in relation to tympanoplasty and toxic gas penetration. *J. Int. Audiol.* **9**, 354-357.

Djupesland, G. (1964a). Discussion. *Acta Oto-Laryngol.* **188**, 207-208.

Djupesland, G. (1964b). Middle ear muscle reflexes elicited by acoustic and non-acoustic stimulation. *Acta Oto-Laryngol. Suppl.* **188**, 287-292.

Djupesland, G. (1965). Electromyography of the tympanic muscles in man. *J. Int. Audiol.* **4**, 34-41.

Djupesland, G. (1967). "Contractions of the Tympanic Muscles in Man." Thesis, Universitets-forlaget Trykningssentral, Oslo.

Djupesland, G. (1969a). Observation of changes in the acoustic impedance of the ear as an aid to the diagnosis of paralysis of the stapedius muscle. *Acta Oto-Laryngol.* **68**, 1-5.

Djupesland, G. (1969b). Use of impedance indicator in diagnosis of middle ear pathology. *J. Int. Audiol.* **8**, 570-578.

Djupesland, G., and Flottorp, G. (1970). Correlation between the Fowler loudness balance test, the Metz recruitment test, and the Flottorp-Opheim's aural harmonic test in various types of hearing impairment. *J. Int. Audiol.* **9**, 156-175.

Djupesland, G., and Zwislocki, J. J. (1971). Effect of temporal summation on the human stapedius reflex. *Acta Oto-Laryngol.* **71**, 262-265.

Does, I. E. S., and Bottema, T. (1965). Posttraumatic conductive hearing loss. *Arch. Otolaryngol.* **82**, 331-339.

Donaldson, J. A., and Selters, W. A. (1961). Unilateral conductive hearing loss without middle ear inflammation. *Arch. Otolaryngol.* **74**, 635-638.

Elbrønd, O. (1970). Defects of the auditory ossicles in ears with intact tympanic membrane. *Acta Oto-Laryngol. Suppl.* **264**.

Ewertsen, H. W., Filling, S., Terkildsen, K., and Thomsen, K. A. (1958). Comparative recruitment testing. *Acta Oto-Laryngol. Suppl.* **140**, 116-122.

Farrant, R. H., and Skurr, B. (1966). Measuring the acoustic impedance of severely deaf ears to test for conductive component. *J. Otol. Soc. Aust.* **2**, 49-53.

Farrior, J. B. (1960). Ossicular repositioning and ossicular prostheses in tympanoplasty. *Arch. Otolaryngol.* **71**, 443-449.

Farrior, J. B. (1969). Tympanoplasty (ossicular repositioning in reconstruction). *Arch. Otolaryngol.* **89**, 220-225.

Favors, A., and Lilly, D. J. (1971). Some effects of anesthesia upon auditory bone-conduction thresholds. Manuscript in preparation.

Fay, R. D., and Hall, W. M. (1933). The determination of the acoustical output of a telephone receiver from input measurements. *J. Acoust. Soc. Amer.* **5**, 46–56.

Fay, R. D., and White, J. E. (1948). Acoustic impedance from motional impedance diagrams. *J. Acoust. Soc. Amer.* **20**, 98–107.

Feldman, A. S. (1963). Impedance measurements at the eardrum as an aid to diagnosis. *J. Speech Hearing Res.* **6**, 315–327.

Feldman, A. S. (1964). Acoustic impedance measurement as a clinical procedure. *J. Int. Audiol.* **3**, 156–166.

Feldman, A. S. (1967). Acoustic impedance studies of the normal ear. *J. Speech Hearing Res.* **10**, 165–176.

Feldman, A. S. (1969). Acoustic impedance measurement of post-stapedectomized ears. *Laryngoscope* **79**, 1132–1155.

Feldman, A. S. (April, 1971). Raw, acoustic-impedance data for 24 patients with clinical otosclerosis, and for 7 patients with ossicular discontinuity. *Personal Communication.*

Feldman, A. S., and Zwislocki, J. (1965). Effect of the acoustic reflex on the impedance at the eardrum. *J. Speech Hearing Res.* **8**, 213–222.

Flisberg, K. (1964). Clinical assessment of tubal function. *Acta Oto-Laryngol. Suppl.* **188**, 29–35.

Flisberg, K., and Floberg, L. E. (1960). Traumatic luxation of the incus in children. *Acta Oto-Laryngol.* **51**, 469–475.

Flisberg, K., Ingelstedt, S., and Örtegren, U. (1963). Controlled "ear aspiration" of air; a "physiological test of the tubal function." *Acta Oto-Laryngol. Suppl.* **182**.

Floberg, L. E., Ivstam, B., and Lundborg, T. (1969). Some experiences with three hundred stapedectomized patients. *Acta Oto-Laryngol.* **67**, 501–510.

Flottorp, G., and Djupesland, G. (1970). Diphasic impedance change and its applicability in clinical work. *Acta Oto-Laryngol. Suppl.* **263**, 200–204.

Franceschetti, A., and Zwahlen, P. (1944). Un syndrome nouveau: La dysostose mandibulo-faciale. *Schweiz. Akad. Med. Wiss.* **1**, 60–66.

Franzen, R. L., and Lilly, D. J. (1970). Threshold of the acoustic reflex for pure tones. *ASHA* **12**, 435.

Freeman, J. (1959). Relief of deafness, following replacement of an incus dislocated 16 years previously. *J. Laryngol. Otol.* **73**, 196–197.

Garrett, H. E. (1953). "Statistics in Psychology and Education," 4th ed. Longmans, Green, New York.

Geffcken, W. (1934). Untersuchungen über akustische Schwellenwerte III. Über die Bestimmung der Reizschwelle der Hörempfindung aus Schwellendruck und Trommelfellimpedanz. *Ann. Phys.* **19**, Ser. 5, 829–848.

Gisselsson, L. (1958). Bilateral luxation of the incudo-stapedial joint. *J. Laryngol. Otol.* **72**, 329–331.

Goodhill, V. (1957). Otosurgical developments and the hard of hearing child. *Trans. Amer. Acad. Ophthal. Otolaryngol.* **61**, 711–722.

Goodhill, V. (1960). Pseudo-otosclerosis. *Laryngoscope* **70**, 722–757.

Goodhill, V. (1966). The fixed malleus syndrome. *Trans. Amer. Acad. Ophthal. Otolaryngol.* **70**, 370–380.

Greisen, O., and Rasmussen, P. E. (1970). Stapedius muscle reflexes and otoneurological examinations in brain-stem tumors. *Acta Oto-Laryngol.* **70**, 366–370.

Guild, S. R. (1944). Histologic otosclerosis. *Ann. Otol. Rhinol. Laryngol.* **53**, 246–266.

Guilford, F. (1963). *In* "Panel on Footplate Pathology, Techniques, and Prognosis," (J. Lindsay, *et al.*). *Arch. Otolaryngol.* **78**, 520–538.

Guilford, F. (1969). Indications for obliteration and closed mastoid operations. *Arch. Otolaryngol.* **89**, 191–195.

Guilford, J. P. (1950). "Fundamental Statistics in Psychology and Education." McGraw-Hill, New York.

Hajek, E. F. (1961). Conductive deafness of congenital origin. *J. Laryngol. Otol.* **75**, 371–386.

Hall, A., and Rytzner, C. (1957). Stapedectomy and autotransplantation of ossicles. *Acta Oto-Laryngol.* **47**, 318–324.

Hammond, V. T. (1962). A case of post-traumatic conduction deafness. *J. Laryngol. Otol.* **76**, 699–702.

Hammond, V. (1964). Conductive deafness following head injury. *J. Laryngol. Otol.* **78**, 837–848.

Harper, A. R. (1961). Acoustic impedance as an aid to diagnosis in otology. *J. Laryngol. Otol.* **75**, 614–620.

Harrison, M. S. (1957). The Treacher Collins-Franceschetti syndrome. *J. Laryngol. Otol.* **71**, 597–604.

Heaviside, O. (1886). *In* "The Encyclopedia of Electronics," (C. Susskind, ed.) 1962. Reinhold, New York.

Hecker, M. H. L., and Kryter, K. D. (1965). A study of the acoustic reflex in infantrymen. *Acta Oto-Laryngol. Suppl.* **207**.

Holborow, C. A. (1962). Deafness associated with cleft palate. *J. Laryngol. Otol.* **76**, 762–773.

Holmquist, J. (1969). Eustachian tube function assessed with tympanometry. *Acta Oto-Laryngol.* **68**, 501–508.

Holmquist, J. (1970). Auditory tubal function in chronic middle ear disease and the role of tubal function in myringoplasty. *J. Int. Audiol.* **9**, 197–202.

Holst, H.-E., Ingelstedt. S., and Örtegren, U. (1963). Ear drum movements following stimulation of the middle ear muscles. *Acta Oto-Laryngol. Suppl.* **182**, 73–83.

Hood, R. B., and Lamb, L. E. (1969). Tympanometry: Reliability and applicability. *ASHA* **11**, 417.

Hough, J. V. D. (1958). Malformations and anatomical variations seen in the middle ear during the operation for mobilization of the stapes. *Laryngoscope* **68**, 1337–1379.

Hough, J. V. D. (1959). Incudostapedial joint separation: etiology, treatment and significance. *Laryngoscope* **69**, 644–664.

House, H. P. (1956). Diagnostic aspects of congenital ossicular fixation. *Trans. Amer. Acad. Ophthal. Otolaryngol.* **60**, 787–790.

House, H. P. (1960). Unfavorable results of stapes mobilization surgery. *Arch. Otolaryngol.* **71**, 312–320.

House, H. P., Linthicum, F. H., and Johnson, E. W. (1964). Current management of hearing loss in children. *Amer. J. Dis. Child.* **108**, 677–696.

Inglis, A. H., Gray, C. H. G., and Jenkins, R. T. (1932). A voice and ear for telephone measurements. *Bell Syst. Tech. J.* **11**, 293–317.

Ithell, A. H. (1963a). The measurement of acoustical input impedance of human ears. *Acustica* **13**, 140–145.

Ithell, A. H. (1963b). A determination of the acoustical input impedance characteristics of human ears. *Acustica* **13**, 311–314.

Ithell, A. H., Johnson, G. T., and Yates, R. F. (1965). The acoustical impedance of human ears and a new artificial ear. *Acustica* **15**, 109–116.

James, G., and James, R. C. (1959). "Mathematics Dictionary." Van Nostrand-Reinhold, Princeton, New Jersey.

400   DAVID J. LILLY

Jepsen, O. (1953). Intratympanic muscle reflexes in psychogenic deafness. *Acta Oto-Laryngol. Suppl.* **109**, 61–69.

Jepsen, O. (1963). Middle-ear muscle reflexes in man. In "Modern Developments in Audiology", (J. Jerger, ed.). Academic Press, New York.

Jerger, J. (1970). Clinical experience with impedance audiometry. *Arch. Otolaryngol.* **92**, 311–324.

Jerger, J. (1971). Reply. *Arch. Otolaryngol.* **93**, 339–340.

Johansson, B., Kylin, B., and Langfy, M. (1967). Acoustic reflex as a test of individual susceptibility to noise. *Acta Oto-Laryngol.* **64**, 256–262.

Keibs, L. (1936). Methode zur Messung von Schwellendrucken und Trommelfellimpedanzen in fortschreitenden Wellen. *Ann. Phys.* **26**, Ser. 5, 585–608.

Kelemen, G. (1943). Otosclerotic focus outside the inner ear capsule. *Laryngoscope* **53**, 528–532.

Kelemen, G. (1944). Fractures of the temporal bone. *Arch. Otolaryngol.* **40**, 333–373.

Kelley, T. L. (1923). "Statistical Method." Macmillan, New York.

Kelly, W. D. (1961). Mobilization of a "fixed" malleus following on head injury. *J. Laryngol. Otol.* **75**, 826–827.

Kennelly, A. E. (1925). The measurement of acoustic impedance with the aid of the telephone receiver. *J. Franklin Inst.* **200**, 467–488.

Kennelly, A. E. and Kurokawa, K. (1921). Acoustic impedance and its measurement. *Proc. Amer. Acad. Arts Sci.* **56**, 1–42.

Klockhoff, I. (1960). Discussion. *Acta Oto-Laryngol. Suppl.* **158**, 236–237.

Klockhoff, I. (1961). Middle ear muscle reflexes in man. *Acta Oto-Laryngol. Suppl.* **164**.

Klockhoff, I. (1963). Middle ear muscle reflex tests for otologic diagnosis. *Trans. Amer. Acad. Ophthal. Otolaryngol.* **67**, 777–784.

Klockhoff, I. H., and Anderson, H. (1959). Recording of the stapedius reflex elicited by cutaneous stimulation. *Acta Oto-Laryngol.* **50**, 451–454.

Klockhoff, I., and Anderson, H. (1960). Reflex activity in the tensor tympani muscle recorded in man. *Acta Oto-Laryngol.* **51**, 184–188.

Klockhoff, I., Ånggård, G., and Ånggård, L. (1965). The acoustic impedance of the ear and craniolabyrinthine pressure transmission. *J. Int. Audiol.* **4**, 45–49.

Kneser, H. O. (1933). The interpretation of the anomalous sound-absorption in air and oxygen in terms of molecular collisions. *J. Acoust. Soc. Amer.* **5**, 122–126.

Knudsen, V. O. (1933). The absorption of sound in air, in oxygen, and in nitrogen-effects of humidity and temperature. *J. Acoust. Soc. Amer.* **5**, 112–121.

Kos, C. M. (1959). Late hearing results in mobilization surgery. *Laryngoscope* **69**, 1066–1070.

Kosten, C. W., and Zwikker, C. (1941). Die Messung von akustischen Scheinwiderständen und Schluckzahlen durch Rückwirkung auf ein Telefon. *Akust. Z.* **6**, 124–131.

Kristensen, H. K., and Jepsen, O. (1952). Recruitment in otoneurological diagnostics. *Acta Oto-Laryngol.* **42**, 553–560.

Kristensen, H. K., and Zilstorff, K. (1967). Modern diagnostic methods in otoneurology. *Acta Oto-Laryngol. Suppl.* **224**, 46–55.

Kurtz, R. (1938). Zur Messung von Absorptions- und Empfindlichkeitskurven des menschlichen Ohres. *Akust. Z.* **3**, 74–79.

Lamb, L. E., and Norris, T. W. (1969). Acoustic impedance measurement. In "Audiometry for the Retarded," (R. T. Fulton and L. L. Lloyd, eds.). Williams and Wilkins, Baltimore, Maryland.

Lamb, L. E., and Peterson, J. L. (1967). Middle ear reflex measurements in pseudo-hypacusis. *J. Speech Hearing Dis.* **32**, 46–51.

Lamb, L. E., Peterson, J. L., and Hansen, S. (1968). Application of stapedius muscle reflex measures to diagnosis of auditory problems. *J. Int. Audiol.* **7**, 188–189.

Lamb, L. E., Hood, R. B., and Norris, T. W. (1969). Pressure-compliance measurements as an aid to audiologic-otologic diagnosis. *ASHA* **11**, 416–417.

Lempert, J., and Wolff, D. (1945). Histopathology of the incus and the head of the malleus in cases of stapedial ankylosis. *Arch. Otolaryngol.* **42**, 339–367.

Lidén, G. (1969a). Tests for stapes fixation. *Arch. Otolaryngol.* **89**, 399–403.

Lidén, G. (1969b). The scope and application of current audiometric tests. *J. Laryngol. Otol.* **83**, 507–520.

Lidén, G. (1970). The stapedius muscle reflex used as an objective recruitment test: A clinical and experimental study. *In* "Sensorineural Hearing Loss", (G. E. W. Wolstenholme and J. Knight, eds.). Churchill, London.

Lidén, G., Peterson, J. L., and Björkman, G. (1970a). Tympanometry. *Acta Oto-Laryngol. Suppl.* **263**, 218–224.

Lidén, G., Peterson, J. L., and Björkman, G. (1970b). Tympanometry. *Arch. Oto-laryngol.* **92**, 248–257.

Lidén, G., Peterson, J. L., and Harford, E. R. (1970c). Simultaneous recording of changes in relative impedance and air pressure during acoustic and non-acoustic elicitation of the middle-ear reflexes. *Acta Oto-Laryngol.* **263**, 208–217.

Lilly, D. J. (1964). Some properties of the acoustic reflex in man. *J. Acoust. Soc. Amer.* **36**, 2007.

Lilly, D. J. (1966). Measurement of the acoustic reflex as an audiometric technique. *Science* **154**, 1228.

Lilly, D. J. (1970). A comparison of acoustic impedance data obtained with Madsen and Zwislocki instruments. *ASHA* **12**, 441.

Lilly, D. J. (1971). Acoustic impedance of an equivalent volume of air. Manuscript in prep.

Lilly, D. J., and Shepherd, D. C. (1964). A rebalance technique for the measurement of absolute changes in acoustic impedance due to the acoustic reflex. *ASHA* **6**, 380.

Lilly, D. J., Sherman, D., Compton, A. J., Fisher, C. G., and Carney, P. J. (1968). Annual review of JSHR Research, 1967. *J. Speech Hearing Dis.* **33**, 303–317.

Lilly, D. J., Mills, J. H., and Kos, C. M. (1969). The acoustic reflex after stapedectomy: Its effect upon temporary threshold shift. *ASHA* **11**, 413.

Lindström, D., and Lidén, G. (1964). The tensor-tympani reflex in operative treatment of trigeminal neuralgia. *Acta Oto Laryngol. Suppl.* **188**, 271–274.

Livingstone, G. (1959). The establishment of sound conduction in congenital deformities of the external ear. *J. Laryngol. Otol.* **73**, 231–241.

Mawardi, O. K. (1949). Measurement of acoustic impedance. *J. Acoust. Soc. Amer.* **21**, 84–91.

McGuckin, F. (1960). Chronic otitis media. *Postgrad. Med. J.* **36**, 256–260.

McLaurin, J. W. (1954). Otitis externa: The facts of the matter. *J. Amer. Med. Ass.* **154**, 207–213.

McPherson, D. L. (1971). Impedance audiometry. *Arch. Otolaryngol.* **93**, 338–339.

Menzel, W. (1940). Messungen der Hörschwelle und der Trommelfellabsorption an gesunden und kranke Ohren. *Akust. Z.* **5**, 257–268.

Metz, O. (1946). The acoustic impedance measured on normal and pathological ears. *Acta Oto-Laryngol. Suppl.* 63.

Metz, O. (1952). Threshold of reflex contractions of muscles of middle ear and recruitment of loudness. *Arch. Otolaryngol.* 55, 536–543.

Metz, O. (1953). Influence of the patulous eustachian tube on the acoustic impedance of the ear. *Acta Oto-Laryngol. Suppl.* 109, 105–112.

Miller, G. F. (1965). Eustachian tube function in normal and diseased ears. *Arch. Otolaryngol.* 81, 41–48.

Møller, A. R. (1958). Intra-aural muscle contraction in man examined by measuring acoustic impedance of the ear. *Laryngoscope* 67, 48–62.

Møller, A. R. (1960). Improved technique for detailed measurements of the middle ear impedance. *J. Acoust. Soc. Amer.* 32, 250–257.

Møller, A. (1961a), Bilateral contraction of the tympanic muscles in man. Report No. 18, Speech Trans. Lab., Roy. Inst. of Tech., Stockholm.

Møller, A. R. (1961b). Bilateral contraction of the tympanic muscles in man. *Ann. Otol. Rhinol. Laryngol.* 70, 735–752.

Møller, A. R. (1961c). Network model of the middle ear. *J. Acoust. Soc. Amer.* 33, 168–176.

Møller, A. R. (1962). Acoustic reflex in man. *J. Acoust. Soc. Amer.* 34, 1524–1534.

Møller, A. R. (1963). Transfer function of the middle ear. *J. Acoust. Soc. Amer.* 35, 1526–1534.

Møller, A. R. (1964). The acoustic impedance in experimental studies on the middle ear. *J. Int. Audiol.* 2, 123–135.

Møller, A. R. (1965). An experimental study of the acoustic impedance of the middle ear and its transmission properties. *Acta Oto-Laryngol.* 60, 129–149.

Morse, P. M. (1948). "Vibration and Sound." McGraw-Hill, New York.

Morton, J. Y., and Jones, R. A. (1956). The acoustical impedance presented by some human ears to hearing-aid earphones of the insert type. *Acustica* 6, 339–345.

Nager, F. R. (1938). Ueber Labyrinthveränderungen bei Otosklerose. *Schweiz. Acad. Med. Wiss.* 68, 85–86.

Nager, F. R. (1941) Ueber Veränderungen der Gehörknöchelchenkette bei Otosklerose. *Schweiz. Acad. Med. Wiss.* 71, 757–761.

Nager, F. R., and Fraser, J. S. (1938). On bone formation in the scala tympani of otosclerotics. *J. Laryngol. Otol.* 53, 173–180.

Nager, G. T. (1969). Histopathology of otosclerosis. *Arch. Otolaryngol.* 89, 341–363.

Nager, G. T., and Nager, M. (1953). The arteries of the human middle ear, with particular regard to the blood supply of the auditory ossicles. *Ann. Otol., Rhinol. Laryngol.* 62, 923–949.

Neergaard, E. B., Rasmussen, P. E., and Jepsen, O. (1965). Measurement of acoustic impedance by a new principle, cross-coupling. *J. Int. Audiol.* 4, 20–24.

Neklepajev, N. (1911). Über die Absorption kurzer akustischer Wellen in der Luft. *Ann. Phys.* 35, 175–181.

Nilges, T. C., Northern, J. L., and Burke, K. S. (1969). Zwislocki acoustic bridge; clinical correlations. *Arch. Otolaryngol.* 89, 727–744.

Noguera, J. T., and Haase, F. R. (1964). Congenital ossicular defects with a normal auditory canal: Its surgical treatment. *Eye Ear Nose Throat Mon.* 43, 37–39.

Nylén, B. (1949). Histopathological investigations on the localization, number, activity and extent of otosclerotic foci. *J. Laryngol. Otol.* 63, 321–327.

Nylén, C. O., and Nylén, B. (1952). On the genesis of otosclerosis. *J. Laryngol. Otol.* 66, 55–64.

Olson, H. F. (1943). "Dynamical Analogies." Van Nostrand-Reinhold, Princeton, New Jersey.

Olson, H. F. (1947). "Elements of Acoustical Engineering." Van Nostrand-Reinhold, Princeton, New Jersey.

Onchi, Y. (1949). A study of the mechanism of the middle ear. *J. Acoust. Soc. Amer.* **21,** 404–410.

Onchi, Y. (1961). Mechanism of the middle ear. *J. Acoust. Soc. Amer.* **33,** 794–805.

Onchi, Y. (1963). Aural reflex indicator. *Tran. Amer. Acad. Ophthal. Otolaryngol.* **67,** 785–789.

Palva, T., and Pulkkinen, K. (1960a). Hearing after surgery in chronically discharging ears, I. atticoantrotomy. *Acta Otolaryngol.* **51,** 123–134.

Palva, T., and Pulkkinen, K. (1960b). Hearing after surgery in chronically discharging ears, II. radical operation. *Acta Oto-Laryngol.* **52,** 175–185.

Perry, E. T. (1957). "The Human Ear Canal." Thomas, Springfield, Illinois.

Pielemeier, W. H. (1945). Observed classical sound absorption in air. *J. Acoust. Soc. Amer.* **17,** 24–28.

Pinto, L. H., and Dallos, P. J. (1968). An acoustic bridge for measuring the static and dynamic impedance of the eardrum. *IEEE Trans. Bio. Med. Eng.* **BME-15,** 10–16.

Plester, D. (1959). Die operative Behandlung der Gehörknöchelchenluxation. *Z. Laryngol. Rhinol. Otol.* **38,** 221–225.

Priede, V. M. (1970). Acoustic impedance in two cases of ossicular discontinuity. *J. Int. Audiol.* **9,** 127–136.

Proctor, B. (1960). Pitfalls in tympanoplasty. *Laryngoscope* **70,** 1433–1447.

Rambo, J. H. T. (1969). Musculoplasty for restoration of hearing in chronic suppurative ears. *Arch. Otolaryngol.* **89,** 210–216.

Randall, R. H. (1951). "An Introduction to Acoustics." Addison-Wesley, Reading, Massachusetts.

Rayleigh, Lord. (1896). "The Theory of Sound," Vol. II. Dover, New York.

Rettinger, M. (1968). "Acoustics: Room Design and Noise Control." Chem. Publ. Co., New York.

Robertson, E. O., Lamb, L. E., and Peterson, J. L. (1967). Relative impedance measurements in young children. *ASHA* **9,** 372.

Robertson, E. O., Peterson, J. L., and Lamb, L. E. (1968). Relative impedance measurements in young children. *Arch. Otolaryngol.* **88,** 162–168.

Robinson, N. W. (1937). An acoustic impedance bridge. *Philo. Mag., J. Sci.* **23,** Suppl. 665–681.

Rosen, S. (1958). Stapes surgery for otosclerotic deafness. *J. Laryngol. Otol.* **72,** 263–280.

Rüedi, L., and Spoendlin, H. (1957). The histology of the otosclerotic ankylosis of the stapes with regard to its surgical mobilization. *Adv. Oto-Rhino-Laryngol.* **4,** 1–84. S. Karger, Basel.

Sadé, J. (1964). Traumatic fractures of the stapes. *Arch. Otolaryngol.* **80,** 258–262.

Sadé, J. (1965). Wedging of the stapes for lenticular process necrosis. *Arch. Otolaryngol.* **82,** 212–216.

Scevola, P. (1938). Il quadro, termico locale fisiologico dell orecchio e le sue variazioni in alcune affezioni infiammatorie. *Arch. Ital. Otol. Rinol. Laringol.* **50,** 333–351.

Schuknecht, H. F., and Davison, R. C. (1956). Deafness and vertigo from head injury. *Arch. Otolaryngol.* **63,** 513–528.

Schuknecht, H. F., and Trupiano, S. (1957). Some interesting middle ear problems. *Laryngoscope* **67,** 395–409.

Schuster, K. (1934). Eine Methode zum Vergleich akustischer Impedanzen. *Phys. Z.* **35**, 408–409.

Schuster, K. (1936). Messung von akustischen Impedanzen durch Vergleich. *Elek. Nachr.-Tech.* **13**, 164–176.

Schuster, K., and Stöhr, W. (1939). Aufbau und Eigenschaften eines veränderbaren akustischen Vergleichswiderstandes. *Akust. Z.* **4**, 253–260.

Scott, P. G. (1964). Report on cases of conductive deafness associated with head injury. *J. Laryngol. Otol.* **78**, 1119–1122.

Seltzer, A. P. (1962). An unusual middle ear injury. *Ann. Otol. Rhinol. Laryngol.* **71**, 170–172.

Sheehy, J. L. (1962). Stapedectomy in the fenestrated ear. *Ann. Otol. Rhinol. Laryngol.* **71**, 1027–1038.

Silverstein, H., Miller, G. F., and Lindeman, R. C. (1966). Eustachian tube dysfunction as a cause for chronic secretory otitis in children. *Laryngoscope* **76**, 259–273.

Simmons, F. B. (1964). Variable nature of the middle ear muscle reflex. *J. Int. Audiol.* **2**, 136–146.

Sivian, L. J., and White, S. D. (1933). On minimum audible sound fields. *J. Acoust. Soc. Amer.* **4**, 288–321.

Sleeckx, J. P., Shea, J. J., and Pitzer, F. J. (1967). Epitympanic ossicular fixation. *Arch. Otolaryngol.* **85**, 619–631.

Söhoel, T., and Arnesen, G. (1962). The choice of probe-tube position and test frequency in determining the intra-aural reflexes. *Acta Oto-Laryngol.* **54**, 233–238.

Sooy, F. A. (1960). The management of middle ear lesions simulating otosclerosis. *Ann. Otol. Rhinol. Laryngol.* **69**, 540–558.

Steinmetz, C. P. (1893) (1962). *In* "The Encyclopedia of Electronics" (C. Susskind, ed.). Van Nostrand-Reinhold, Princeton, New Jersey.

Stewart, G. W. (1926). Direct absolute measurement of acoustic impedance. *Phys. Rev.* **28**, 1038–1047.

Stewart, G. W. (1932). "Introductory Acoustics." Van Nostrand-Reinhold, Princeton, New Jersey.

Stewart, G. W., and Lindsay, R. B. (1930). "Acoustics." Van Nostrand-Reinhold, Princeton, New Jersey.

Stewart, J. L. (1960). "Fundamentals of Signal Theory." McGraw-Hill, New York.

Stokes, G. G. (1868). On the communication of vibration from a vibrating body to a surrounding gas. *Phil. Trans. Roy. Soc. London* **158**, Part II, 447–463.

Tabor, J. R. (1970). Reconstruction of the ossicular chain. *Arch. Otolaryngol.* **92**, 141–146.

Terkildsen, K. (1960a). An evaluation of perceptive hearing losses in children, based on recruitment determinations. *Acta Oto-Laryngol.* **51**, 476–484.

Terkildsen, K. (1960b). Acoustic reflexes of the human musculus tensor tympani. *Acta Oto-Laryngol. Suppl.* **158**, 230–238.

Terkildsen, K. (1964). Clinical application of impedance measurements with a fixed frequency technique. *J. Int. Audiol.* **3**, 147–155.

Terkildsen, K., and Scott Nielsen, S. (1960). An electro-acoustic impedance measuring bridge for clinical use. *Arch. Otolaryngol.* **72**, 339–346.

Terkildsen, K., and Thomsen, K. A. (1959). The influence of pressure variations on the impedance of the human ear drum. *J. Laryngol. Otol.* **73**, 409–418.

Thomsen, K. A. (1955a). Case of psychogenic deafness demonstrated by measuring impedance. *Acta Oto-Laryngol.* **45**, 82–85.

Thomsen, K. A. (1955b). Employment of impedance measurements in otologic and otoneurologic diagnostics. *Acta Oto-Laryngol.* **45**, 159–167.

Thomsen, K. A. (1955c). Eustachian tube function tested by employment of impedance measuring. *Acta Oto-Laryngol.* **45**, 252–267.

Thomsen, K. A. (1955d). The Metz recruitment test. *Acta Oto-Laryngol.* **45**, 544–552.

Thomsen, K. A. (1957). Studies on the function of the eustachian tube in a series of normal individuals. *Acta Oto-Laryngol.* **48**, 516–529.

Thomsen, K. A. (1958a). Investigations on Toynbee's experiment in normal individuals. *Acta Oto-Laryngol. Suppl.* **140**, 263–268.

Thomsen, K. A. (1958b). Investigations on the tubal function and measurement of the middle ear pressure in pressure chamber. *Acta Oto-Laryngol. Suppl.* **140**, 269–278.

Thomsen, K. A. (1961). Objective determination of the middle-ear pressure. *Acta Oto-Laryngol. Suppl.* **158**, 212–216.

Thorburn, I. B. (1957). Post-traumatic conduction deafness. *J. Laryngol. Otol.* **71**, 542–545.

Tröger, J.(1930). Die Schallafnahme durch das äussere Ohr. *Phys. Z.* **31**, 26–56.

Turner, J. L. (1969). Hearing results in malleostapediopexy. *Arch. Otolaryngol.* **89**, 83–87.

Ulrich, K. (1926). Verletzungen des Gehörorganes bei Schädelbasisfrakturen. *Acta Oto-Laryngol. Suppl.* **6**.

Varner, W. R. (1947). "The Fourteen Systems of Units." Vantage Press, New York.

Waetzmann, E. (1936). Über symmetrie- und Erblichkeitsfragen am menschlichen Gehörorgan. *Z. Tech. Phys.* **17**, 549–553.

Waetzmann, E. (1938). Absorptionsmessungen am Trommelfell mit der Schusterschen Brücke. *Akust. Z.* **3**, 1–6.

Waetzmann, E., and Keibs, L. (1936). Hörschwellenbestimmungen mit der Thermophon und Messungen am Trommelfell. *Ann. Phys.* **26**, Ser. 5, 141–144.

Ward, W. D. (1962). Studies on the aural reflex. II. Reduction of temporary threshold shift from intermittent noise by reflex activity; implications for damage-risk criteria. *J. Acoust. Soc. Amer.* **34**, 234–241.

Webster, A. G. (1919). Acoustical impedance, and the theory of horns and of the phonograph. *Proc. Nat. Acad. Sci.* **5**, 275–282.

Wedenberg, E. (1963). Objective auditory tests on non-cooperative children. *Acta Oto-Laryngol Suppl.* **175**.

Wegel, R. L. (1932). Physical data and physiology of excitation of the auditory nerve. *Ann. Otol. Rhinol. Laryngol.* **41**, 740–779.

West, W. (1928). Measurements of the acoustical impedances of human ears. *P. O. Elect. Eng. J.* **21**, 293–300.

Wever, E. G., and Lawrence, M. (1954). "Physiological Acoustics." Princeton Univ. Press, Princeton, New Jersey.

Wilber, L. A., Goodhill, V. G., and Hogue, A. C. (1969). Diagnostic implications of acoustic impedance measurements. *ASHA* **11**, 417.

Wilber, L. A., Goodhill, V., and Hogue, A. C. (1970). Comparative acoustic impedance measurements. *ASHA* **12**, 435.

Williams, R. A. (1958). Head injury with fracture of stapes. *J. Laryngol. Otol.* **72**, 666–670.

Wilmot, T. J. (1969). Auditory analysis in some common hearing problems. *J. Laryngol. Otol.* **83**, 521–527.

Wilson, J. G. (1935). Fissula ante fenestram and adjacent tissue in the human otic capsule. *Acta Oto-Laryngol.* **22**, 382–389.

Wullstein, H. (1956). The restoration of the function of the middle ear, in chronic otitis media. *Ann. Otol. Rhinol. Laryngol.* **65**, 1020–1041.

Wustrow, F. (1956). Die Knochenbildung in den Gehörknöchelchen. *Z. Laryngol. Rhinol. Otol.* **35,** 487–498.

Zöllner, F. (1957). Prognosis of the operative improvement of hearing in chronic middle ear infections. *Ann. Otol. Rhinol. Laryngol.* **66,** 907–917.

Zwislocki, J. (1957a). Some measurements of the impedance at the eardrum. *J. Acoust. Soc. Amer.* **29,** 349–356.

Zwislocki, J. (1957b). Some impedance measurements on normal and pathological ears. *J. Acoust. Soc. Amer.* **29,** 1312–1317.

Zwislocki, J. (1961). Acoustic measurement of middle ear function. *Ann. Otol. Rhinol. Laryngol.* **70,** 599–606.

Zwislocki, J. (1962). Analysis of the middle-ear function. Part I: Input impedance. *J. Acoust. Soc. Amer.* **34,** 1514–1523.

Zwislocki, J. (1963a). Acoustics of the middle ear. *In* "Middle Ear Function Seminar," (J. L. Fletcher, ed.). Report No. 576. U.S. Army Med. Res. Lab., Ft. Knox, Kentucky.

Zwislocki, J. (1963b). An acoustic method for clinical examination of the ear. *J. Speech Hearing Res.* **6,** 303–314.

Zwislocki, J. (1964). Introduction. *J. Int. Audiol.* **3,** 121–122.

Zwislocki, J. (1965). Summary by the moderator: The acoustic impedance of the ear. *J. Int. Audiol.* **4,** 18–19.

Zwislocki, J. J. (1968). On acoustic research and its clinical application. *Acta Otolaryngol.* **65,** 86–96.

Zwislocki, J., and Feldman, A. S. (1963). Post-mortem acoustic impedance of human ears. *J. Acoust. Soc. Amer.* **35,** 104–107.

Zwislocki, J. J., and Feldman, A. S. (1970). Acoustic impedance of pathological ears. *ASHA* Mono. No. **15.** Amer. Speech and Hearing Assoc., Washington.

Chapter 11

Electroencephalic Audiometry

ROBERT GOLDSTEIN

University of Wisconsin, Madison

I. Introduction

Electrophysiologic audiometry differs from behavioral audiometry in that the response to acoustic stimulation manifests itself by some change in the observed electrical properties of the person under test, while in behavioral audiometry the response is some overt bodily reaction. Ongoing electrical activity can be observed on an oscilloscope or in a graphic recording. An electrophysiologic response is a relatively abrupt change in the ongoing activity associated with an acoustic stimulus.

In behavioral audiometry the overt responses can be voluntary or involuntary, but the listener has little or no control over his electrophysiologic responses. Electrophysiologic audiometry has often been dubbed "objective" because the response mechanism is not under the "subjective" control of the listener. Since audiometry is a procedure and not merely a response, the term *objective* can apply only if the technique as well as the response is objective. Objectivity will be discussed later.

Clinical use of electrophysiologic responses has focused on threshold audiometry. Because of this clinical emphasis, much of the discussion will center around threshold measures. Specific techniques of electrophysiologic audiometry and instrumentation are not of concern in this chapter except as they relate to the particular topic under discussion.

Most clinical studies in audition have employed some measure of autonomic function or of the ongoing electrical activity of the central nervous system (CNS). Muscle and cochlear potentials have also been used, as well as changes in corneoretinal potentials brought about by searching movement of the eyes during sound localization.

The most common index of autonomic activity used in audiometry is a change in the state of the sweat glands. The activity can be reflected as alterations in resistance to a small current flow or in changes of potential between two points on the skin (electrodermal responses). Perspiration can be measured directly, but such measurements have not been adapted to practical clinical audiometry. Changes in cardiac rate have been used in many experimental studies and in some clinical studies, as have modifications in respiratory rate, but neither response index has been adapted in a consistent way for audiometry.

Transient changes in the electrical activity of the CNS in response to sound are most commonly observed in the electroencephalogram (EEG). The background EEG is usually of greater magnitude than the transient changes elicited by acoustic stimuli. Detecting transient responses within a background of electrical noise has been accomplished in at least two ways. Originally, segments of the ongoing electrical activity following the onset of each of a series of identical stimuli were superimposed photographically, or were recorded over each other on a continuous loop of paper. Now, the commonly used procedure is to add the EEG segments electronically. The background activity cancels itself through successive additions because, presumably, it is random with respect to the onset of the stimuli, while the small, time-locked responses grow into an identifiable pattern.

This chapter emphasizes changes in the electrical activity of the brain in response to sound (electroencephalic responses). None of the other electrophysiologic responses except electrodermal have had sufficient clinical application to have produced adequate generalizations. Electrodermal audiometry has declined in popularity in recent years and is not generally used in most clinical settings. The treatment of electrodermal responses and electrodermal audiometry in the first edition of this book is still essentially valid and will not be extended here.

The body of literature relevant to this chapter is too vast to permit citations of each reference pertinent to the topic under discussion. The material presented is based largely on common observations reported in the literature and on my own experimental and clinical experience.

An electroencephalic response (EER) in the context of audiometry is any distinct change in the ongoing electroencephalic activity brought about by acoustic stimulation. The response can be viewed as a change in the ongoing EEG during or following a single test sound, or it can be an average of responses to repetitions of a given sound. Little stress will be placed on the significance of the details of electroencephalic response configurations, and illustrations of actual responses will not be presented. Illustrations of representative response patterns and details of how they were derived are found in many of the references cited later.

Electroencephalic audiometry (EEA) in which responses are observed within the raw EEG is rarely performed clinically today. Nevertheless, an extended discussion of this technique is warranted because it provides background for and insight into EEA in which the averaged electroencephalic response (AER) is used as the response index. In addition, the technique is still viable, is relatively inexpensive, and can yield information not yet attainable from the averaged responses.

Electrical activity of the cochlea and auditory nerve will also be considered. The cochlear microphonic and the auditory nerve action potential are detected by instruments similar to those used for EEA and provide information about the overall functioning of the auditory system.

II. Electroencephalic Response (EER)

A. Method of Recording

Electrical activity of the brain can be recorded from small disc electrodes applied to the scalp or from fine needles under the scalp. Electrodes have been placed directly on or in the brain in some patients who have undergone craniotomies, but obviously, this is not a feasible technique for routine EEA. The electroencephalic activity can be recorded between two electrodes on the scalp (bipolar) or between one scalp electrode and another electrode located on a presumably neutral spot such as the earlobe, mastoid, or nose (monopolar). The electrodes are usually capacitance-coupled to the amplifiers and associated oscillograph and thus the EEG machine records only ac activity.

B. Nature of Subjects and Patients

Electroencephalic responses to sound have been observed in persons of all ages. Most clinical EEA studies, however, have concentrated on young children because ordinarily they cannot be tested by other audiometric techniques which are easily applied to older children and adults. These young children must usually be asleep when tested because their restless behavior renders the EEA procedure impractical. Few young normal children therefore, have been put through the procedure, mainly because sedation or anesthesia is often required.

Most of the young children studied by EEA have been deaf or have had another disorder of communication. Responses from persons with disorders of communication may differ according to the nature of the disorder, and as a group their responses may differ from those of normal subjects. However, the descriptions of EER to follow are generally applicable to all subjects.

C. Nature of Responses

The kind of EER elicited by sound will depend largely on the ongoing EEG pattern at the time of stimulation. The EEG in turn depends largely on the age of the person, state of alertness, if awake, and stage of sleep, if asleep. It depends somewhat, too, on the portion of the head from which the recording is being made.

In the awake adult and older child, the most prominent feature of the EEG is a rhythmic activity occurring at the rate of about 10 per second. This so-called alpha(α)-rhythm is most evident from the occipital region, and is largest when the subject is alert but relaxed with his eyes closed. In this state the response to acoustic stimulation is usually a reduction in the α-rhythm starting about 150–300 msec after the onset of the stimulus.

A person with little α-rhythm usually has brain waves of faster rate and of small amplitude. An acoustic stimulus may further reduce this activity but because of the initial low amplitude further reduction may not be obvious. A person who normally shows a prominent α-rhythm may also have low-voltage, fast activity when drowsy and going to sleep. A stimulus may elicit an EER in the form of a return of the α-rhythm.

Another common EER is the K-complex. It is a combination of large, slow waves with faster activity superimposed and following the slow waves. The latency of the slow component is usually between 100 and 500 msec. The K-complex generally is not large for a person who is awake, and often only a small, slow component is evident. It is more prominent in the record of a sleeping person. In deep sleep, however, the K-complex is not easily elicited.

The background EEG in sleep differs greatly from that of a person who is awake. Frequencies are diverse, and often large, slow waves are evident that are not seen in the record of an awake subject. Because the EER represents a change in the ongoing activity, EER's in sleep are also diverse. In addition to the K-complex, other changes may take place, such as reduction of some or all of the components of the ongoing activity, introduction of new frequencies, increase in some components of the ongoing activity, or a generalized change in the ongoing pattern.

D. Time Course

Latency of response is shortened as the intensity of the stimulus is increased. This is not a very predictable relation, however, because many subject and stimulus variables influence latency. Duration of the response is also variable and depends upon those conditions which affect latency as well as upon the length of the stimulus itself.

The refractory period for an EER has not been adequately determined. In addition, not all components of the response are equally refractory. As a clinical precaution, at least 20 sec should elapse between the termination of one stimulus and the onset of the next.

E. Stimulus Parameters

The clarity of responses and the likelihood of responding (responsivity) are directly related to stimulus intensity. However, other stimulus parameters, differences in test conditions, and individual variability in responsivity restrict the value of an intensity–response function. A weak sound of one quality may elicit an EER after complete adaptation or habituation to a much stronger stimulus of a different quality. The nature of the EER does not seem to be predictably related to stimulus intensity.

The rise time of a stimulus such as a pure tone influences responsivity to a minor extent: For most patients the shorter the rise time, the more effective the stimulus in evoking a response.

No clear relation has been established between electroencephalic responsivity in sleep and such stimulus parameters as frequency, complexity, or meaningfulness. At times, however, speech will elicit responses when pure tones appear to be ineffective.

F. Evaluation of Responses

Electroencephalic changes can be effected not only by the onset of the stimulus but by the steady-state portion and by its termination, if the sound persists for several seconds. Derbyshire and Farley (1959) outlined a practical system for describing and scoring changes in each of the three EEG segments as part of a system for objective identification of responses and determination of threshold. Other objective techniques for determining whether an EER occurred are electronic analysis of frequency changes, and planimetric determination of changes in area under the EEG waves.

III. Averaged Electroencephalic Response (AER)

The EER's to individual stimuli are often too small or too obscure to be seen or evaluated. A technique has been developed to extract small EER's from the background of the larger EEG. The technique is predicated on the assumptions that the EER's to successive repetitions of the same stimulus maintain a constant form and latency, and that the background EEG is random in time with respect to stimulus onset. Short segments of EEG following each stimulus are summed electronically. The small EER's which are time-locked to the stimuli grow through this summing process while the random background EEG tends to disappear. When the resulting EER is divided by the number of stimuli which produced it, the resultant pattern is considered an averaged electroencephalic response (AER).

A. Basic Description

The initial descriptions of the AER resembled descriptions of the "K" response to a single stimulus. Most investigators have noted that the clearest response is recorded from the vertex of the skull; the same was observed for the K-complex as a result of a single stimulus in the standard EEG tracing.

The AER is not a unitary response. It is a composite or a sequence or some other combination of electrical potentials reflecting the activity of much of the brain. Figure 1 presents an idealized or "average" AER. The temporal dividing lines between the early components, late components, and contingent negative variation (CNV) are arbitrary. They might be shifted in either direction. Current research in our own laboratory, for example, suggests that what we have called the early components may not extend beyond 40 msec after the onset of the stimulus. It is also possible that the three major components shown in Figure

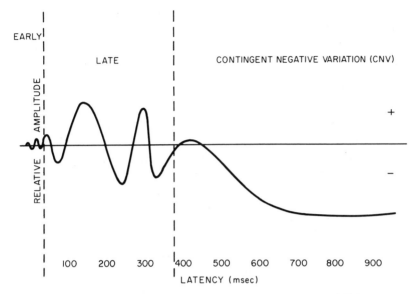

FIG. 1. Schematic averaged electroencephalic response (AER).

1 can be further divided into segments, each with its own distinctive or unique properties. For example, most descriptions of the late components focus on a vertex-negative wave at about 80 msec and a vertex-positive wave at about 170 msec; the segment of the response between 200 and 400 msec may have different properties. The early component may also have to be fractionated. Recent evidence points to possible brain stem responses recorded extracranially with latencies between 2 and 7 msec (Jewett *et al.*, 1970; Moore, 1971). Each segment or component of response probably reflects different functions or activities. It is unlikely that one component of the AER is more important than another for the understanding of auditory function or dysfunction.

Studies of AER have proliferated greatly during recent years and so have the terms and designations by which AER's are identified, defined, and described. What one investigator calls "P_1," for instance, may be designated as "P_2" or "P_b" by others. Whenever possible, therefore, I shall refer to various peaks by latency rather than by a numerical or literal subscript.

Except for some electrophysiologists, most persons follow the convention of plotting the magnitude of time-related phenomena in the first and fourth quadrants of the Cartesian coordinates. Time is plotted from the origin along the x-axis in the positive direction; positive magnitudes are plotted above the x-axis and negative magnitudes are plotted below the x-axis. It seems advisable, therefore, that positivity at one specified electrode relative to another (for example, vertex relative to earlobe) be shown as an upward deflection, and negativity by a downward deflection, as in Figure 1.

B. Recording Parameters

The late components of the AER are most prominent from an electrode on the vertex referred to an inactive, or at least less active, electrode on the mastoid, earlobe, or nose. AER's to visual and to somatosensory stimulation are also seen best with these electrode combinations. Early components of the AER in the visual and somatosensory modalities are more prominent when the active electrode is placed over the corresponding primary reception area of the cortex. Early components of the AER to sound, however, seem to be as prominent with a vertex-earlobe combination (C_z-A_1 or C_z-A_2) as they are with a temporal-earlobe combination (T_3-A_1 or T_4-A_2). Because of the short latency of the initial waves, it is likely that some of the earliest activity recorded from the vertex-earlobe combination originates from subcortical structures.

Each time domain of the AER has its own properties, including that of spectrum. In general, the earlier the component, the higher the frequency composition. At the late end, the CNV is virtually a direct current change. Response amplitudes also vary with the time segments; in general, the earlier the component, the smaller the amplitude. Spectral and amplitude differences as well as some other differences to be discussed later usually make it impractical to study all components of the AER under identical recording conditions. Extensive high-frequency filtering particularly to eliminate 60-Hz artifact, has little effect on the late components whose energy lies mainly in the range of 2–7 Hz. The same filtering can reduce the amplitude of the early components whose energy extends significantly above as well as below 60 Hz. Furthermore, conventional filtering produces phase shifts which can be misinterpreted as latency shifts when comparing peak latencies of the filtered and unfiltered responses. Greater amplification is ordinarily needed for the early than for the late components. With extensive amplification, the background noise level is also increased, but noise below about 150 Hz cannot be filtered without altering some aspects of the early components. Beyond the use of low-noise amplifiers and low-resistance electrode contacts, clarity of the early components of the AER usually has to be achieved by the averaging of many responses (for example, 250–500) to stimuli presented at relatively rapid rates (for example, 5–15 per second).

C. Stimulus and Procedural Parameters

These parameters will be discussed mainly as they relate to conventional audiologic measures. Therefore, the discussion will emphasize the late components of the AER because these components have been the ones used most frequently in clinical EEA. Attention will also be given to the effect of the same parameters on the early components with the expectation that these components will gain wider clinical use in the near future. Inasmuch as threshold determination has been a major goal of clinical EEA and pure tones are the most commonly used stimuli for threshold determination, the parameters of pure-tone stimulation will be the focus of this section.

Pure-tone frequency has only a minor influence on AER amplitude; apparently the higher the frequency, the smaller the response elicited (Evans and Deatherage, 1969; Rothman, 1970).

AER amplitude bears a general relation to stimulus magnitude: the greater the stimulus, the larger the AER. Conversely, latencies of the major peaks tend to decrease with increasing stimulus magnitude. Response amplitude does not continue to grow indefinitely with stimulus magnitude; it can reach a maximum and can even diminish while stimulus magnitude and loudness continue to grow. The response curve is not necessarily monotonic; in some individuals under some circumstances (not fully defined), a weak stimulus can elicit a larger AER than a stronger stimulus. The lack of a clearly lawful relation between stimulus magnitude and AER amplitude makes it risky to extrapolate to threshold from an amplitude–response curve.

AER amplitude and latency are also affected by rise time of pure tones: in general, the shorter the rise time, the shorter the latency, and the larger the amplitude. Between 3 and 50 msec, close to the practical lower and upper limits of rise time for pure-tone audiometry, latency and amplitude do not vary appreciably with rise time (Onishi and Davis, 1968).

There appears to be a direct relation between stimulus duration and AER amplitude for stimulus durations (plateaus of the tone bursts) of less than 30 msec, probably because of temporal summation. Prolonging the stimulus beyond 30 msec has a negligible effect on response amplitude.

The late components of the AER require about 10 sec for full recovery. Recovery is nearly complete, however, at about 2 sec. Difference in recovery at 1 sec compared to 2 sec is not great. A long interstimulus interval, for example, 2 sec (or a slow rate of stimulation, for example, 1 per 2 sec) may elicit a slightly larger and more definable AER than can be evoked by the same number of stimuli presented at a faster rate, for example, 1 per second. The advantage of the faster rate is shortened test time for a fixed number of stimuli. On the other hand, if test time is not a major consideration, then with a faster rate, twice as many stimuli can be presented within a given time segment, serving to reduce further the noise of the non-time-locked activity. Stimulus rate and regularity, however, seem to affect response configuration as well as amplitude (Vaughan and Ritter, 1970); therefore, criteria for response identification for threshold audiometry should be compatible with the temporal sequencing of the stimuli.

The tendency of the late components of the AER to habituate or adapt with repetitive stimulation can be offset partially by randomizing the interstimulus interval; however, the resultant increase in AER amplitude may not be sufficient to warrant, for clinical purposes, the inconvenience or the additional timing equipment required for irregular spacing of stimuli.

The later the event in time, the more susceptible it is to modification and manipulation. It has been shown that the magnitude of a segment of the late components can be altered through conditioning even though there is no apparent relation between the nature of the instrumental conditioning and the response component manipulated (Rosenfeld *et al.*, 1969).

Masking of the late components of the AER has not been studied extensively. Nevertheless, it appears that the AER follows the same rules as voluntary behavioral responses, and that masking of the nontest ear in EEA is feasible.

The amplitude of the late components may be greater from the side of the brain opposite the stimulated ear than from the ipsilateral hemisphere. This observation has no immediate practical relevance to threshold audiometry. In the future, however, it may be considered when the totality of responsivity is used to assess the totality of auditory function or dysfunction.

Little clinical use has been made of the early components of the AER. Nevertheless, some of their properties (for example, long-term stability, resistance to habituation, persistence during sleep) make it probable that the early components will be incorporated into clinical EEA.

Clicks have been used in most studies on the early components. Thresholds for clicks have been found in a variety of experimental subjects to be the same when measured by voluntary responses and by the early components. Similar correspondence for pure tones has not yet been found because pure tones do not seem to elicit early components that are as identifiable at low sensation levels. Some of the differences in the clarity of responses to the two stimuli are undoubtedly related to differences in stimulus characteristics. Pure tones differ from clicks in rise time, duration, and spectrum. It is not certain which of these parameters has the greatest effect on responsivity, although it is probable that rise time is more influential than spectrum and duration (Kupperman, 1970). Laboratory experience is showing that modifications in pure-tone envelope and in response filtering can improve the identifiability of the early components to tones, and that pure-tone audiometry with the early components probably will be feasible.

Just as with the late components of the AER, the amplitude of the early components grows with increasing stimulus magnitude, and latency correspondingly decreases. However, the amplitude of the early components seems to be more nearly linearly related to stimulus magnitude in decibels. Even within the first 50 msec, the earlier the peaks, the more nearly related to stimulus magnitude are the peak-to-peak amplitudes (Madell, 1969). Despite the relative linearity of the group data, it is difficult to extrapolate to threshold for an individual from an amplitude-response curve of the early components of the AER to clicks.

Absolute amplitudes of early and late components for a given stimulus magnitude differ considerably. For a 50-dB sensation level (SL) click the peak-to-peak amplitude of N_{80}-P_{170} averages about 9 microvolts (μV); for the N_{22}-P_{32} waves, the largest of early components, the amplitude usually averages about 1 μV.

While there appears to be some short-term equilibration or habituation or adaptation of the early components, long-term effects do not seem to occur, at least with interstimulus intervals as long as 65 msec. Regardless of rate stimulation, equilibration of the early components appears to be complete after 1000 clicks. Continuous stimulation even at 9.6/sec produces no further response decrement over periods as long as 7 hours (Mendel and Goldstein, 1971).

No clear earedness or brainedness is obvious for the early components of the AER. Subtle differences in latency, amplitude, or configuration, if they do exist, have not yet been reported.

Systematic studies on masking of the early components have not been reported. Preliminary experience in our own laboratory suggests that the early components, as the late components, of the AER follow the same rules of masking as do behavioral responses (Smith, 1971).

D. Relation to Loudness Functions

Attempts to relate amplitude of the late components of the AER and loudness have, in general, been unsuccessful. The positive results reported by Keidel and Spreng (1965) apparently have not been replicated. AER amplitude grows at a slower rate than the equivalent loudness curve, reaches a maximum value while loudness continues to grow, and seems to bear no systematic relation to any loudness scale.

In at least one study on the early components, a relation was shown between loudness and the amplitude of the AER to clicks (Madell, 1969). Slopes of loudness functions and of AER amplitudes were not equal nor were they correlated. Significant correlation was found, however, between group loudness magnitude estimates and peak-to-peak voltage values as a function of sensation level; and the earlier the peaks, the higher the correlation.

The difference limen (DL) for intensity apparently can be determined by a paradigm similar to that employed in the clinical SISI test, that is, changes in the level of the continuous background tone have to serve as the stimuli to elicit the AER. Stimulus increments as small as 5 dB have been able to elicit identifiable late components (McCandless and Rose, 1970).

E. Effects of State

Sleep greatly modifies the late components of the AER. During the beginning stage of sleep, the response is often characterized by a large negative wave between 300 and 325 msec. If this light sleep stage persists, N_{300} usually remains detectable and can be used as a response index for threshold audiometry. Late components become more variable (or are less identifiable) as sleep deepens. During the REM stage (rapid eye movement stage), late components cannot be elicited, or at least cannot be identified with any certainty.

Many children for whom EEA is required cannot be restrained for adequate testing while they are awake, and will not ordinarily remain in natural sleep long enough for definitive testing. In addition, waiting for a child to fall asleep can make the entire procedure prohibitively long. Induced sleep, therefore, must frequently be considered. Barbiturates in particular, and some other drugs to a lesser extent, modify the late components of the AER. Although responsivity may persist even with barbiturates, the pattern of responses during induced sleep may vary enough to limit the certainty with which responses can be identified for threshold audiometry.

The amplitude of the late components of the AER can also vary in the subject who is awake. Responses from a person sitting in a dark room with his eyes closed can differ measurably from those derived when he is in a lighted room with his eyes open. Attention to the signal, distraction from it by reading or other tasks, reverie, etc., all influence the amplitude and, to a lesser degree, the configuration of the AER. Hypnotic suggestion of deafness, however, apparently has no effect on response amplitude (Halliday and Mason, 1964).

By contrast, the early components of the AER are characterized by consistency and stability. Simple changes in test conditions (room darkened, eyes closed; room lighted, eyes opened; silent reading) have no apparent effect on the pattern or peak-to-peak amplitudes of the early components (Mendel and Goldstein, 1969a). The configuration and amplitude remain constant over prolonged periods of wakefulness during which the state of the subject must change considerably (Mendel and Goldstein, 1969b).

Configuration and peak-to-peak amplitudes remain constant during brief periods of natural sleep (Mendel and Goldstein, 1969b). Amplitude of response is affected by changes in the depth of sleep during a full night of natural sleep: the deeper the sleep, the smaller the response. During REM sleep, however, responses are as clear as they are during the awake state and almost as large. The response configuration through the first 40 msec, at least, does not vary significantly with sleep stage despite the moderate changes in response amplitude (Mendel and Goldstein, 1971). AER's to clicks during sleep have been observed at levels corresponding to thresholds previously determined by voluntary behavioral responses.

Effects of induced sleep on the early components have not been studied extensively. The few studies on humans which have been reported, however, do suggest that drugs, including barbiturates, have negligible effect on the early components (Celesia and Puletti, 1969; Horwitz et al., 1966). Similarly, early components of the AER to somatosensory stimulation appear resistant to the effects of barbiturates (Allison et al., 1963). Thus, the prospects are favorable for clinical use of the early components under conditions of natural or induced sleep.

I do not know of any definitive reports on the effects of concentrated attention, hypnosis, conditioning, etc., on the early components. Studies in other modalities suggest that none of these manipulations will significantly affect the early components to sound.

F. Subject Parameters

Most of the properties of the AER discussed so far are generally applicable to all subjects. Several aspects of response, however, do vary with age. Late components are present at birth even in premature infants. Latencies tend to shorten with age and appear to reach their mature limits at 7 or 8 years, while response amplitude decreases with age through puberty, and then slowly increases thereafter. Amplitude changes may reflect anatomical differences (for example, thickness of skull) more than physiological differences, whereas latency differences probably are related to physiological maturation. Amplitude and latency variations with age may be of little consequence for threshold audiometry except as they broaden or blur the criteria for response identification. Deviation from amplitude and latency norms, however, may eventually provide insight into the central nervous system function of patients with undefined auditory disorders.

Differences in amplitudes of the late components of the AER have also been noted as a function of race and sex. These differences are inconsequential in terms of threshold audiometry, and may possibly be too small for practical application to other aspects of audiometry. Studies have not been reported on the relation between race or sex and the early components.

A provocative study by Chalke and Ertl (1965) pointed out significant differences in the latency of both early and late components of the AER to visual stimulation as a function of a particular measure of intelligence. Those persons with distinctly subnormal IQ scores showed longer latencies than those subjects with distinctly superior scores. The latencies for persons with average scores fell between the other two groups. The relation between any measure of intelligence and the latencies of the various peaks of the acoustically evoked AER has not, to my knowledge, been established.

Studies on maturation of the early components have not been reported. Engel (1971), however, has found that a vertex-negative peak at about 34 msec can be elicited within the first week of life.

G. Contingent Negative Variation (CNV)

No clear definition can be given at this time of those phenomena which trail after or which perhaps overlap the late components of the AER. One point of agreement emerges from among those who have studied the contingent negative variation or expectancy wave: the CNV is not related to the sensory aspects (for example, loudness, pitch) of the messages which trigger it, but to the contingencies of the set of sensory signals, to expectancy, to differentiation, etc. In other words, the CNV is related to some psychic aspect or aspects (for example, cognition) beyond the elemental sensory level.

Two stimuli are needed to develop the CNV. The first is a conditional signal, the second an imperative one demanding a specified reaction. After several pairings, a response develops in anticipation of the second signal. Mental processes without overt response may be sufficient to maintain the CNV. Once established, the CNV does not adapt as long as the conditional situation is maintained. The CNV dissolves quickly, however, if the imperative signal is removed.

The CNV is at least as large from a vertex-mastoid electrode combination as from any other pair of leads. The activity, however, seems to sweep over time in a frontal-to-posterior direction.

The CNV may not be totally a direct current shift, but the time course of its polarity change is slow. The temporal course depends in part on the interval between the conditional and imperative stimuli. A majority of the studies reported have used a 1-sec interstimulus interval. The activity which initiates the total response ordinarily lumped under CNV begins with a vertex-positive wave about 300 msec after the onset of the conditional stimulus. The rise time of the large, slow negative variation appears to vary with individuals, taking either a rectangular or a ramp form. The CNV reaches its maximum in 500–900 msec.

Amplitude of the CNV, usually 20–25 μV, seems unrelated either to stimulus modality or magnitude. Averaging is not always necessary to obtain an identifiable response, but when averaging is done, 10–12 samples usually suffice. Although a voluntary response is not necessary for its elicitation, the CNV is usually larger when a voluntary response is required. Amplitude may also be related to the rapidity of the voluntary response (Hillyard and Galambos, 1967). Area under the CNV curve (that is, total energy) may be a more appropriate measure of response magnitude than baseline-to-peak or peak-to-peak voltage (Low, 1969).

Children less than 5 years old generally do not yield a clear CNV, nor is the CNV evident in some young children, even under circumstances in which they can perform the task that elicits a CNV in older children and adults.

The CNV is not easily adaptable to threshold audiometry because amplitude of CNV bears little relation to stimulus magnitude. It is also doubtful that the CNV could be used practically in assessing loudness and pitch dysfunctions. It might be used as an index in a test of speech intelligibility, but such a test would have particular value only for adults or older children incapable of oral and written responses. One might well speculate that the CNV could be adapted to distinguish restricted linguistic deficits from general intellectual deficits.

The apparent age limitation seems to prevent the audiologic application of the CNV to an important group of patients whose higher level linguistic potentialities need to be assessed. This shortcoming might be circumvented by studying the relation of the CNV to the other components of the AER, with the possibility that information derived from

the CNV may also be extrapolated from certain properties of the early
and late components. A parallel to this approach is seen in the use
of pure-tone thresholds to predict, with some restrictions on certainty,
speech discrimination capacity in children too young to give verbal responses for conventional speech discrimination tests.

IV. Objectivity in Threshold Audiometry

Audiometry is a procedure, not a response. An objective response does
not guarantee objective audiometry. A procedure which employs subjective responses can be quite objective while one employing objective responses can be quite subjective. The first situation is seen in most forms
of pure-tone audiometry. The tester usually asks the patient to raise
his finger each time a tone is heard and to lower it when the tone
disappears. The patient is further instructed to raise his finger regardless
of the faintness of the sound and to signal even if he thinks he hears
a tone.

The patient is seated so that he cannot observe the facial expressions,
or the movements of the audiologist's hands. He has no way of knowing
when a test sound will be presented, when it will be discontinued, or
when it will be altered in character (intensity, frequency, ear). The
patient, therefore, operates solely on a fixed set of instructions and is
cued only by the stimulus.

The audiologist has structured the test situation to limit the response
repertory of his patient to a simple, identifiable gesture. That gesture
is usually unequivocal in response to sounds above a given intensity
level, but rarely made at levels distinctly below that same point. Thus
the audiologist has a series of yes–no observations from which he can
plot a curve (usually in his own mind) of the percentage of responses
as a function of the magnitude of the stimulus. His criterion for threshold
is predetermined, and is customarily that magnitude at which the patient
responds at least 50% of the time. The practicality of this particular
threshold criterion is reinforced by the nature of the patient's response
to stimuli at or close to threshold: considerable hesitation in raising
his finger at the onset of the tone, and less hesitation in lowering his
finger at the termination of the tone. The patient's hesitation near the
threshold level and the clarity of response at suprathreshold levels reflect
his introspection. Despite the subjectivity of the patient's response, the
test itself is quite objective because of the identifiable nature of the
response and the predetermined criterion for threshold. The objectivity
is also strengthened by a system of stimulus presentations which is ordi-

narily predetermined and applied in a similar way from patient to patient.

The predictability of the patient's behavioral response is ordinarily so great that he appears to be only a passive participant in the procedure. The patient raises and lowers his finger as if a string were tied to it, with the opposite end of the string controlled by the audiologist. When the audiologist presents the stimulus, in effect he exerts a pull on the string in proportion to the magnitude of the stimulus. The weight of the patient's finger corresponds to his hearing loss. When the pull on the string barely exceeds the inertial effects of the weight, the finger rises slowly, but drops quickly when the string is released. With greater pull (stronger auditory stimulus) the finger rises consistently and quickly, and again drops quickly when the pull is terminated.

This analogy presumes, of course, that the audiologist has the cooperation of his patient. The presumption is indeed true for the large majority of patients, and for them audiometry is quite objective despite the subjective nature of their responses. When patients cannot or will not cooperate, however, validity as well as objectivity of behavioral audiometry is open to considerable question. It is for such patients (for example, young children, malignerers) that electroencephalic audiometry is usually recommended.

Most clinicians who have described their procedures for electroencephalic audiometry have followed a scheme similar to the one for behavioral audiometry just described. In the past they observed changes in the ongoing EEG as indicators of responses to sound, and now they look for certain positive and negative peaks in the AER. Since the AER is an objective response, why should not electroencephalic audiometry automatically be considered objective audiometry?

First of all, the AER is not as uniform a response as the raising and lowering of a finger. Second, the amplitude of the AER (corresponding to the definiteness with which a finger is raised and lowered) does not always bear a direct relation to the magnitude of the auditory stimulus. Although there is a crude relation between AER amplitude and stimulus magnitude, sometimes the weaker of two sounds elicits a larger reaction. A third difference relates to the small number of false positives and false negatives in behavioral audiometry. A patient seldom raises his finger when a test sound has not been presented and seldom fails to respond when the stimulus is clearly audible. By contrast, clear peaks resembling responses often occur in the averaged electroencephalogram when no test stimuli have been presented. Conversely, deflections in an averaged EEG can appear to be completely random even when the sound is known to be audible. If an audiologist uses a procedure similar to that described for behavioral audiometry, he must make an immediate judgment whether a response occurred to the set of test stimuli when in fact the form of the response can be changing, the clarity of the response may not be related to the stimulus level, and the deflections in the tracing may be unrelated to the test stimuli. The next set of stimuli which he presents will depend on this immediate subjective judgment. Thus the EEA *procedure* can be quite subjective because of the tester, despite the objective nature of the response.

Subjectivity intrudes itself in another way. As mentioned previously, patients referred for EEA are usually those for whom behavioral audiometry has not been satisfactory. The audiologist who performs EEA on these patients often has prior knowledge about their communicative behavior. If a patient's behavior during previous audiometry suggests better hearing than can be established with certainty, the audiologist may be willing to accept a small or unusually patterned AER to a set of weak stimuli as substantiation of that better hearing. If prior behavioral audiometry suggests poorer hearing than had been suspected from the patient's reactions to environmental sounds, then the small and questionable AER to the weak stimuli might be regarded as too small and questionable to be a response.

Finally, the full objectivity of electroencephalic audiometry is not achieved if the audiologist does not establish a criterion for threshold. The 50% response point commonly used in behavioral audiometry is generally too time-consuming to achieve in EEA. The audiologist, therefore, often accepts as threshold the weakest stimulus level at which any identifiable AER is elicited. While this liberal criterion does not negate the objectivity of the test procedure, it does seriously limit the validity of the clinical inferences drawn from the threshold data.

How does one make EEA objective? Objectification is best accomplished by a series of steps, the first of which is programming the stimuli to be used before beginning the test.

Practical limitations of time do not allow the audiologist to determine as complete or precise threshold measurements as he can obtain on cooperative adults during behavioral audiometry. He is compelled to sample the auditory sensitivity of his patient rather than to explore it in detail. He must, therefore, decide in advance which results will be most helpful in his evaluation of the patient. On this basis, the audiologist selects appropriate stimulus conditions in terms of hearing level, frequency, and ear. For example, during a single test session he may be able to present stimuli at only two frequencies (for example, 500 and 3000 Hz) and at three widely spaced hearing levels (for example, 20, 60 and 100 dB). When the audiologist decides in advance which stimuli are to be presented, he does not have to depend upon an immediate yes-or-no decision during the test to determine what the next stimulus condition should be.

The sequence of the predetermined stimuli should be randomized. A pattern of sequencing in terms of hearing levels (for example, weak to strong), frequency (for example, low to high), and ear (for example, right always first) could be recalled at the time that the tracings are being analyzed. Knowledge of the stimulus condition can bias one's judgment. If the audiologist knows, for example, that the stimuli associated with a questionable tracing were intense, he may be influenced to call that tracing a response. Had the stimulus been weak, the questionable tracing would be likely to be dismissed as a random occurrence.

In order to maintain the "anonymity" of the stimulus condition, each scheduled set of stimuli is numbered in advance. That number is entered on the recording paper next to its signal averager readout. Only after decisions of response or no response have been completed are the judgments paired with the stimulus conditions by reference to the original schedule. Response analysis should be done by someone other than the person who performed the EEA; or if the audiologist who performed the EEA also analyzes the records, he should allow sufficient time to elapse to forget which tracings and stimulus conditions correspond.

Silent controls add another element to the total objectivity of EEA. The control conditions are prescheduled, numbered, and randomized along with the stimulus conditions. Sounds are not presented, but the background EEG is averaged as if stimuli had been presented. The resultant tracing is judged blindly at the conclusion of the test along with tracings derived during actual stimulation. Thus when the audiologist looks at a tracing, he has no clue to which ear had been stimulated, what frequency had been used, whether weak or strong stimuli were given, or whether any stimuli had been given at all.

One presentation of a given stimulus condition does not allow the audiologist to determine with certainty whether a seemingly positive AER was truly a response to the test sounds or whether it was a coincidental time-locking of the background EEG. Silent controls help to establish a rate of chance occurrence, in essence, a zero baseline. The criteria for what is significantly more than chance occurrence should be determined in advance for the EEA procedure to be completely objective. Any stimulus level at which significantly more than chance responses are elicited can be considered at or above a patient's auditory threshold. Although particular circumstances may later force alterations in the predetermined criteria for significant differences, failure to establish even tentative criteria before the test opens the way for subjectivity

when the audiologist makes inferences about his patient's thresholds.
Prior to analysis of test records, criteria should be established for
identification of the response itself. Some persons use AER's to high-
intensity stimuli as templates for judging responses to weaker stimuli,
and some use the pattern of the AER to light or vibration as a template.
A "typical" AER validated on normals or on calibrated hearing-impaired
subjects can also be used as a guide. One should not forget, however,
that most patients for whom EEA is required are not typical, and their
patterns of response may not fit a classic mold.

Comparison of a patient's AER patterns with some universal norm
for purposes of response identification can be a questionable procedure
even if the patient is a "typical" responder. Amplifier characteristics,
coupler time constants, and the nature and extent of filtering differ from
one clinic or laboratory to another. These physical differences can produce disparate patterns in terms of relative amplitude of peaks, latency
of peaks, interpeak intervals, and addition or exclusion of some peaks.
Within a given clinic, when an individual's own response is used as
a template, response identification based on pattern is more feasible.
Even this procedure, however, has some limitation. Physiological noise
not related to the response may change from time to time and cause
basically similar responses to look different. Perhaps when the temporal
and spectral characteristics of the various aspects of the AER are better
understood, amplification, coupling, and filtering can be adjusted to yield
more reproducible responses for recognition and comparison. At the
present, however, the objectivity, reliability, and validity of response
identification are limited, particularly for the late components of the
AER. For this reason little attention has been given in this chapter
to the precise details of response configuration, and illustrations of actual
responses have been omitted.

Future developments in electronics and computer systems may lead
to other means of objective response identification and analysis. For
example, responses may be judged in terms of power spectrum differences
between stimulus and silent periods, or perhaps simple differences in
total energy will provide the response index.

V. Functional and Clinical Significance of the Averaged Electroencephalic Response

The AER recorded from scalp electrodes probably reflects direct activity of the higher brain, speculatively the thalamic level and above. However, with certain electrode arrays and with appropriate amplification

and filtering, some components of response can be seen within the first 8 msec after stimulus onset, probably reflecting activity of lower brain structures. This section will deal only with the early components of the AER as previously described, the late components, and with the CNV. It is probable that conclusions drawn from the higher level activity can be generalized to all levels of the CNS.

The speculations presented are derived from my own clinical and laboratory experience, and are strongly influenced by the concepts of others, particularly those of Bishop (1959, 1961), Sokolov (1960), and Broadbent (1958). The generalities are based mainly on my interpretations of auditory responses and functions, but they probably apply to the visual and somatosensory modalities as well.

For the discussion, the tripartite division of the AER will be continued with full recognition of the tentativeness of the dividing lines.

The early components of the AER reflect activity of the primary projection systems, including the primary projection area in the cerebral cortex, for example, Heschl's gyrus in the case of hearing. The properties of the early components are compatible with large fiber pathways containing relatively few synapses and having a relatively rapid recovery time.

The properties of the late components argue that they emerge from a system with relatively small nerve fibers, many synapses, and slow recovery time. The brain stem reticular formation qualifies for this system. It is not clear whether the late components, so prominent at the vertex, reflect activity of the cortex triggered by reticular formation activity, or direct response of the reticular formation, or both.

The CNV reflects activity of much of the cortical mantle, particularly the frontal and central portions. The intrinsic properties of the structures contributing to the CNV are not easily surmised because this response depends so heavily on test conditions.

One can debate my speculations on the anatomical origin of the components of the AER, but at least the structural concepts can be described by a fairly well-understood vocabulary. It is more difficult, however, to find commonly agreed-upon words to formulate speculations about the reflected *functions* of the various components of the AER. I hope that the concepts which I offer will emerge despite the inadequacy of the descriptive vocabulary.

The early components of the AER reflect a gating mechanism or "perceptual filter" to prepare the cortex to react to the stimulus selectively or in an organized way. The late components reflect "sensation," defined crudely for present purposes as conscious awareness of the stimulus. The CNV reflects "cognition" by which I imply appropriate recognition of the stimulus. The CNV may also be an index of the conceptualization of the stimulus situation.

I do not suggest that the functions just described are the only ones attributable to the anatomical units which give rise to the various components of the AER. Nor do I imply that only the upper levels of the brain negotiate the functions. In all probability, all of these functions take place within equivalent systems at all levels of the brain, but increase in sophistication with each successively higher level of the brain.

In essence, I am speculating that we "hear" with our reticular formation, that a *prior* signal to the temporal lobe tells us how to deal in an organized way with what we are going to hear soon via the reticular formation, and that the organized message is elaborated by a large portion of the cortical mantle. This reverses the traditional view of the reticular formation as an alerting mechanism and the primary projection system as the conveyer of sensation.

On the assumption that my speculations are correct, how can the components of the AER be used to evaluate central auditory function? Any speculation must be tempered by the probability that the various components of the AER are not independent of each other. It is most unlikely that either the late components or the CNV would be normal if early activity were faulty. It is possible, however, to conceive of components in one sensory modality to be abnormal without concomitant abnormalities in the other modalities.

In a simple approach, one could speculate that aberrations in the early components to sound point to aphasia, dysphasia, or possibly just diminished discrimination of distorted speech. Abnormalities in the late components may represent faulty reticular formation function and some disturbance in auditory sensitivity provided, of course, that the abnormalities were not secondary to malfunction of the primary projection system. Aberrations in the CNV, when sound is used as the conditional or imperative stimulus, may reflect the inability of the frontal and central cortex to refine spoken messages into appropriate understanding or response.

It is doubtful that many patients with significant, generalized, organic impairment of the reticular formation are seen for audiologic evaluation. Such patients are probably comatose; and if not comatose, then unreactive to stimuli in all modalities. It is also doubtful that malfunctioning of the anterior half of the cerebral cortex could lead to aberrations of the CNV only in the auditory modality. Faulty interaction, however, between the early and late components of activity in any modality could prevent the emergence of the CNV in that modality, even with a normal-functioning cortex.

These last comments reflect my opinion that central auditory function cannot be adequately evaluated without looking at responses in several modalities. Figure 2 displays a grid that can be used for such a total evaluation. As mentioned earlier, the dividing lines on the latency grid may be shifted as more is learned about the properties of the AER, and perhaps additional time lines will have to be incorporated. Likewise, modalities such as olfaction may have to be added, or we may have to look at the submodalities of the somatosensory domain. Or, experience may show that only the auditory and visual modalities need to be explored.

Once the two-dimensional grid is established, it should be swept along the z-axis which could be a temporal, spatial, spectral, or intensive aspect of stimulation. Perhaps all of these z-dimensions should be explored unless experience proves that information derived from one will be sufficiently predictive of the others.

To illustrate how the three-dimensional grid might be used to evaluate central auditory function, let us assume that for any given stimulus condition all three major components in the auditory modality are abnormal, and that these components are normal in the two other modalities. One could assume that the CNS is normal but that the peripheral auditory mechanism is impaired, and this assumption could be verified by sweeping the two-dimensional grid along the intensive dimension primarily for a threshold determination. Or, suppose that the response abnormality was in the CNV and that it cut across all modalities. Regardless of how poorly this patient reacts behaviorally to auditory stimuli, he will most likely also react inappropriately to stimuli in all modalities. In this case, his problem may be quite pervasive, such as mental subnormality, rather than specifically a verbal disorder.

The scheme as presented, if valid, could be of enormous value in assessing the central auditory function of young children for whom be-

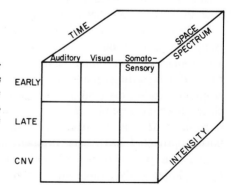

Fig. 2. Three-dimensional grid for evaluation of CNS function by means of AER. The z-axis can be any one parameter involving temporal, spatial, spectral, or intensive aspects of the stimulus.

havioral audiometry now yields either limited or no information. The results of the AER analysis could help to predict educational and communicative development, and to provide guidelines for habilitation. With sufficient refinement the three-dimensional grid could probably be employed to determine the site and nature of circumscribed or generalized lesions.

VI. Responses of the Peripheral Auditory Mechanism Recorded Extracranially

Responses from the cochlea and auditory nerve are not encompassed by an arbitrary narrow definition of "electroencephalic" as electrical activity originating in the brain. Nevertheless, discussion of cochlear microphonics and whole nerve action potentials in this chapter is justified by broadening the definition of "electroencephalic" to mean electrical activity originating in the head, by acknowledging the contribution of peripheral activity to the totality of evaluation of hearing by electrophysiologic audiometry, and by recognizing that instrumentation for eliciting and recording peripheral electrical activity is virtually the same as that used for eliciting and recording electrical activity from the brain.

I have seen no reports of the use of peripheral responses as a method of choice to derive clinical information not obtainable from behavioral audiometry or from other forms of electrophysiologic audiometry; nor are there any clear indications that peripheral responses from humans will yield information about the normal physiology of the auditory system which cannot be obtained from animal studies. Therefore, this topic will be treated in a general way only, but with the expectation that the results of current and future studies will eventually justify more extensive exposition of the subject.

Cochlear microphonics (CM) and whole-nerve action potentials (AP) can be detected in man by extracranial electrodes remote from the end organ. The summating potential (SP) may also be detectable but this phenomenon has not been studied in detail.

Early attempts at recording CM and AP were made on patients whose tympanic perforations allowed insertion of electrodes and placement on the promontory, or on or near the round and oval windows. The first successful recordings made outside of an intact middle ear were derived from electrodes inserted in the skin of the external auditory meatus close to the tympanic annulus. Subsequent attempts have been made to record CM and AP from electrodes outside of the ear canal. Although both approaches have been dubbed "nonsurgical," use of the ear canal electrode is presently feasible only under medical advisement. The procedure is basically simple and benign, and the proximity of the electrode to the end organ permits definition of the responses not yet possible with more remote electrodes. Instrumental refinements, however, will probably improve the quality and resolution of responses detected by electrodes outside of the ear canal, and may promote greater use of the simpler procedures in which the so-called surface electrodes are used.

Various reference electrodes have been paired with the electrode placed in the ear canal, or with the more remote electrode on the earlobe or mastoid. A reference electrode on the bridge of the nose is the most common choice. Both electrodes appear to contribute to the response and thus bipolar recording is advisable. An electrode on the opposite ear often serves as the ground lead.

The AP is smaller than the AER recorded from the vertex, has more high-frequency energy, and is shorter in duration. Consequently, response identification of AP requires: a larger number of response samples (generally 1024 or more) than is required for the AER; amplifier and filter characteristics that will allow recording of frequencies as high as 2000–4000 Hz; and signal averager analysis times of short duration (10–12 msec) to allow sufficient visual resolution of the brief phenomenon.

The N_1 spike of the AP has a latency of about 1.8 msec for clicks at 60 dB SL. Its presence can be detected close to or at the level of the voluntary threshold when an electrode is inserted deep in the ear canal (Salomon and Elberling, 1971), but ordinarily not below 40 dB SL when a surface electrode (for example, earlobe, mastoid) is used.

The properties of the AP from humans seem to be identical to those obtained from lower animals with electrodes within or in the immediate vicinity of the cochlea. The same seems to be true for the human cochlear microphonic, except that CM is even more difficult than AP to identify clearly at weak and moderate levels of stimulation (Moore, 1971).

When CM and AP are elicited by a given stimulus, they are highly reproducible within a given subject. In general, their amplitude and latency change quite predictably with changes in stimulus parameters. These properties appear to make CM and AP ideal response indices for objective audiometry.

One must be alert, however, to the clinical limitations of these responses. The AP reflects activity mainly of the basal turn of the cochlea (Deatherage et al., 1959) and cannot easily be used to measure thresholds for low-frequency sounds. By contrast, CM recorded from remote electrodes may originate from any portion of the cochlea, and not specifically from the area most sensitive to the frequency of the stimulating tone. Although CM may be related to the spectrum of the acoustic signal, it is less validly related than AP to the audibility of the signal.

TABLE I

SUMMARY OF PROPERTIES OF THE AVERAGED ELECTROENCEPHALIC RESPONSE (AER) TO SOUND, ACTUAL AND SPECULATIVE

Components of AER	Amplitude	Spectrum	Stability	Habituation	Source	Reflected function
Early (8–50 msec)	0.2–2 μV	20–150 Hz (?)	High intra- and intersubject stability. Affected very little by sleep and probably little by drugs.	Little habituation over long periods of time with interstimulus intervals in as short as 65 msec.	Primary auditory projection system (?)	Gating mechanism or "perceptual filter" (?)
Late (51–400 msec)	1–15 μV	2–7 Hz	Considerable intra- and intersubject variability. Greatly affected by sleep and drugs.	About 10 sec for full recovery. Amplitudes greatly reduced with interstimulus intervals less than 1 sec	Reticular formation (?)	Sensation (?)
Contingent negative variation (CNV) (greater than 400 msec) (?)	20–25 μV	DC (?)	Depends upon experimental conditions and set. Requires conditional and imperative stimuli.	Response persists unless imperative stimulus is withdrawn.	Frontal cortex (?)	Cognition (?)

432

It is possible to have CM without subsequent neural discharge (Peake et al., 1962). Thus, while absence of CM at a given stimulus level may possibly be construed as evidence of cochlear dysfunction, presence of CM at any level does not necessarily imply that the patient can hear the sound.

VII. Summary

Electroencephalic audiometry (EEA) initially used a stimulus-related change in the ongoing EEG as an index of response for threshold determination. More recently, the averaged electroencephalic response (AER) to consecutive presentations of a given sound has been used as the response index. The AER, which is seen most clearly from an electrode on the vertex of the skull referred to the earlobe or mastoid, is a composite phenomenon expediently described in three segments: early components, late components, and contingent negative variation (CNV). These segments are depicted schematically in Figure 1 and their properties are summarized in Table I. These segments are probably not functionally independent. If speculations about the functional significance of the components and their interactions are valid, a powerful clinical tool can be developed for evaluating peripheral and central auditory disorders using all components of the AER and the AER to stimuli in other modalities as well. It is probable that cochlear microphonics and whole-nerve action potentials as detected by extracranial electrodes will also be used in this comprehensive scheme for audiometry.

As ordinarily performed, EEA is not an objective procedure for threshold audiometry even though an objective response is used. EEA can be made more objective and valid by preprogramming stimulus conditions, randomization of stimulus conditions, use of silent controls, multiple presentations of a given stimulus condition, predetermination of threshold criteria, predetermination of criteria for response identification, and blind posttest analysis of tracings.

ACKNOWLEDGMENT

Preparation of this chapter was supported in part by Public Health Service Training Grant No. NS05499 and by Public Health Research Grants Nos. NS07417, NS09278, and NS09355 from the National Institute of Neurological Diseases and Stroke. Extreme gratitude is expressed to Leslie B. Rodman for her extensive help in the preparation of this chapter.

References

Allison, T., Goff, W. R., Abrahamian, M. A., and Rosner, B. S. (1963). The effects of barbiturate anesthesia upon human somatosensory evoked responses. *Electroencephalogr. Clin. Neurophysiol. Suppl.* **24**, 68–75.
Bishop, G. H. (1959). The relation between nerve fiber size and sensory modality:

Phylogenetic implications of the afferent innervation of the cortex. *J. Nerv. Ment. Dis.* **128**, 89–114.

Bishop, G. H. (1961). The organization of the cortex with respect to its afferent supply. *Ann. N.Y. Acad. Sci.* **94**, 559–569.

Broadbent, D. E. (1958). "Perception and Communication." Pergamon, Oxford.

Celesia, G. G., and Puletti, F. (1969). Auditory cortical areas of man. *Neurology,* **19**, 211–220.

Chalke, F. C. R., and Ertl, J. (1965). Evoked potentials and intelligence. *Life Sci.* **4**, 1319–1322.

Deatherage, B. H., Eldredge, D. H., and Davis, H. (1959). Latency of action potentials in the cochlea of the guinea pig. *J. Acoust. Soc. Amer.,* **31**, 479–486.

Derbyshire, A. J., and Farley, J. C. (1959). Sampling auditory responses at the cortical level. *Ann. Otol. Rhinol. Laryngol.* **68**, 675–697.

Donald, M. W. Jr., and Goff, W. R. (1971). Attention-related increases in cortical responsivity disassociated from the contingent negative variation. *Science,* **172**, 1163–1166.

Engel, R. (1971). Early waves of the electroencephalic auditory response in neonates. *Neuropaediatrie,* **3**, 147–154.

Evans, T. R., and Deatherage, B. H. (1969). The effect of frequency on the auditory evoked response. *Psychonomic Sci.,* **15**, 95–96.

Halliday, A. M., and Mason, A. A. (1964). The effect of hypnotic anaesthesia on cortical responses. *J. Neurol. Neurosurg. Psychiat.* **27**, 300–312.

Hillyard, S. A., and Galambos, R. (1967). Effects of stimulus and response contingencies on a surface negative slow potential shift in man. *Electroencephalogr. Clin. Neurophysiol.* **22**, 297–304.

Horwitz, S. F., Larson, S. F., and Sances, A. Jr. (1966). Evoked potentials as an adjunct to the auditory evaluation of patients. *Proc. Symp. Biomed. Eng.,* **1**, 49–52.

Jewett, D. L., Romano, M. N., and Williston, J. S. (1970). Human auditory evoked potentials: Possible brain stem components detected on the scalp. *Science,* **167**, 1517–1518.

Keidel, W. D., and Spreng, M. (1965). Neurophysiological evidence for the Stevens power function in man. *J. Acoust. Soc. Amer.* **38**, 191–195.

Kupperman, G. L. (1970). Effects of three stimulus parameters on the early components of the averaged electroencephalic response. Doctoral Dissertation, Univ. of Wisconsin, Madison.

Low, M. D. (1969). Discussion. *In* "Average Evoked Potentials: Methods, Results, and Evaluations," pp. 163–171. National Aeronautics and Space Administration, Washington, D.C.

Madell, J. R. (1969). Relation between loudness and the amplitude of the averaged electroencephalic response. Doctoral Dissertation, Univ. of Wisconsin, Madison.

McCandless, G. A., and Rose, D. E. (1970). Evoked cortical responses to stimulus change. *J. Speech and Hearing Res.* **13**, 624–634.

Mendel, M. I. (1970). Early components of the averaged electroencephalic response during sleep. Doctoral Dissertation, Univ. of Wisconsin, Madison.

Mendel, M. I., and Goldstein, R. (1969a). The effect of test conditions on the early components of the averaged electroencephalic response. *J. Speech and Hearing Res.* **12**, 344–350.

Mendel, M. I., and Goldstein, R. (1969b). Stability of the early components of the averaged electroencephalic response. *J. Speech and Hearing Res.* **12**, 351–361.

Mendel, M. I., and Goldstein, R. (1971). Effect of sleep on the early components of the averaged electroencephalic response. *Arch. Klin. Exp. Ohren-, Nassen- U. Kehlk. Heilk.* **198,** 110–115.

Moore, E. J. (1971). Human cochlear microphonics and auditory nerve action potentials from surface electrodes. Doctoral Dissertation, Univ. of Wisconsin, Madison.

Onishi, S., and Davis, H. (1968). Effects of duration and rise time of tone bursts on evoked V potentials. *J. Acoust. Soc. Amer.* **44,** 582–591.

Peake, W. T., Goldstein, M. H. Jr, and Kiang, N. Y-S. (1962). Responses of the auditory nerve to repetitive acoustic stimuli. *J. Acous. Soc. Amer.* **34,** 562–570.

Rosenfeld, J. P., Rudell, A. P., and Fox, S. S. (1969). Operant control of neural events in humans. *Science,* **165,** 821–823.

Rothman, H. H. (1970). Effects of high frequencies and intersubject variability on the auditory-evoked cortical response. *J. Acoust. Soc. Amer.* **47,** 569–573.

Salomon, G., and Elberling, C. (1971). Cochlear nerve potentials recorded from the ear canal in man. *Acta Oto-Laryngol.* **71,** 319–324.

Smith, L. L. (1971). Influence of background noise on the early components of the averaged electroencephalic response to clicks. Master's Thesis, Univ. of Wisconsin, Madison.

Sokolov, E. N. (1960). Neuronal models and the orienting reflex. *In* "Central Nervous Systems Behavior Trans. Conf." 3, 187–278. Josiah Macy, Jr. Foundation, New York.

Vaughan, H. G., and Ritter, W. (1970). The sources of auditory evoked responses recorded from the human scalp. *Electroencephalogr. Clin. Neurophysiol.* **28,** 360–367.

Chapter 12

The Theory of Signal Detectability and the Measurement of Hearing

FRANK R. CLARKE

Stanford Research Institute

ROBERT C. BILGER

University of Pittsburgh

I. Introduction

The theory of signal detectability (TSD) describes the performance of an ideal observer in the detection of signals in noise. As a mathematical ideal it does not attempt to describe the human observer per se, but rather it describes the best performance theoretically possible for the detection of specified signals in specified noise backgrounds. Thus, it defines the inherent detectability of signals in noise and specifies how detectability varies as a function of signal parameters and decision goals.

The theory of signal detectability was introduced into psychophysics in the mid 1950s (Birdsall, 1955; Tanner, 1955; Tanner and Swets, 1954). Since that time is has provided a powerful tool for the study of human performance in the detection and recognition of acoustic signals and in the development of descriptive models of the auditory system. As a broad and systematic approach to the description of detection systems, it has contributed greatly to the understanding of the human detection process. As one index of its importance, Egan (1967) compiled a bibliography of several hundred papers in the field of psychophysics that dealt with or were influenced by the theory.

The theory of signal detectability can no longer be considered a new and somewhat controversial approach in psychophysics. It may remain a specialized study for many years, but several of its basic concepts and empirical findings have proved valuable to the nonspecialist. This chapter describes some aspects of the theory which are particularly important in the measurement of hearing. It does not provide a detailed development of the theory. Fortunately, authoritative secondary texts are now available. For another, more specific introduction to the subject, see Egan and Clarke (1966). For a detailed but elementary mathematical treatment of ideal performance in representative signal detection tasks, see the first edition of this chapter (Clarke and Bilger, 1963). Swets' (1964) *Contemporary Readings* incoprorates 33 of the germinal papers covering a broad range of topics in signal detection by human observers. Finally, Green and Swets (1966) in their excellent text, *Signal Detection Theory and Psychophysics*, provide a detailed and extensive introduction to the subject.

II. Some Comments on the Measurement of Hearing

In any discussion of the measurement of hearing, an immediate problem is the lack of a single, widely accepted definition of "hearing" which is at once broad and precise. Although for most purposes, a general and rather vague definition may serve, in a particular experiment, a very narrow but precise operational definition of "hearing" may be required. The class of phenomena typically included under this heading consists of those functional relationships between the auditory input and the inferred properties of the hearing mechanism which remain essentially invariant over the class of methods for measuring these relationships.

Any attempt to take measurements relevant to such a loosely defined class of phenomena presents certain inherent difficulties. For example, suppose the absolute threshold of hearing at a given frequency is measured by numerous methods only to yield results which vary over a range of 10 dB. Should it then be concluded that all methods measure the same thing ("hearing"), and are relatively "more or less" invariant? Or, should it be assumed that such a range of results is *not* more-or-less invariant and that some measures were contaminated by other factors? The decision is difficult, but if one method of measurement proves easily influenced by variables external to the loosely defined realm of hearing, whereas a second method is not so influenced, then it may be concluded that other things being equal, the second method yielded a more precise measure of hearing than the first. The choice between two methods differing in precision, in a given situation will depend upon external considerations. In some instances, an imprecise measurement may yield sufficiently accurate data for the task at hand, and, for purposes of convenience, such a method may be employed deliberately. The present authors argue, however, that in basic research into the human organism's processing of and response to auditory stimuli, the accuracy bounds of conventional measurement techniques are usually inadequate. The fact that measures of absolute threshold are often influenced by nonauditory processes may encourage misleading inferences regarding the functioning of the auditory mechanism.

It is emphasized here that the procedures of the experimental audiologist merely allow specification of a relation between an acoustic input to the auditory system and an output, usually behavioral, from a motor subsystem of the organism. On the basis of this relationship, inferences relevant to the auditory system, or to any other subsystem in the chain from input to output may be made. The appropriateness of such inferences depends not only upon the particular manner in which the input–output relation is determined, but also upon what performance measure is derived from the input–output function.

Because of the human organism's complexity, it is extremely difficult to make valid inferences from simple input–output functions. Presumably, such inferences relate accurately to the auditory system. However, aside from the end organ itself, there are higher centers which include what can be termed a "decision-making" system as well as the motor subsystems involved in responding to the input. Most traditional psychophysical measures do not provide the necessary data to distinguish between variables which affect the auditory system per se and those which may conveniently be thought of as affecting biases in the decision-making system. Relative to this point, the listener's criterion for deciding "I heard something" is heavily dependent both upon his past experience and upon the instructions used to bring the response to be observed under control. For example, an observer may report detection of a signal only if he judges it to have a definite tonal quality; or, on the other hand, he may report that he heard a tone when he detected "something different from nothing." Pollack (1948) has shown that, depending on frequency, instructions in this regard produce differences of 2.5–6.5 dB in the determination of absolute threshold. Yet, even under some particular set of instructions, where does the observer set his criterion for "a tonal quality" or "something different from nothing"? How dependent upon the observer's criterion are these measures of threshold?

Many of the procedures for obtaining absolute thresholds do not permit a description of the sensitivity of the auditory system in terms of parameters uncontaminated by criterial variables. Consider, for example, a procedure with a number of discrete observation intervals in each of which a tone is presented. If the observer were asked when he heard the tone, it could be assumed that, in most cases, he would make every effort to follow the instructions conscientiously. In such a procedure there is no question of the actual presence of a signal input and often the observer knows that the signal is always there. However, if he is a cooperative observer he must make a decision as to whether or not he "heard" the tone. Now, hearing is as poorly defined for the observer as it is for most students of the subject. In the enthusiasm to use operational definitions, the burden of definition is placed on the observer, who must employ some criterion to determine whether he does or does not "hear" something. It is only in a vague way, through the observer's verbal report of his criterion (or the experimenter's assumption that the observer followed instructions), that the experimenter can know the nature of this criterion. With such an experimental procedure there is no known way of separating criterial variables from parameters describing the sensory mechanism.

Audiologists and psychoacousticians have long been aware that criterial variables and procedural variations have important effects upon their data. By careful clinical procedure and experimental design they attempt to minimize the degree to which these variables affect their inferences regarding the auditory mechanism. However, the complicated interrelations among these variables and those being studied are often improperly evaluated because there is no comprehensive theory of hearing which ensures that all factors are appropriately weighted.

To defend against wide variations in criteria, the experimenter may introduce "catch trials" in which no signal is present. If the observer reports that he "heard" a signal when no signal was present, the experimenter may simply inform the observer of this fact and ask him to be more careful in responding. Alternatively, he may introduce a sufficient number of catch trials to estimate the observer's probability of guessing. Then, without having to ask the observer to change his behavior, the experimenter would apply a correction for guessing to the observer's responses on those trials which did, in fact, contain a signal. In either case, the experimenter will believe that he has taken account of criterial variables and made a fairly accurate measure of the absolute threshold. We shall, toward the end of this chapter, present some illustrative data which suggest that the first method for controlling criteria may actually increase the criterial involvement in the measure, while the second method has but a slight corrective property.

Thus far, we have argued that when a signal is always present in an observation interval, the burden of defining hearing falls upon the observer. We have also argued that with this procedure we do not know of any way of separating variables affecting the observer's criterion from those describing his sensory processes. Where there are a large number of trials with no signal presented, traditional methods for controlling criterial variables are, at best, inadequate. However, in this latter case, where we obtain an external correlate for the decision "I did not hear anything," it is possible to obtain a measure of performance relatively independent of the observer's criterion for stating that he heard a signal. This is one of the important contributions of the theory of signal detectability and will be discussed fully in the subsequent pages.

The word threshold has been used several times in this discussion. Audiologists are aware that this word has two distinct meanings. In one case it is a performance measure with an operational definition. For example, threshold may be defined as that signal strength necessary to elicit the response "I heard the signal" on 50% of the trials in which the observer was presented with the signal. (Of course, a complete operational definition would require an exact specification of the experimental procedures utilized in obtaining this response.) On the other hand, the word threshold sometimes refers to an inferred property of the human auditory system. It has been suggested (Stevens, 1951) that at any moment in time there exists a critical value of signal intensity such that if the input is below this intensity, the auditory system does not respond to the signal; whereas, if the input is above this intensity, the auditory system does show a response. This latter notion is easily refuted by experimental data and few are willing to maintain strongly that such a simple sensory threshold actually exists. Due to a lack of adequate theory, the concept of a sensory threshold persists, and, in fact, the methods for controlling the "guessing behavior" of an observer stem from this concept. In this chapter we hope to provide a more adequate framework for viewing human performance in auditory detection and recognition tasks. We also wish to indicate the inadequacies of the threshold as a performance measure.

III. Some Comments about the Theory of Signal Detectability

The main virtue of the theory of signal detectability is the simplicity with which it handles a wide variety of factors that affect the detection and recognition of signals. It deals simultaneously with information that the observer may have before the actual presentation of the signal, with the informational content of the signal, with the properties of the sensory mechanism under investigation and with some motivational variables that affect the responses of the observer. Consequently it often provides us with a means of separating the parameters of the system under study from those that might describe other aspects of the total system. Furthermore, it is able, in one comprehensive theory, to incorporate both sets of parameters as well as some of their interrelations.

Despite the fact that this approach provides a simple framework for dealing with a broad class of variables, one of the major complaints often heard is that the theory is too complicated; it is difficult to learn. Let us stop at this point and discuss briefly some of the problems that have led to this difficulty.

Perhaps one of the major sources of difficulty has been the fact that the theory of signal detectability did not evolve from earlier work in psychophysics. It is a mathematical theory developed without reference to data from any substantive investigation in psychoacoustics or audiology. The initial emphasis was on the inherent detectability of signals, not upon the detection of signals by any man-made device or human observer. This approach has its roots in decision theory and in the mathematics dealing with the analysis of waveforms. Classical work in psychophysics has not utilized this mathematical background, and different ways of viewing similar problems have often resulted in difficulties in communication between the two groups of workers.

The major task which the developers of the theory of signal detectability set for themselves was to determine the ideal manner in which a complex input space (which might consist of voltage waveforms arising from a signal in a background of noise or of noise alone) might be mapped into a simple output space consisting of the decision "yes, there was a signal present" and "no, there was not a signal present." They developed the concept of the ideal observer. An ideal observer (a mathematical concept) is one that, for some particular set of decision alternatives, utilizes all of the relevant information in the input to arrive at a best choice among the alternatives as dictated by a consideration of external criterial variables.

One source of confusion to the student arises from the fact that the theory of signal detectability has been utilized in two distinct ways in the development of a model of human signal detection and recognition. The concept of the ideal observer served initially as an approximation of a descriptive model of human performance. Second, this theory has provided the mathematical tools by which the original concept of the ideal observer has been modified to arrive at a more adequate descriptive model of human performance. We shall comment briefly on each of these uses of the theory.

Tanner and his associates recognized that the ideal observer was essentially a behavioristic model. The theory specified changes in the performance of an ideal observer as a function of signal strength, noise level, criterial variables, *a priori* information, knowledge concerning the precise waveforms of the signals, and many other factors. In some ways the behavior of the ideal observer paralleled that of the human observer as determined experimentally. Consequently, at the very outset the concept of the ideal observer provided a descriptive model of human performance. It was recognized to be an inadequate descriptive model in that, quantitatively, the ideal observer always did better than the human observer and in many cases curve shapes showing the performance of the ideal observer as a function of some variable were quite different than those obtained with human observers. But, of the inadequate models of human performance available, this one had particular advantages: first, it was based on carefully stated assumptions and provided a complete statement of the conditions which must be met if ideal performance were to be attained; and, secondly, the theory of signal detectability provided the mathematically tools necessary for analyzing experimental data to determine the specific properties of the ideal observer that were not shared by the human observer.

The precise manner in which the theory of signal detectability is used as a tool in developing a more adequate model of human performance is too complex to describe at this point. However, it takes the following form. Experiments are conducted with human observers in situations where the performance of an ideal observer is known. The specific manner in which the human performance is inferior to that of the ideal observer is determined. Then, an attempt is made to identify those information-bearing aspects of the signal which are lost in the transmission of the signal through the human auditory mechanism or in the decision process itself. For purposes of analysis we can introduce various types of uncertainty in the signal-generating equipment, determine the performance of an ideal observer on this degraded signal, and compare this performance to that of the human. If this very same signal degradation does not affect the performance of the human observer, we may then conclude that the human observer does not utilize these particular information-bearing aspects of the signal. This then leads directly to a mathematical description of the uncertainty introduced by the human observer and serves as a more adequate mathematical model of human performance in signal detection.

This dual use of the theory of signal detectability, as a descriptive model and as a mathematical tool, understandably often leads to confusion on the part of the reader. Unless one is well aware of the problem (and sometimes even then) it is difficult to know when the detectability theorist is talking about ideal observers and when he is talking about a descriptive model of human performance.

A remaining source of difficulty is that many workers in psychoacoustics and audiology have little formal training in mathematics. A detailed understanding of many papers applying the theory of signal detectability requires a fairly sophisticated background in mathematics but a general understanding of the theory requires only some elementary probability theory, some elementary statistics, and some elementary signal analysis. Those aspects of the theory that might currently affect techniques of measurement in audiology require little in the way of mathematics and this chapter will be written without recourse to mathematical derivations.

IV. The Theory of Signal Detectability

The theory of signal detectability[1] views signal detection as a problem in the testing of statistical hypotheses. If, because of the noise in a system, any particular observed waveform may arise either from signal plus noise or from noise alone, then the observer must distinguish between alternative hypotheses on the basis of statistical information. In such a situation, the total set of all possible inputs must be divided into two classes: (1) those inputs which the observer should decide arose from signal plus noise; (2) those which the observer should decide arose from noise alone. In other words, a region in some decision space must be defined such that an observation falling in this region will result in the acceptance of one of the two hypotheses under test, while an obser-

---

[1] The theory of signal detectability had at least four independent developments. This section is based on the work of Peterson *et al.* (1954). It was their work which provided the stimulus for the application of this theory to psychophysics.

vation falling in the complement of this region will result in acceptance of the alternative hypothesis. Selection of the particular boundary between these two regions is always dependent upon external considerations. For example, the boundary chosen to maximize the probability of a correct decision is usually quite different from that chosen to limit the occurrence of the response "signal" when no signal is present.

A. Decision Theory in TSD

Consider a sample drawn from one of two possible distributions. On the basis of this sample, which is here termed an observation, the observer must identify the distribution from which the sample was drawn. For notational convenience—though with no intention of restricting the generality of the problem—suppose that one of the distributions is associated with noise alone and the other with signal plus noise. In the present notation, upper- and lowercase letters refer to observer's responses and physical events respectively. There are four possible outcomes to the experiment. (1) The observation is drawn from the signal-plus-noise distribution and the observer accepts the hypothesis signal plus noise. This outcome will occur with some probability, here denoted $P(s \cdot S)$. (2) The observation is drawn from the signal-plus-noise distribution and the observer accepts the hypothesis noise alone. Here the associated probability is noted by $P(s \cdot N)$. (3) With probability $P(n \cdot S)$, the observation will be drawn from the noise alone distribution and the observer will accept the hypothesis signal plus noise. (4) With probability $P(n \cdot N)$, the observation will be drawn from the noise-alone distribution and the observer will accept this hypothesis. As these are the only possible outcomes of the experiment,[2] then:

$$P(s \cdot S) + P(s \cdot N) + P(n \cdot S) + P(n \cdot N) = 1.0. \qquad (1)$$

Conditional probabilities are of particular interest; clearly, too, the possible outcomes of the experiment may also be defined by the following three equations:

$$P(s) + P(n) = 1.0 \qquad (2)$$

$$P(S|s) + P(N|s) = 1.0 \qquad (3)$$

$$P(S|n) + P(N|n) = 1.0. \qquad (4)$$

---

[2] It is possible to derive results from the situation in which the observer is allowed to defer his decision pending one or more repeated observations. In such cases the decision axis can be shown to be likelihood ratio, but the determination of criterial boundaries is relatively difficult. In this chapter we shall only treat situations in which the observer must make a decision "signal present" or "no signal present" following each observation interval.

The observer's behavior may be defined in terms of the probabilities in Eqs. (3) and (4), for the probabilities in Eq. (2) are not under his control. Furthermore, as both Eqs. (3) and (4) sum to one, the behavior of the observer may be specified with only two probabilities, $P(S|s)$ and $P(S|n)$, referred to as the hit rate and the false-alarm rate, respectively.

In judging the presence or absence of a signal during some observation interval, a mathematically ideal observer must consider two distinct factors: (1) the observed waveform itself; and (2) the criterion, or decision function which is to be maximized in determining the signal's presence or absence. A number of possible criteria might be used in reaching a decision. For example, it may be desirable (1) to maximize the probability of a correct decision (that is, to minimize error), (2) to maximize the expected value associated with the decision, (3) to minimize the probability of ruin, (4) to maximize information transmitted, or (5) to maximize the hit rate while maintaining some fixed false-alarm rate. Mathematically all of the above criteria can be characterized by their positive weighting of "hits" and negative weighting of "false alarms." Thus, all possible observations are divided into two classes, "signal" and "noise," in such a way that

$$P(S|s) - \omega P(S|n) = \text{a maximum},\qquad(5)$$

where ω is the absolute value of the ratio of the weight given a false alarm to the weight given a hit. Equation (5) is satisfied if the response is S on all observations, x, for which $P(x|s) - \omega P(x|n) \geq 0$, and N on all observations for which $P(x|s) - \omega P(x|n) < 0$. Thus, the ideal observer accepts the hypothesis signal plus noise on those observations for which $P(x|s)/P(x|n) \geq \omega$. This ratio is called the likelihood ratio, $l(x)$, and may be calculated both for discrete probabilities as above and for continuous probability density functions $f(x|s)$ and $f(x|n)$. In its simplest and most general form, the decision rule for this ideal observer is:

Accept the hypothesis signal plus noise when $l(x) \geq \omega$.   (6)

Note that this says nothing about the form of the input waveform. Knowledge of signal and noise parameters is necessary to compute likelihood ratio for any given observation, but it is the likelihood ratio as such that is used in the decision. As this is the only information in the observation, per se, which is relevant to a decision regardless of the dimensionality of the actual signals to be observed, the decision process reduces to a number on a single-dimension axis. If the observed likelihood ratio is greater (less) than some critical value, then the ideal observer must accept the hypothesis that signal plus noise (noise alone) was present. Although likelihood ratio is the basic decision variable, any monotonic transformation of likelihood ratio will serve equally well. If the decision rule states that a particular decision should be made when $l(x) \geq \omega$, then the same decision will be made if a particular monotonic transformation of $l(x)$ is required to be greater than the same monotonic transformation of ω.

Let us examine this value of likelihood ratio, ω, in greater detail and for some simple cases determine the manner in which this "decision threshold" is computed. The specific value of ω selected depends upon the particular criterion of decision. For example, if the aim is to maximize the proportion of correct responses, then

$$P(C) = P(s \cdot S) + P(n \cdot N) = \text{a maximum.} \tag{7}$$

By simple manipulation, Eq. (7) may be rewritten in the form of Eq. (5) to yield

$$P(S|s) - \frac{P(n)}{P(s)} P(S|n) = \text{a maximum.} \tag{8}$$

Thus, to maximize correct identifications (minimize error), the criterion cutoff, ω, is equal to the ratio of *a priori* probabilities, $P(n)/P(s)$.

As a further example, consider the case in which the four possible outcomes mentioned above have different values and costs associated with them. Then, it is readily demonstrable that the criterion cutoff (decision threshold) is

$$\omega = \frac{P(n)(V_{n \cdot N} + K_{n \cdot s})}{P(s)(V_{s \cdot s} + K_{s \cdot N})} \tag{9}$$

where $P(n)$ and $P(s)$ are the *a priori* probabilities of noise alone and signal plus noise, $V_{n \cdot N}$ is the value associated with a correct identification of noise alone, $K_{n \cdot s}$ is the cost associated with identifying noise alone as signal plus noise, and $V_{s \cdot s}$ and $K_{s \cdot N}$ are similarly defined.

These examples should illustrate a most important fact. A mathematically ideal observer when making a decision must consider *a priori* probabilities and any other factors which may arise from the decision function to be maximized as well as the observation itself.

There are other bases for evaluating performance, but insofar as they evaluate correct responses as being good in some sense, and incorrect responses as bad in some sense, they may all be reduced to the form of Eq. (5). However, the examples discussed above are those which have greatest application in psychoacoustics.

It may be noted that any dichotomous or discrete response required of the observer discards information which is available to him. Only by a statement of likelihood ratio, or equivalently by a statement of a posteriori probability given that the a priori probabilities are known, does the observer convey the full extent of information available to him.

B. The Detectability of a Signal Known Exactly

The following experimental paradigm illustrates several important aspects of the theory of signal detectability. An observation interval, O to T, is defined during which a voltage waveform, $x(t)$, is presented. With some given probability, $P(s)$, $x(t) = s(t) + n(t)$, where $s(t)$ is the signal to be detected and $n(t)$ is noise. With probability $P(n) = 1 - P(s)$, $x(t) = n(t)$. The waveform of the signal is precisely specified and known by the observer. On the basis of the observation, $x(t)$, the observer must state whether or not a signal was present in the interval, that is, whether $x(t)$ arose from noise alone or from signal plus noise.

In most problems of interest, any particular waveform, $x(t)$, could have arisen either from the event signal-plus-noise or from noise alone. Thus the two hypotheses cannot be distinguished with certainty. However, in most instances the probabilities that the waveform consisted of $s(t) + n(t)$ or $n(t)$ alone will be different. Thus, the waveform itself provides information relevant to the two hypotheses. As noted above, for a large class of criteria an ideal observer should base his decision on likelihood ratio. No process will result in better performance. Thus, the specification of an ideal observer's detection performance is equivalent to the specification of the inherent detectability of the signal in the noise.

Much of the theory of signal detectability deals with the specification of the inherent detectability of various types of signals in various types of noise. These derivations are not detailed in this chapter. However, some results are instructive. Consider the detection of a signal known exactly in a background of white Gaussian noise. "A signal known exactly" here signifies that the ideal observer knows the precise waveform of the signal which may or may not be added to the noise on any particular trial. He must merely state whether an observed waveform contained this signal added to noise or noise alone. Likelihood ratio can be calculated in this case. Because the sample of noise changes from trial to trial, the observed waveform will likewise vary. Thus, too, likelihood ratio will vary from trial to trial and will in fact be a random variable. In the case of a signal known exactly in white Gaussian noise, it is most convenient to work with a particular monotonic transformation of likelihood ratio as a decision variable. With an ap-

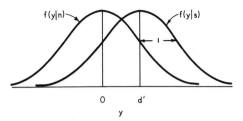

Fig. 1. The distributions of a transformation of likelihood ratio conditional upon noise alone and upon a signal specified exactly in noise. For convenience we have labeled the decision axis y, where y is a monotonic transformation of likelihood ratio:

$$y = \frac{\log l(x) + E/N_0}{\sqrt{2E/N_0}}.$$

Given noise alone, y is distributed normally with a mean of zero and unit variance, $N(0,1)$. Given signal plus noise, y is $N(d',1)$.

propriate choice of the transformation, it can be shown that for those events consisting of noise alone, y (the decision variable) is a normally distributed random variable with mean zero and unity standard deviation. For those events consisting of signal plus noise, y is a normally distributed random variable with mean d' and unity variance. These distributions are shown in Figure 1. The value d' depends only upon the energy of the signal and the noise power per unit bandwidth: $d' = (2E/N_0)^{1/2}$. The detailed structure of the signal is important only insofar as it determines the signal's energy and the actual calculation of likelihood ratio. Thus far, only the performance of the ideal observer has been considered. In this context d' serves as a measure of the inherent detectability of a signal specified exactly and presented in a background of white Gaussian noise. In other contexts, and in much of the literature, d' is used as an index of human performance and reflects the apparent separation between the two hypotheses "signal plus noise" and "noise alone" as inferred from listener performance in a detection task. Some performance measures are later defined in Section V,A.

C. The Receiver-Operating Characteristic

Thus far, the index of detectability has been determined for the ideal observer. However, his performance in this detection task is not yet completely specified. To do so, not only the detectability of the signal but also the criterion of the observer must be considered.

In Section IV,A it was shown that two probabilities were necessary to specify the behavior of the ideal observer, $P(S|s)$ (a hit) and $P(S|n)$

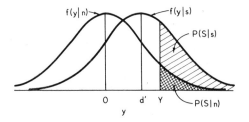

FIG. 2. The hit rate, $P(S|s)$, and the false-alarm rate, $P(S|n)$, for some particular value of d' and of the decision threshold Y.

(a false alarm). These two values are affected by both the detectability of the signal and the criterion of the observer.

To illustrate the relation between these variables and d', reference is made to the distributions in Figure 1. For some value Y (that is, some particular transformed value of ω) on the decision axis y, the probability of a hit is given by the equation $P(S|s) = P(y > Y|s)$, and the probability of a false alarm by $P(S|n) = P(y > Y|n)$ (see Figure 2).

With a constant d' both $P(S|n)$ and $P(S|s)$ may vary from zero to unity, depending upon the criterion of the observer. It is clear from Figure 2 that as the cutoff value Y varies from $+\infty$ to $-\infty$, both $P(S|n)$ and $P(S|s)$ will increase monotonically, though at different rates, from 0 to 1. The relation between these two variables for various values of d' is shown in Figure 3. These curves are called ROC-curves or receiver-operating characteristics.

For the ideal observer, as d' changes, there is a shift from one curve to the other. For a fixed value of d', performance may fall anywhere on a particular ROC-curve. The particular point will depend upon *a priori* probabilities and the decision function to be maximized. With values of these variables which require a very strict criterion, the ideal observer will operate toward the lower left of Figure 3. As conditions

FIG. 3. A family of ROC-curves showing the relation between the hit rate and the false-alarm rate for various values of d'.

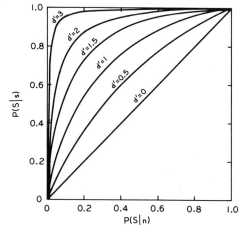

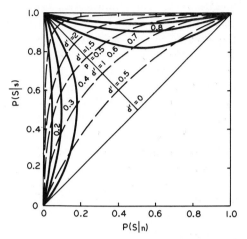

FIG. 4. Constant-criterion contours for various *a priori* probabilities.

require increasingly lax criteria, the point describing the ideal observer's performance will move along one of these curves toward the upper right of the figure. Assuming that the observer is attemtping to maximize the proportion of correct responses, Figure 4 shows constant-criterion cutoffs for various *a priori* probabilities. Thus, for example, for an ideal observer operating on a signal with a d' equal to 1 and an *a priori* probability equal to 0.2, his false-alarm rate and hit rate will be described by the point of intersection of that receiver-operating characteristic for d equal to 1 and the constant-criterion contour labeled 0.2.

One final point regarding ROC-curves: the ROC-curves shown in Figure 3 were derived for a signal specified exactly and presented in a background of white Gaussian noise. They represent the performance of an

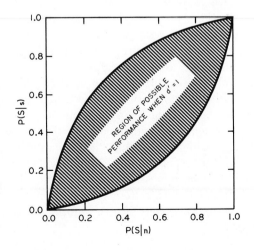

FIG. 5. The region of possible performance when $2E/N_o = 1$.

ideal observer in response to a signal with energy E and a noise power per unit bandwidth of N_0. In plotting these curves it was assumed that the ideal observer was attempting to respond correctly. If, for some reason, values and costs were such that it was more profitable to always be, or attempt to be, wrong, then the performance of an observer who could utilize all of the information content in the signal and noise waveforms would fall on a ROC-curve that is the mirror image (around the diagonal) of the one in Figure 3. This is illustrated in Figure 5 for $d' = 1$. Consequently, the region between these two curves defines the region of possible performances of any nonideal observer. That is, any nonideal observer who fails to utilize all the information in the waveform, or who utilizes some improper decision process, must generate a performance point between these two curves.

D. Other Cases

The detection of a signal known exactly in a background of white Gaussian noise was dealt with above. A single observation interval occurred in which a representative of one of the two hypotheses under test was presented and the observer's task was to state which of the two events occurred.

Of course, many other cases have been studied. These include cases in which the properties of the signal or noise, or the experimental paradigm were different. Examples of the former include the detection of a signal specified except for phase, the detection of a sample of white Gaussian noise, amplitude discrimination for signals known exactly, and the detection of signals in noise other than white Gaussian. Examples of the latter include two-alternative forced-choice experiments (and, more generally, n-alternative forced-choice experiments) and experiments in which the observer must specify whether two stimuli are representatives of the same or different events. Not all cases result in the normal distributions of Figure 1, nor the ROC-curves of Figure 3. Commonly encountered distributions include chi-square and Rayleigh-Rice.

In all instances the result is well worth obtaining. In studying the human organism's processing of auditory information, the informational content at the input to the organism is one of the most important parameters to be considered. If the experimental paradigm is such that this parameter cannot be specified, it would suggest that, in the absence of conflicting design requirements, the experimental procedure should be changed. If this is not done, it will be impossible to distinguish between changes in performance variables resulting from properties of the organism and changes attributable to variations in the informational content of the input to the organism.

V. Some Substantive Results with Human Observers

The bulk of the chapter thus far has dealt with the normative model of the ideal observer. Some of the ways in which this development might be applicable to the study of human observers have been suggested. In this section, some illustrative examples of the application of the theory of signal detectability to the study of the human detection process are presented.

A. Performance Measures

First, three performance measures are defined.

In the detection of a signal specified exactly, $d' = (2E/N_0)^{1/2}$ refers to the separation between the two conditional distributions of a transformation of likelihood ratio for the ideal observer. In this case, early studies quickly demonstrated that the human observer behaved as though he were testing two statistical hypotheses, both of which were distributed normally with approximately equal variances. The separation between these inferred distributions acts as a performance measure for the human observer. The quantity d' used for this measure is given a more general definition and now refers to the value of $(2E/N_0)^{1/2}$ required by the ideal observer to match the performance of the human observer. The value of d' may be calculated by simply looking at the observer's hit and false-alarm rates and determining the separation between two normal distributions of unit variance required to produce these response rates for an ideal observer (as in Figure 2).

We are interested in the separation of the two hypotheses, as well as the criterion of the observer. As a performance measure value, d' indicates which ROC-curve the observer is operating on, but we need an additional measurement specifying the exact location of the data point on this curve. Here we shall use the observer's false-alarm rate, $P(S|n)$ as a measure of criterion although it lacks certain desirable properties.

Since the performance measure d' changes from one situation to another for the ideal observer and the human observer, it is convenient to refer the performance of the human observer to the performance which would have been realized by the ideal observer. Consequently, we introduce an additional performance measure, η, the efficiency of the observer (Tanner and Birdsall, 1958). We shall define η in the following manner. Consider an experiment in which the human observer attempts to detect some well-specified signal with energy E_0. He will perform with some hit rate and some false-alarm rate. In making a mathematical calculation we maintain all experimental parameters constant, with the single exception of the signal energy and solve for the energy, E_i, required by

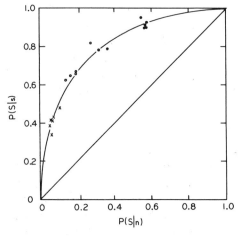

Fig. 6. An ROC-curve for a signal observer detecting a signal in a background of noise. See text for details of the experiment. [This figure is adapted from data reported by Egan et al. (1959).]

an ideal observer to match the performance of the human observer. The ratio of these two energies E_i/E_0 defines η. This measure of efficiency results in a value ranging from zero, at chance performance, to unity with performance equal to that of the ideal observer. The performance measure d' may be obtained with knowledge of a measure of the observer's hit rate and false-alarm rate. In order to determine the efficiency of the observer, a measure of d' for the observer and knowledge of ideal performance in the same situation are essential.

B. Some Illustrative Data

With these performance measures obtained, we can now look at some illustrative data. The ROC-curve of Figure 6 is taken from Egan et al. (1959). These data points were obtained with a single subject detecting a signal in a background of noise at a constant signal-to-noise ratio. In this experiment observation intervals were well defined and the observer knew that the a priori probability of the presence of a signal (a 500-msec, 1000-Hz tone) in the background of noise was one-half, that is, $P(s) = 0.5$. The observer's task was to state whether or not he heard the signal. Each point in Figure 6 is based on 240 observations. For those data points indicated by an X, the observer was instructed to be "strict," that is, to maintain a low false-alarm rate. Those data points indicated by a solid circle were obtained under instructions to be "lax," that is, to maintain a very high hit rate regardless of the false-alarm rate. The open circles occurred when the observer was instructed to adopt a "medium" criterion.

The data from the experiment of Egan et al. are closely fit by an ROC-curve of the type shown for the ideal observer in Figure 3. The curve in Figure 6 has the parameter $d' = 1.30$. Even though the ideal observer would have been on a higher ROC-curve the important finding is that the human observer operates with a fairly constant d'. The effect of the instructions in this experiment are reflected primarily in the measure of the observer's criterion and not in the measure of his sensitivity. Because of the nature of the instructions one would expect the observer's criterion to change but not the observer's sensory capacity. Yet, measures typically used in the clinic and in psychoacoustic experiments are affected not only by changes in signal strength or changes in the sensitivity of the organism but by such instructional variables as the above.

Let us consider three such measures which are often reported in the literature. The first of these is simply $P(S|s)$, the observer's hit rate with no account taken of his false-alarm rate. The second is the observer's hit rate corrected by his false-alarm rate, usually by the familiar correction for guessing. We shall call this measure P, where

$$P = \frac{P(S|s) - P(S|n)}{1 - P(S|n)}. \tag{10}$$

A third measure which is sometimes used is the observer's proportion of correct responses considered over both intervals containing a signal and those which contain noise alone. We shall call this measure $P(C)$, where

$$P(C) = P(s \cdot S) + P(n \cdot N). \tag{11}$$

The data in Figure 6 are typical of those obtained with human observers in the detection experiment. [For many more examples of such curves for different observers and at different signal-to-noise ratios see Egan et al. (1959, 1961a).] Consequently, we can, by way of example, illustrate the manner in which the three performance measures listed above vary as a function of the observer's false-alarm rate. Consider the situation where the observer's index of detectability is a constant, $d' = 1$. The change in these performance measures as a function of the observer's criterion is shown in Figure 7. In calculating the curve for $P(C)$ it was assumed that the a priori probability of a signal was one-half. More extreme values of $P(s)$ would result in larger changes in $P(C)$ as a function of false-alarm rate.

We have now illustrated a point made in the opening section of this chapter. Typical methods for controlling for the criterion of the observer are generally inadequate. Joint consideration of the data shown in Figure 6 and the curves shown in Figure 7 illustrates that the typical "correction

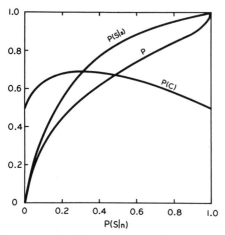

Fig. 7. Changes in three performance measures as a function of change in the observer's criterion.

for guessing" has but small corrective value, while instructing the observer to operate with a very low false-alarm rate only serves to force the observer to operate on that part of the curve where the usual performance measures vary most radically with small changes in criterion.

A further illustration of the use of d' as a performance measure is provided by a consideration of data reported by Fairbanks et al. (1956). In this experiment an observation interval might contain noise alone or signal (a 1-sec, 1500-Hz tone) plus noise, where $P(s) = P(n) =$ 0.5. Observers were run in pairs. The two members of each pair were instructed separately and did not communicate. Instructions were identical, with the following exception. One of the pair, termed the "positive observer" was instructed "press the signal key if the noise contained a tone," while the "negative observer" was instructed to "press the signal key if the noise did not contain a tone." The experiment was carefully controlled with subjects responding to 100 trials at each of three signal-to-noise ratios. The authors conclude, "it is interesting to note that the difference in instructions produced of difference of about 2 dB in the statistical threshold of signal detection and a corresponding difference in null detection. The differences between subgroups are large, approximately equal for both signal and no-signal samples, reasonably constant at the three voltage levels, and are statistically significant." After further discussion they add: "it should be possible to manipulate the statistical threshold of signal detection by various combinations of set and attitude over a range of 6 dB."

Fairbanks and his co-workers ascribe this change in the threshold measure to changes in the observer's criterion for making a decision. We see clearly that their hypothesis is supported if we plot their data on ROC-curves. Even though their data do not provide enough points

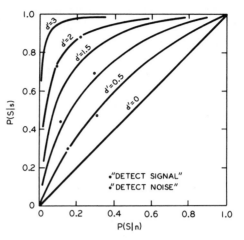

FIG. 8. Changes in performance as a function of signal-to-noise ratio under each of two sets of instructions. [Data taken from Fairbanks *et al.* (1956).]

to trace out entire curves, the two points at each signal-to-noise ratio come very close to falling on ROC-curves of the type shown in Figure 3. Figure 8 shows their data superimposed on the curves of Figure 3. It is apparent that the "negative observers" have about the same index of detectability as do the "positive observers," while at the same time they have a very different "false-alarm rate." As is seen most clearly in Figure 9a, the index of detectability is affected by the signal-to-noise ratio but is not significantly changed by the instructional variable. On the other hand, as seen in Fig. 9b, the instructional variable has markedly affected the observers' criterion. Although changes in signal-to-noise ratio have had little effect upon the measure $P(S|n)$ there are many experimental situations for which this is not the case, either for the human or for the ideal observer.

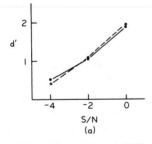

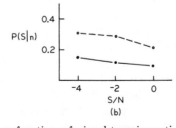

FIG. 9. Changes in d' and $P(S|n)$ as a function of signal-to-noise ratio under each of two sets of instructions. A. The measure d' shows marked changes as a function of signal-to-noise ratio but is not influenced by changes in instructions. B. The effect of the different sets of instructions is reflected in $P(S|n)$ which serves as a measure of the observer's criterion. [Data taken from Fairbanks *et al.* (1956).]

The foregoing data illustrate the commonly observed fact that, in the detection of a well-specified signal, conventional performance measures are often affected by criterial variables whereas the performance measure d' is not confounded with the criterion of the observer. A further advantage to be realized from the utilization of the theory of signal detectability is reflected in the fact that the human observer demonstrates a relatively constant efficiency in many types of experiments. By way of example let us compare the procedure in which a signal is randomly presented in one of two fixed observation intervals [two-alternative temporal forced-choice (2ATFC) experiment] with the procedure in which the signal is either presented or not presented during a single, fixed observation interval (the single-interval experiment, sometimes called the "yes–no" experiment). In comparing these two methods, the typical finding is that the threshold from the 2ATFC experiment is from 3 to 6 dB more sensitive than the threshold obtained in a single-interval experiment. Are we to explain this result on the basis of the sense organ, the nervous system, the difference in experimental design, or the decision process of the human? We can, of course, give this result a name and treat it as an independent phenomenon, but we are in danger of wasting much time and energy. A careful analysis will show us that at least two of the following factors are operating. First of all, if we analyze the informational content of the signal inputs, we will find that the 2ATFC experiment provides the observer with twice as much energy per decision as was available in the single-interval experiment. Thus, if the human observer were to show a constant efficiency in both types of experiments, the difference of the information available to him at the input could account for a 3-dB change in his performance. A second factor which leads to lower thresholds in 2ATFC experiments relates to the fact that the typical human observer does not show a response bias toward either observation interval (at least over a broad range of time intervals between the two observations). Consequently, if the signal appears about half the time in each of the two intervals, the human observer is operating at a point on his ROC-curve that tends to maximize his percentage of correct responses. In a single-interval experiment, on the other hand, the human observer often has a conservative bias. That is, he tends to avoid the "hallucinatory" response of saying "signal present" when the sample is really noise alone. This can be noted by comparing the points obtained with the "positive observers" in Figure 8 with the $P(s) = 0.5$ criterion contour in Figure 4.

Swets (1959) provides a direct comparison of these two experimental paradigms. He reports data for three observers tested at each of three signal-to-noise ratios. Changes in the observers' efficiencies are less than 1 dB from one method to the other. This is to be contrasted with the

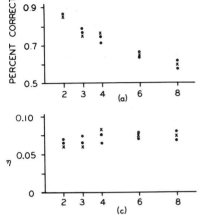

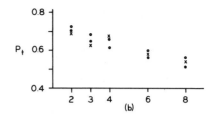

FIG. 10. The influence upon performance measures of the number of alternatives in an n-alternative temporal forced-choice experiment. [Data taken from Swets (1959).]

typical shift in threshold as we move from one method to the other.

In the second experiment Swets compared performance in nATFC experiments were n varied from 2 to 8. In these experiments the signal to be detected was presented in one of n observation intervals. Following the n observation intervals it was the observer's task to state which of these temporal intervals contained the signal in the background of noise. In Figure 10a we see the percentage of correct identifications for each of three observers as a function of the number of observation intervals involved in the nATFC procedure. As would be expected, the percentage of correct responses falls off as the number of intervals is increased. If we make a threshold-type correction for guessing, we may approximate the probability of the signal being above threshold, P_t, by the formula

$$P_t = \frac{P(C) - 1/n}{1 - 1/n}. \tag{12}$$

This "corrected" response measure is shown in Figure 10b. Although this second response measure has definitely tended to flatten out the curves, a marked and significant downward trend is still apparent. On the other hand, as we see in Figure 10c, η shows but slight and insignificant evidence of change as a function of the number of observation intervals. The finding that the efficiency of the observer is fairly constant over various experimental designs constitutes an additional argument for the adoption of performance measures derived from the theory of signal detectability.

C. Summary

With the development outlined in this chapter we have been able to account for some of the changes in the performance of the human observer (as typically measured) in terms of changes in the observer's criterion and changes in the information available at the input to the observer. Obviously, these few simple observations do not lead us immediately to a comprehensive theory of hearing. Thus far, we have merely emphasized those situations where the performance of the human auditory system may be described by the equation $d' = (n2E/N_0)^{1/2}$. Considering the complexity of the human auditory mechanism, it is not surprising that such a simple equation is inadequate. But the point to be made is that with proper measurement techniques we stand a much better chance of arriving at a reasonable description of the auditory mechanism than if we continually confound our measures.

The foregoing does not exhaust the evidence which leads us to prefer performance measures based on the theory of signal detectability to measures rooted in the concept of a sensory threshold. However, it should be sufficient for an introduction to the subject. Let us stop at this point to summarize briefly some of the advantages we have noted in approaching the measurement of hearing from the point of view of the theory of signal detectability. First, we have seen that, unlike traditional approaches to this subject, the theory of signal detectability provides a method of analyzing the input information available to the observer. Second, this theory also provides the mathematical tools necessary to analyze and describe human performance. Third, this approach leads to performance measures which distinguish between the criterion of the observer and the detectability of the signal. Finally, the resultant measure of detectability is relatively invariant with instructional variables and over different experimental paradigms.

VI. Some Implications for Audiology

The theory of signal detectability has thrived as a specialization within psychoacoustics. Much of this research may be characterized by (1) detailed mathematical analysis of the properties of signal and noise waveforms, (2) detailed mathematical analysis of the manner in which various ideal and nonideal detection systems would process these waveforms, and (3) critical comparison of human performance with the performance that would be realized by these theoretical processing systems. This research effort in combination with much excellent research not so obviously influenced by the theory of signal detection has resulted in significant advances in our understanding of the manner in which the human auditory system processes acoustic information. However, most of this effort has been expended on the study of the normal ear and there has been relatively little progress of a substantive nature emanating from the theory of signal detectability that would directly influence the clinical audiologist in the performance of his duties. Efforts by experimental audiologists to expand this research to include comparative data for the normal auditory system and various pathological systems are sorely needed and should prove rewarding.

There are, however, several generally applicable concepts and findings, mostly methodological in nature, which should be of concern to the audiologist. We shall briefly discuss: (1) the role of the listener's criterion in arriving at his response, and (2) the specification of the stimulus that elicited the listener's response.

A. The Role of the Criterion and Psychophysical Methods

We have discussed the fact that methods based on TSD result in measures of sensitivity that are relatively uncontaminated by criterial variables. Consequently, given adequate testing time and cooperative listeners, such measures typically have greater validity and greater reliability than methods traditionally used in the clinic. In many clinical situations this is not important. For example, a diagnosis would rarely be affected by changes of a few decibels in measured absolute threshold. On the other hand, the experimental audiologist may often require the most precise and accurate measures he can get. This is particularly important in the development of diagnostic measures that may rely on small differences in performance or on the estimation of the slope of a function. In general, both the clinician and the experimenter should estimate the degree of precision and accuracy that they require of their measures and chose that method of measurement that will most efficiently provide such precision and accuracy.

In some instances it is possible that one does not want an index of sensitivity independent of criterion. If one is interested solely in the question "Does the listener respond to the signal?" then traditional measures are adequate. If the question is to be followed by the further question, "Why does the listener fail to respond normally to many signals?" then the distinction between sensitivity and criterion may be important. For instance, different types of treatment are indicated for a hearing loss of 40 dB resulting from damage to the auditory system and a hearing loss of 40 dB due to functional (criterial) causes.

In many instances where "criterion-free"[3] measures are desirable, it

---

[3] We use the term "criterion-free" as a convenient abbreviation for the phrase "relatively independent of criterial involvement in most cases." The quotes are to remind the reader that our abbreviation is somewhat of an overstatement. A "criterion-free" method is a method for obtaining "criterion-free" measures.

is simply not possible to use the required methods. Such methods are fairly time-consuming and usually require alert and cooperative subjects. Often the clinical audiologist (and sometimes the experimental audiologist) suffers severe time limitations and may have to test many patients not sufficiently motivated or capable of performing properly using criterion-free methods. Furthermore, the nature of the experimental question may make it extremely difficult to obtain criterion-free measures. Such measures are usually based on the assumption that the sensitivity of the listener is not changing during the time required to obtain the measure. This assumption may be obviously violated in some cases, for example, the acquisition of and the recovery from auditory fatigue in one form or another.

Despite these limitations, there are many instances in which criterion-free methods are directly applicable to audiological research and indirectly applicable to clinical testing. Probably the single best criterion-free method to use in most cases is the two-alternative temporal forced-choice method (2ATFC). Here, a signal is presented in one of two intervals usually separated by 0.5 to 1.0 sec and the task of the observer is to state which interval contained the signal. The observer is required to respond on every trial. His performance on any given condition is scored in terms of percentage of correct responses, that is, $P(c) = \#\text{cor}/\#$ total. There is nothing inherently criterion-free about this method when scored in this way, but (1) as an empirical finding in most situations most listeners show little bias on this task, that is, they do not seem to have a decided preference for responding to one or the other intervals; (2) small biases have little effect on the measured $P(c)$ (see Figure 7); (3) if a large bias exists it is easily detected by separately scoring those cases in which the signal appeared in the first interval and those cases in which the signal appeared in the second interval; and finally (4) if the shape of the underlying ROC-curve is known, an accurate correction for bias may be applied.

The 2ATFC method is typically used in one of two manners. Sometimes the experimenter wishes to obtain functions showing how performance varies as a function of some physical parameter. Here it is common to run some fixed number of trials[4] at each of several values of the experimental parameter and to plot the resultant performance score as a function of the parameter. The psychometric function showing $P(c)$ as a function of the intensity of a given signal is a common example. In other instances the experimenter wishes to obtain functions

---

[4] An informative discussion of experimental techniques is provided in Appendix III of Green and Swets (1966).

showing how some physical parameter varies as a function of a second parameter in order to maintain fixed performance. An example of this is the absolute threshold contour in which the experimenter determines the intensity of a tone as a function of frequency that is required for some fixed performance level (usually 75% in 2ATFC). Such data may be obtained by getting the psychometric function and interpolating to determine the intensity required for 75% correct judgments or by using adaptive psychophysical techniques.

Adaptive psychophysical procedures incorporate the sequential testing procedures developed by Wald (1947). The PEST (point estimation by sequential testing) technique advanced by Taylor and Creelman (1967) represents a noteworthy effort along these lines. In the PEST procedure, signals are presented at a specific level (typically in a 2ATFC format) only as often as is necessary to determine at some specified level of confidence that the listener is above or below the point that is being estimated on the psychometric function. When a decision is made, the intensity of the signal is changed in the appropriate direction. In accordance with prescribed rules, step sizes are changed from time to time to hasten the process of reaching the estimate of threshold, usually defined as 75% correct responses in 2ATFC. When some minimum step size is reached, the procedure is terminated and the last signal level is used as an estimate of the threshold value. According to Taylor and Creelman about 2 minutes and fewer than 50 signal presentations are required to reach the threshold estimate. Recently one of us (RCB) compared critical ratios obtained by a PEST-like procedure to those obtained using fixed-frequency Békésy tracking. In this comparison masked thresholds were estimated at three frequencies (250, 1000, 4000 Hz) on a group of 12 hard-of-hearing patients. The critical ratios based on the adaptive forced-choice procedures were significantly less variable than and significantly smaller than those based on a tracking procedure. These data are shown in Table I. It is interesting to note that the critical ratios obtained with these patients using the adaptive sequential

TABLE I

MEANS AND STANDARD DEVIATIONS (IN DECIBELS) OF CRITICAL-RATIOS FOR
12 HARD-OF-HEARING PATIENTS AS OBTAINED BY TWO METHODS

	250 Hz	1000 Hz	4000 Hz
Adaptive sequential procedure	15.4	19.6	24.4
	(2.2)	(2.7)	(2.5)
Békésy tracking	20.5	21.8	27.0
	(3.1)	(3.0)	(3.6)

procedure are within a decibel of those obtained by Hawkins and Stevens (1950) using trained observers and a method of adjustment.

We have recognized that criterion-free methods are not sufficiently fast and convenient to replace traditional methods in the audiological clinic. However, they may prove to be a valuable adjunct to the traditional methods. We would suggest that roughly one out of the ten data points obtained by traditional methods be checked by use of a criterion-free method. If results were within a few decibels of one another, the clinician could feel quite confident that the data accurately reflected the state of the listener's auditory system. Large discrepancies in the two types of measures would serve to warn the clinician that he was not obtaining accurate information about the auditory system per se and that the data were probably affected by criterial variables or failure to cooperate fully in the testing procedure.

B. Specification of the Stimulus

Performance in the detection of sinusoids is affected by at least three physical parameters of the signal: Frequency, amplitude, and duration. Performance is also affected by the observer's knowledge of the values of these parameters on any given observation (Green and Swets, 1966, p. 283f; Tanner, 1961) and in addition by his knowledge of the starting time of the observation interval (Egan et al., 1961a,b). In many traditional techniques not only are the values of the parameters not known to the listener, but they are not known to the experimenter. For example, in the method of adjustment a listener controls an attenuator to set the intensity of the signal to a level where he reports that he can just hear the signal. In this case the effective duration of the signal leading to his report is unknown and furthermore, it is possible that the amplitude of the signal was changing during the time he was making his judgment. For some practical applications such methods are adequate since precise measures are not required and, for normal listeners at least, duration is not an important variable in affecting performance as long as it exceeds approximately 250 msec.

For shorter duration tones the auditory system acts much more like an energy detector than like an amplitude detector. Thus, as the duration of the signal is increased, the measured threshold for the signal is decreased. For the normal ear,[5] the threshold is lowered from 10 to 15

---

[5] The sensorineural ear often shows much less threshold shift as a function of duration (Miskalczy-Foder, 1959, 1960; Wright, 1968). This difference between the normal ear and the sensorineural ear may be of diagnostic significance but at the moment there are unresolved methodological problems (Chamberlain and Zwislocki, 1970).

dB as the duration of the signal is increased from 10 msec to 320 msec (Watson and Gengel, 1969; Zwislocki, 1965). Obviously, when short-duration signals are employed it is important that duration be controlled and specified. As duration is increased above 250 msec there is little further improvement in performance.

Recently, N. T. Hopkinson (1970) pointed out to us that she has noted relatively large differences in the hearing loss measures obtained on certain patients when controlled durations of 300 msec followed by 3.5–4.0 sec of off-time were used, as opposed to the relatively uncontrolled durations characteristic of most audiometric techniques. Specifically, among patients who exhibit excessive tone decay, measures of hearing loss arrived at using conventional audiometric procedures indicate greater losses in sensitivity than hearing losses measured with the 300-msec signal. The tentative explanation of this difference is that duration of tones used when the audiologist controls signal duration with the manual interrupter switch tends to be long enough and the off-interval between tones brief enough so that measured hearing loss is contaminated by tone decay. There would appear to be some basis for recommending that routine threshold determination employ signals of from 300 msec to 500 msec and that a separate test be used to determine tone decay.

The phenomenon reported to us by Hopkinson is probably similar to that relating off-time for periodically interrupted tones to the extent of tone decay in patients with acoustic neuromas as reported by both Dallos and Tillman (1966) and Jerger and Jerger (1966). Audiometric technique already has been modified to prevent a moderate decay or adaptation of threshold (Carhart and Jerger, 1959). Carhart and Jerger recommended a modified Hughson–Westlake technique employing relatively short signals (1–2 sec) and an ascending method of limits. With normal listeners (Carhart and Jerger, 1959) and with patients suffering sensorineural hearing loss (Jerger, 1962), this technique results in thresholds comparable but slightly higher than obtained with more traditional techniques. This small difference is probably due to the fact that the signal is not well defined for the listener. With most trials conducted "below threshold" the listener does not have good information regarding the parameters of the signal. This technique, however, is inadequate for determining threshold sensitivity in patients who exhibit exaggerated tone decay. A technique employing short-duration signals, 2ATFC, or some other accuracy indicator of performance, and well-defined observation intervals, should yield lower thresholds, uncontaminated by accelerated adaptation phenomenon, critical variables, and inadequate specification of the stimulus.

ACKNOWLEDGMENT

Revision of this chapter was supported in part by grants from the U.S. Public Health Service; Department of Health, Education, and Welfare; National Institute of Neurological Diseases and Stroke.

References

Birdsall, T. G. (1955). The theory of signal detectability. In "Information Theory in Psychology," (H. Quastler, ed.), pp. 391–402. Free Press, Glencoe, Illnois.

Carhart, R., and Jerger, J. (1959). Preferred method for clinical determination of pure-tone thresholds. J. Speech Hearing Dis. 24, 330–345.

Chamberlain, S. C., and Zwislocki, J. (1970). Threshold of audibility as a function of tone duration: Is there a frequency effect? (A) J. Acoust. Soc. Amer. 48, 71.

Clarke, F. R., and Bilger, R. C. (1963). The theory of signal detectability and the measurement of hearing. In "Modern Developments in Audiology." (J. Jerger, ed.), pp. 371–408. Academic Press, New York.

Dallos, P. J., and Tillman, T. W. (1966). The effects of parameter variations in Békésy audiometry in a patient with acoustic neurinoma. J. Speech Hearing Res. 9, 557–572.

Egan, J. P. (1967). Signal detection theory and psychophysics: A topical bibliography. NAS–NRC Committee on Hearing, Bioacoustics, and Biomechanics.

Egan, J. P., and Clarke, F. R. (1966). Psychophysics and signal detection. In "Experimental Methods and Instrumentation in Psychology." (J. Sidowski, ed.), pp. 211–246. McGraw-Hill, New York.

Egan, J. P., Schulman, A. I., and Greenberg, G. Z. (1959). Operating characteristics determined by binary decisions and by ratings. J. Acoust. Soc. Amer. 31, 768–773.[6]

Egan, J. P., Greenberg, G. Z., and Schulman, A. I. (1961a). Interval of time uncertainty in auditory detection. J. Acoust. Soc. Amer. 33, 771–778.[6]

Egan, J. P., Schulman, A. I., and Greenberg, G. Z. (1961b). Memory for waveform and time uncertainty in auditory detection. J. Acoust. Soc. Amer. 33, 779–781.[6]

Fairbanks, G., House, A. S., and Melrose, J. (1956). Auditory detection of the presence and absence of signals in noise. J. Acoust. Soc. Amer. 28, 614–616.

Green, D. M., and Swets, J. A. (1966). "Signal Detection Theory and Psychophysics." Wiley, New York.

Hawkins, J. E., Jr., and Stevens, S. S. (1950). The masking of pure tones and of speech by white noise. J. Acoust. Soc. Amer. 22, 6–13.

Hopkinson, N. T. (1970). Personal communication.

Jerger, J. (1962). Comparative evaluation of some auditory measures. J. Speech Hearing Res. 5, 3–17.

Jerger, J., and Jerger, S. (1966). Critical off-time in VIIIth nerve disorders. J. Speech Hearing Res. 9, 573–583.

Miskolczy-Foder, F. (1959). Relation between loudness and duration of tonal pulses. I. Response of normal ears to pure tones longer than click-pitch threshold. J. Acoust. Soc. Amer. 31, 1128–1134.

Miskolczy-Foder, F. (1960). Relation between loudness and duration of tonal pulses. III. Response in cases of abnormal loudness function. J. Acoust. Soc. Amer. 32, 486–492.

---

[6] This article is reprinted in Swets (1964).

Peterson, W. W., Birdsall, T. G., and Fox, W. C. (1954). The theory of signal detectability. *Trans. IRE Prof. Group Inf. Theory, PGIT-4*, 171–212. Also in "Readings in Mathematical Psychology" (Luce, Bush, and Galenter, eds.) Vol. I. Wiley, New York, 1963.

Pollack, I. (1948). The atonal interval. *J. Acoust. Soc. Amer.* **20**, 146–149.

Stevens, S. S. (1951). Mathematics, measurement, and psychophysics. *In* "Handbook of Experimental Psychology," (S. S. Stevens, ed.), pp. 1–49 (see esp. p. 33). Wiley, New York.

Swets, J. A. (1959). Indices of signal detectability obtained with various psychophysical procedures. *J. Acoust. Soc. Amer.* **31**, 511–513.[6]

Swets, J. A. (ed.) (1964) "Signal Detection and Recognition by Human Observers." Wiley, New York.

Tanner, W. P., Jr. (1955). On the design of psychological experiments. *In* "Information Theory in Psychology," (H. Quastler, ed.), pp. 403–414. Free Press, Glencoe, Illinois.

Tanner, W. P., Jr. (1961). Physiological implications of psychophysical data. *Ann. N.Y. Acad. Sci.* **89**, 752–765.[6]

Tanner, W. P., Jr., and Birdsall, T. G. (1958). Definitions of d' and η as psychophysical measures. *J. Acoust. Soc. Amer.* **30**, 922–928.[6]

Tanner, W. P., Jr., and Swets, J. A. (1954). A decision-making theory of visual detection. *Psychol. Rev.* **61**, 401–409.

Taylor, M. M., and Creelman, C. D. (1967). PEST: Efficient estimates on probability functions. *J. Acoust. Soc. Amer.* **41**, 782–787.

Wald, A. (1947). "Sequential Analysis." Wiley, New York.

Watson, C. S., and Gengel, R. W. (1969). Signal duration and signal frequency in relation to auditory sensitivity. *J. Acoust. Soc. Amer.* **46**, 989–997.

Wright, H. N. (1968). Clinical measurement of temporal auditory summation. *J. Speech Hearing Res.* **11**, 109–127.

Zwislocki, J. (1965). Analysis of some auditory characteristics. *In* "Handbook of Mathematical Psychology, Vol. III." (R. D. Luce, R. R. Bush, and E. Galanter, eds.), pp. 3–97. Wiley, New York.

---

[6] This article is reprinted in Swets (1964).

Chapter 13

Research Frontiers in Audiology

University of Pittsburgh

I. Introduction

The word *frontier* denotes a boundary, as that between the known and unknown in science. It also has the connotation of a rudimentary stage of development and an unsophisticated mien. Expansion of a frontier represents progress during this early stage in the development of a society. Sooner or later, however, expansion must give way to maturation of the way of life. Audiology has reached the point in its development at which, if expansion of its frontiers is to continue, it must devote some effort to maturing scientifically.

Two characteristics of present-day audiology can be used to illustrate its lack of scientific maturity. First, the study of auditory function is fragmented among researchers trained in many different disciplines. In addition to those trained as audiologists, who may be in the minority, others have been trained as physiologists, psychologists, engineers, educators, etc. Although such diversity could be a source of vigor, that vigor has not been realized in that the field of audition has not developed a vocabulary with which workers with different backgrounds can communicate effectively. At the present time, engineers still talk and write in engineering terms, psychologists in psychological terms, etc. Attempts to circumvent these vocabulary barriers often lead to dilution of the concepts; even when a word or concept comes into general use in audiology, none of the strength that concept has in its primary context is transferred with it.

The fact that workers from so many different fields are interested in the auditory system reflects, in large part, practical problems that they have encountered which involve the auditory system. Since their initial motivation is so often applied in nature, it should not be surprising that audiology is so pragmatic in its outlook. The question, "What works?" has always had precedence over such questions as "Why? What does it mean?" or "How does it relate?" While this practical bent is understandable, it is surprising how often theory is rejected by audiologists. They seem to have a strong tendency to look on theories as a source of bias and an unnecessary encumbrance in their search for truth. This attitude is reflected in the absence of theories in audiology.

The heterogeneous backgrounds of those who do research in audiology and the practical bent they share are reminiscent of the frontier. The consequent lack of a common vocabulary and of theories is evidence of scientific immaturity. The purpose of this undertaking is to consider the nature of scientific theories and their role in science, to assess the effects of nontheory to audiology, and to suggest a basis for theorization that might profit audiology.

II. Theory and Scientific Progress

Since a precise and thorough discussion of scientific theory would require a book in itself (cf. Braithwaite, 1953), the detail of this treatment will be commensurate with the space available. No science can progress if it rests, as audiology tends to, on simple generalizations concerning directly observable phenomena. Such first-level generalizations about data are merely descriptive. There is a second level of generalization at which the descriptions of the first level can be "explained" in terms or more general hypotheses (Braithwaite, 1953). The third level of generalization involves hypotheses that are no longer properties of anything that can be observed directly. At this level, deductions of phenomena not previously observed can occur, and these deductions might be called predictions. There is an obvious ordering of description, explanation, and prediction.

As one proceeds up the hierarchy of theory, several difficulties arise. For example, highly general hypotheses are difficult to accept or reject. Braithwaite (1953) indicates that an incorrect hypothesis is sensed and finally is rejected only when a replacement has been generated. In addition, at higher levels of abstraction mathematical logic becomes more tortuous. Above all, once past the ground level of generalization, scientific theories tend to become formal and explicit. To formalize a theory, it is necessary to identify any undefined terms and to list all of the assumptions that underlie the theory. Finally, the hypotheses themselves must be identified.

The role of such explicit theories should be obvious. They guide the experimenter in where to look and in how to look for previously unobserved facts that will ultimately bring down the theory. That is, when the theory leads to an incorrect prediction or when it is incapable of explaining a new phenomenon, it must be revised or rejected. The more abstract a theory is, as noted previously, the more difficult it is to modify.

Many of the advantages to formal theories are implicit in the brief description presented here, but one advantage must be made explicit. By their very nature, formal theories shed light on what is potentially their weakest point, underlying assumptions. Active experimentation obviously can go on in the absence of formal theories, but it cannot progress with undefined terms, assumptions, and hypotheses. Such unstated assumptions and hypotheses are *covert theories*. A discipline whose experiments are based on covert theories will probably be stalled somewhere between the first and second level of generalization until its theories are formalized because of the unavailability of the sources of error to other workers in the field.

With few exceptions, the study of the auditory system is based on covert or private theories (Licklider, 1959). The exceptions are worth noting. First, Wever's (1949) attempt to encompass existing knowledge in a single theoretical statement should be acknowledged, especially since it is probably more timely now than when it was published. Second, the work in signal detection by Tanner and his associates should be mentioned in light of the correctness of their approach to theorization, even though it is not strictly a theory of hearing. Other theories related to audiology will be mentioned later in this presentation.

III. Covert Hypotheses in Audition

What were called "theories of hearing" in the past were, in essence, explanations of pitch perception or frequency resolution in terms of hypotheses about peripheral mechanisms. That these were relatively low-level generalizations is reflected in the current names, "place principle and periodicity principle." Most other existent theories, called part theories by Licklider (1959), also are low-level generalizations about directly observable results in Braithwaite's terms (1953), for example, Fletcher's critical-band hypothesis. Even though theorization in audiology is still in the primitive stages, these part theories do not impede progress. The impediments are the covert hypotheses that guide individual experimenters in the design, conduct, analysis, and interpretation of their experiments. These tacit assumptions are affected unconsciously in most cases, which is the true source of their power to impede progress.

Although covert hypotheses are basically private to the experimenter, the audiological literature is large enough to show their signs many times over to one who looks for them. Ten such covert assumptions can be identified. Seven of these ten are clearly tacit assumptions about the characteristics of the auditory system, two are clearly assumptions about how to do experiments, and one is a little of each. Of course, the tacit assumptions about how the ear works influence how data are collected and those concerning research strategy affect our knowledge of the auditory system. Finally, this is not the first discussion of many of the ten covert hypotheses.

A. The Ear

The seven tacit hypotheses concerning the characteristics of the auditory system, taken together, lead to the inescapable conclusion that audiologists deal with the "ear" rather than with auditory system itself. Thus, this section is labeled "The Ear" rather than the more appropriate, "Auditory System."

1. SENSORY THRESHOLD

The concept of sensory threshold is very old and very pervasive (cf. Green and Swets, 1966, pp. 117–148). It was formalized by Fechner (1860) who made it the cornerstone of his theory of psychophysics. Interestingly enough, those who reject the remainder of Fechner's theories cling to the sensory-threshold hypothesis, while those who reject the sensory-threshold hypothesis usually retain the rest of Fechner. The lesson to be learned is that to reject a theory, one must be prepared to reject all of it, not just the parts he does not like.

Recently the concept of sensory threshold has come under prolonged, systematic scrutiny by signal-detection theorists (Green and Swets, 1966; Swets, 1961). The results show that estimates of threshold can be affected by many factors, including motivation (that is, risk), detection tasks, signal characteristics, signal probability, and number of signals. For some combinations of these factors the data will appear to indicate the existence of thresholds, but not all combinations of them will support a threshold. Therefore, one must conclude that threshold is a characteristic of certain kinds of data and not a characteristic of the sense organ. Clarke and Bilger (1972) point out that only by careful analysis of the detection task confronting the listener and consideration of how the data are to be interpreted can an experimenter safely use "threshold." In light of the evidence against the validity of the assumption that threshold is a characteristic of the sense organ or sensory system, the casual use of thresholds (because it will tend to generate data contaminated by many unknown, nonauditory factors), cannot lead audiology from its frontier level.

2. PURE-TONE STIMULI

The most obvious characteristic of audiological research is its dependence on pure tones as stimuli. Since technology has been able to provide us with signal generators for pure tones on a reliable and economical basis, and since sine waves are so easy to generate, control, and specify, this dependence on pure tones is not surprising. In contrast to the complete specification of pure-tone signals and the spectra of gated sinusoids, note that noise must be described statistically (that is, its mean is zero and its standard deviation is called the rms voltage of the noise) and speech can be described only approximately in anything approaching real time. Also note that perception of complex tones is indexed under "subjective tones" in the *Journal of the Acoustical Society of America.*

To use pure-tone signals because they are readily available is one thing; but to assume that they are correct and sufficient is a covert hypothesis of considerable force. This hypothesis need not be covert, since it can be inferred from Ohm's Acoustic Law, which contends that the "ear" perceives a complex tone by analyzing it into its Fourier components, that is, pure tones (Bekesy, 1960). When Ohm's Acoustic Law is coupled with Helmholtz's claim that the phase of higher harmonics does not influence perception of complex tones (Helmholtz, 1885), the theoretical justification of the pure-tone oscillator as the primary signal source in audiology is complete. Still, the unquestioned acceptance of this assumption for over 100 years is a strong reflection of the lack of theoretical introspection by audiologists.

If one notes that the first recorded mention of a source for a reasonably pure tone probably was Shore's "pitch fork" in 1714 (Boring, 1942) and assumes that natural signals are to be preferred to artificial ones, then the case for pure tones should lose its appeal, since the human auditory system evolved without the benefit of pure-tone signals. Nor is the auditory system likely to reveal its secret to those who use only pure tones.

Two consequences of the excessive use of pure-tone signals might be noted here. In studies of the organization of the auditory pathways by neurophysiologists, a tremendous amount of work has produced a consistent conclusion that the auditory system is organized, at least in part, on a tonotopic basis. Viewed anatomically, this demonstration that there is level-to-level integrity in the nervous system is comforting. In other contexts this correspondence between points at the periphery and more central locations of the nervous system has been called "specific nerve energies." This result, regardless of its name, is little more than a confirmation of the master plan. It does not, however, tell us anything about the functioning of the auditory system.

In perceptual studies, experiments that use pure-tone signals are, in essence, correlations between the spectrum of the input and the perception. The correlations are of necessity high since the pure-tone signal affords the auditory system little opportunity to interfere. As a result of the system's minimum influence on a pure-tone signal, attempts to use listeners with hearing loss as a basis for gaining new knowledge about the system are fraught with frustration. Both of these examples will be elaborated subsequently.

3. ATTRIBUTES OF AUDITORY SENSATION

Some introductory comments on the reason for this heading are required. Almost as obvious a characteristic of faulty audiological research as the use of pure tones can be found in the simplistic view of audition held by most experimenters. As psychophyscists their general view is that the relevant parameters of audition are pitch, loudness, durational effects, and timbre. Timbre is obviously too complicated to study, so that audition has only three parameters. Essentially all these parameters are attributes and harken back to the beginnings of experimental psychology as an academic discipline (Boring, 1942). The assumption underlying the early theories of attributes was that if the proper set of attributes was invented, then the same attributes could be used to describe all sensation. These attributes were required to be independently manipulable and to all vanish if the value of any one attribute went to zero (threshold again).

A correspondence can be noted between the attributes of audition and vision. Pitch corresponds to hue, since both have wavelength as a physical correlate. Loudness corresponds either to brightness of direct light or lightness of reflected light. Finally, timbre corresponds to saturation. From the standpoint of progress in visual research, the fact that the underlying physical parameters of these attributes have never been brought under economical, reliable, electronic control has been a blessing since it forced researchers to deal with more realistic and thus more profitable situations, while their audiological confreres were being seduced by an oscillator.

That most auditory stimuli can be described by a reasonably intelligent listener in terms of pitch and loudness is not debatable. To stop with these descriptors, however, is to remain at the edge of nowhere. First, one should note Stevens' (1934a,b) work on the attributes of tones, which indicated that loudness and pitch can be replaced by volume and density without injustice to the theory of attributes. A second look will show that the simplistic notion of attributes relates conveniently to pure-tone signals. Listening to the world around you, however, will be more informative. When you hear speech, you can, if you choose, assign pitch and loudness to it; but how often is the pitch or loudness more relevant than the message? Further, can that message be encoded or decoded auditorily in terms of pitch and loudness? If you listen further, then you will hear and identify sounds (a vireo singing, a faucet dripping, an airplane, etc.) to which these attributes are meaningless. The fact that one's sensorium can assign values to attributes should not lead us to believe that the sensory system was designed to hear those attributes.

Another kind of oversimplification that confuses issues and encumbers our progress can be related to the theory of attributes. Once the notion of attributes is given value as a tacit assumption, it is quite easy to think, for example, that all intensive difference limina are the same. One famous issue in clinical audiology, the difference limen for intensity as an indirect test for recruitment, might never have been raised except for the unwarranted assumption that two different signal ensembles (a signal ensemble is a carrier tone to specify level plus an increment of intensity added to the carrier) are the same thing. In studies of the difference limen for frequency too, audiologists generally assume that Shower and Biddulph's (1931) technique of frequency modulating the carrier is not different from discriminating between two tone bursts of different frequency. In fact, there is no reason other than unquestioned acceptance of attributes to think that two such different methods are measuring the same capacities of the auditory system.

Finally, it should be noted that pitch (Sekey, 1963) and loudness (Zwislocki, 1969) judgments are influenced strongly by the duration of the signal, especially for brief durations. That is, pitch and loudness require the listener to cumulate (integrate) information about the signal over its duration. Such temporal dependencies do tell us something about the correlation between spectrum and perception for the human ear. These temporal dependencies also tell us that preoccupation with the concepts of pitch and loudness reflects a tendency on the part of audiologists to think of the auditory system as having one function, that of integrating the input to provide an optimum signal for evaluating the attributes of tones. (This integrative assumption is probably the major shortcoming of the theory of signal detectability.) Sooner or later, audiologists must recognize that the auditory system does more than integrate temporally. For example, the converse operation, differentiation, is adequate to explain many cases of modulation detection, and some instances of adaptation.

Since audiologists are unable to provide data that are appropriate to explain how speech is processed auditorily, consider the effect of the universal auditory integrator on a speech signal. Remember, speech is characterized by rapid changes in its spectrum. If the auditory system only integrates and cannot detect rapid changes in the input (that is, differentiate), then the rapid changes would be averaged out. An auditory system such as this cannot hear speech, a conclusion already reached by some theorists.

4. Sensation Level

Sensation level is the intensive metric used in many clinical and laboratory situations either to set the intensity parameter of a test or an experiment or to describe the magnitude of a level set to another criterion. The hypothesis that it is an appropriate .metric rests on several assumptions that seldom are brought out into the open. Obviously, its use assumes either existence of a sensory threshold or a situation in which threshold is an adequate index of performance. Less obviously, its use is most convenient when pure-tone signals are used, since irregularities in a listener's sensitivity as a function of frequency can lead to confusing results for a broad-band signal, such as speech.

The seldom-discussed assumptions underlying the use of sensation level involve the fact that in most audiological work intensity levels are really specified in terms of the voltage across the transducer or, at best, in terms of sound pressure level at the tympanum. The first hidden assumption then, is that the transfer of energy from the diaphragm of the earphone or from the drum to the stapes footplate is the same from frequency to frequency for all listeners. Confronted with inconsistencies in their data for the response of single units in the auditory nerve, Kiang et al. (1967) recalibrated their experiments in terms of displacement of the stapes footplate. When they replotted tuning curves for single units against the logarithmic displacement in the stapes footplate, the previous inconsistencies in the low-frequency portion of the tuning curves disappeared. In other words, for Felis libyca domestica, are presumably for man, the assumption that energy transfer from the drum membrane to the footplate of the stapes is trivial and cannot be supported. Given the existence of this problem, there are two more assumptions to be considered.

Even if displacement of the stapes footplate were the intensity-level control, one must ask if equal movements of the stapes footplates of two different listeners or for the same listener at two different frequencies result in an equal amount of energy being transferred into the cochlear duct and in equal displacements of the basilar membrane. If, for example, Glorig and Davis (1961) are correct in assuming that the basilar membrane stiffens with age, then the assumption that equal displacement of the stapes footplate causes equal displacement of the sense organ must be questioned. Finally, in using sensation level as the intensive metric, one assumes that equal displacements of the basilar membrane and of the sensory cell result in equivalent inputs to the nervous system. At this point it should be obvious that this third assumption is not always tenable. Its lack of tenability is the basis on which Wever (1949) explains loudness recruitment.

If an experimenter has a homogeneous group of listeners who also have very good hearing, then sensation level, although unnecessary, could be used safely. Whenever heterogeneity, in terms of sensitivity, creeps into the sample, sensation level becomes of doubtful validity. From a statistical point of view, for example, a ratio score such as sensation level makes unwarranted assumptions about the relationship between two variables, and a covariance technique becomes necessary.

Among listeners with hearing loss, use of sensation level with listeners who have conductive lesions might seem safe and actually be safe in a 10-dB ballpark. Their conductive lesion, however, is going to uniquely alter the transfer of energy from the drum to the stapes footplate so that in situations for which 3–5 dB is critical, sensation level may be inadequate. For listeners with sensorineural loss, the use of sensation level will introduce obvious distortions into the data. Suffice it to say, among clinical tests in audiology that are useful and that use sensation level, the test works because it is really testing the assumption that sensation level can be used as an intensive metric and not because the test deals with loudness, pitch, etc.

5. LINEARITY

Ohm's Acoustic Law has withstood every attack in the past because it assumes the ear is a linear device and that any deviation from it can be explained in terms of the generation of distortion products at frequencies other than the input frequency. This assumed linearity fitted well with engineering concepts at the beginning of the era of electro-acoustic devices, so that Wegel and Lane (1924) were able to explain the complex tonal interactions they observed in terms of distortion products. Later, data reported by Wever and his associates (cf. Wever, 1949) for cochlear microphonics recorded at the round window of the cat and by Davis *et al.* (1958) for differential electrodes implanted in the cochlea of the guinea pig indicated that the ear was linear electrically through a wide dynamic range. Further, in his observations on models of the cochlea, Tonndorf (1962) has reported the appearance of eddies at high levels that could serve to transmit distortion products along the cochlea.

The assumption that the ear is a linear device subject to harmonic distortion at high input levels has provided the basis for explaining many auditory phenomena, including the asymmetry of the masking audiogram (Bilger and Hirsh, 1956), the aural harmonic (Lawrence and Yantis, 1956), and combination tones (Boring, 1942). Further, the assumption that listeners with sensorineural hearing losses exhibit more than normal harmonic distortion has seemed attractive (Jerger *et al.,* 1960; Lawrence and Yantis, 1956).

Only two points need to be made here, since the topic of linearity and distortion will be reexamined later. Most obvious is the point that recent data show the ear (cochlea) to be decidedly a nonlinear device. The other point is to note the assumption, first reported by Wegel and Lane (1924), that the ear can be described in terms of engineering concepts.

6. PLACE THEORIES

The role of the cochlea as a mechanoacoustic sound analyzer has been described thoroughly by Békésy. In addition to the description of the frequency-dependent traveling wave, Békésy also has quantified the parameters of the system that controls this frequency analysis (Békésy, 1960). In spite of Békésy's monumental work, there are still several gaps in our knowledge of place mechanisms in audition. One such gap deals with the exact manner in which the mechanical movements are converted into neural activity. (Note that the word *transduce* was not used here since its use implies reciprocity, that is, that neural activity also could be converted back into mechanical activity.) The second gap concerns the distribution of nerve fibers in the organ of Corti and their exact pattern of connection to hair cells. Given such information, it is still possible that place of stimulation is as broadly defined as Békésy's (1960) data indicate, or almost as broad (Rhode, 1971).

It is important to note that when one uses pure tones as the input to the cochlea, it is impossible to differentiate place from periodicity effects because for pure tones the place and periodicity information have exactly the same value. In the context of our present knowledge of the step from the mechanical to the neural and of the exact patterns of innervation of a place on the organ of Corti, it behooves audiologists to be more open minded about the contribution of place of stimulation to auditory phenomena.

7. SIGNAL PROCESSING

One implication of the concept of tonotopic organization, mentioned earlier, is that the auditory pathway is a passive connection between a series of relay stations (nuclei) whose function is to transmit information from the organ of Corti to the cerebral cortex. While the human brain is a fantastically complex and sophisticated information storage and processing device, it may not be reasonable to assume that information can be extracted only at the cortical level. The impracticality of this deferred processing was not apparent from the early ablation studies of the auditory system, which tended to give indecisive results until Neff introduced spatial and temporal complexity to the discrimination tasks (Diamond and Neff, 1957).

The need for subcortical processing, however, was apparent to workers in the area of binaural localization (Moushegian *et al.*, 1964), who settled on the superior olivary complex as the site for extraction of binaural time-intensity relationships. Perhaps the concept of neural sharpening at the sense organ (Spoendlin, 1970), or in the auditory nerve (Békésy, 1960) can be considered to provide an example of peripheral signal processing, although such categorization might surprise those who deal with these concepts.

The major drawback of assuming passive transmission of intact information from cochlea to cortex is that it is so consistent with the concept of the ear as a linear device that it is best tested with pure tones. The assumption that signals are processed all along the auditory system does not preclude the passive pathway. Instead, it suggests that the fact that each higher level of the nervous system is more complex than the immediately lower level is more than another application of Parkinson's Law.

B. Design of Audiological Experiments

The seven issues discussed in the preceding section, of course, could influence what experiment is performed and even how it is performed; but the two factors to be discussed here influence experiments in audiology quite directly and perhaps independently of what assumptions one makes about how the ear works.

1. Deficit

Thus far, the word audiology has been used in its broadest sense, that is, to include everyone who studies the auditory system. Use of the word *deficit* immediately restricts audiology to those who were trained as audiologists. Though this restriction will occur, it is unfortunate since, in the proper context, the listener with impaired hearing represents a potentially significant experiment. In animal experimentation, of course, one is free to vary the site, nature, and extent of lesion, but the experiment has limited value because of the animal's limited response repertoire. Since humans have speech and animals do not, it must be assumed that the human auditory system is different from that of animals. The fact that a summary of the nonspeech research in audition shows humans and animals as being comparable is a devastating criticism of the broad field of audiology.

Although the concept of deficit is central to the practice of audiology, it has become an impediment to research in audiology. For example, in most studies of speech perception the varible of record has been the number or percentage of words correctly repeated. Unfortunately, at the present state of our knowledge, words repeated correctly are of least value; words for which the response is incorrect carry the information. A mere tabulation of the number of errors, however, effectively discards that information. To extract the information in such errors, one must evaluate them in relation to the signal that was presented.

The present goal is not to present a new method for speech audiometry; that will be undertaken later. Instead, the goal here is to stress the point that, to use a listener with impaired hearing efficiently, the emphasis should be on what he hears when sounds have been made loud enough. Determination of what the listener perceives, however, is much more of a challenge to the experimenter than charting what he does not hear.

2. Averaging Data

All of us have been inculcated with the power and virtue of averaging data across subjects. If, however, audiologists are going to utilize effectively listeners with impaired hearing in the search for new knowledge, then they must be prepared to reconsider the process of averaging. This, in turn, will force them to scrutinize their present methods of data collection because those methods mandate averaging as a control for error. Perhaps two points will be sufficient to establish the case against averaging.

In an earlier era, much audiological research was reported on listeners with otosclerosis. As a clinical category, otosclerosis probably provided as homogeneous a group as audiologists ever will see. Averages of data for such a group are interpretable, especially since the metric for intensity level is not critical in their case. Patients with retrocochlear (brain stem) lesions are at the other extreme, however. Lesions that are quite comparable from a surgical standpoint are vastly different in their effect on the auditory system, so that some persons show little or no involvement of the auditory system while others show profound involvement. Average data for a group of such patients would be relatively meaningless. Because it is not reasonable to assume that all sensorineural losses are the same in nature, averages for groups of such patients also should be viewed with skepticism.

If one assumes that data may be averaged legitimately, then, unfortunately, he will overlook a major deficiency in most of our experiments. That deficiency is that the average score for a group of listeners really can be interpreted as the criterion against which one of the nonsubject variables of the experiment can be evaluated. A concrete example may be offensive, but it also will be informative. The attempts to devise a method of predicting who is most susceptible to noise-induced hearing loss have been unsuccessful. Note that this is a question about people. The experiments from which an indices of susceptibility were derived, however, were experiments in which people were used as the criterion against which noises were evaluated, and, as such, have little or no information about people. This experimental literature can be used successfully to set damage-risk criteria but not to define susceptibility.

C. The Communication Paradigm

The interest that the communications industry has in hearing should be obvious. In pursuing this interest, actually in both hearing and speech, their influence has been more profound and longer lasting than is acknowledged generally. (Note that Fletcher and Békésy both worked for a telephone company at the time their interests in hearing emerged.) This influence can still be seen across most of audiology and is evident in at least four different guises. Although these influences may be ephemeral and difficult to document, they should be considered here.

Since the phone companies' major concern is transmitting speech from one place to another, we must assume that maximizing the efficiency with which speech is transmitted motivates much of their research. Consider a hypothetical experiment designed to determine whether system B transmits speech signals more effectively than system A. The experiment requires a sample of speech to be transmitted, the two systems, and a group of listeners. Since the listeners' average score is the criterion against which the communication systems are to be evaluated, listeners must be assumed to constitute a random sample. Since listeners are a random variable, the experiment will provide us with no information about differences among listeners but only about variability. This simple paradigm, designed quite well from the standpoint of evaluating speech transmission, is the basic paradigm for testing speech discrimination in patients. One might argue, further, that this experimental paradigm is the one audiologists usually use. It is a fine experiment for evaluating communication systems (audiometers instead of telephones). It also can be used effectively to test message sets, signal sources (talkers), and signals themselves. The purpose this paradigm serves most poorly, providing information about the listeners, is the purpose audiologists use it for most often. With this experiment, averages are not inappropriate.

A second way that the influence of communication industries is felt in audiology is in terms of the constructs that we now use routinely to explain experimental results. That the performance of the ear is often described in terms of filters, transmission lines, etc., is often a consequence of the fact that people who work in research positions in telephone installations generally have a background in electrical engineering. The constructs are probably quite valid, but, if they were not, then we still might use them. That is, given the present state of knowledge in audiology, it may be more efficient to study hearing in terms of other than electrical constructs.

If the third influence can be described at all, then this whole effort must be deemed successful. The point is that as audiologists, we study hearing rather than audition, that is, the ear instead of the whole of the auditory system. Since the communication system can be evaluated without considering how the message is used, we restrict ourselves to studying only one part of audition. From this background it is difficult to specify fully the distinction between hearing and audition, but that distinction will include a consideration of how auditory inputs are used by the person in real situations.

IV. Unsolved Problems in Audiology

The unsolved problems facing audiological researchers are no different than those facing them 10 or 20 years ago. Since the thesis of this presentation is that these difficult problems will tend to remain unsolved as long as audiological thinking is influenced by untenable and tacit assumptions, these problems will be discussed in terms of the hypotheses described in the previous section. Not all of the so-called covert hypotheses have contributed equally to each problem area, so that only the major impediments in each area will be discussed.

A. Auditory Imperception

Auditory imperception can be defined in terms of what a listener with impaired hearing perceives when sounds are made loud enough for him to hear. That we have little or no information about this problem seems obvious. From the vast literature available, we do not know how the auditorily impaired listener perceives the test signals we use to test his hearing, let alone how he perceives the real-life sounds that he must audit every minute of every day.

This lack of real knowledge about auditory imperception in the face of a voluminous literature is a consequence of several faulty assumptions. Two, however, are major contributors—preoccupation with hearing deficit by the researcher and use of the universally accepted but incorrect experimental paradigm. Even if audiologists are concerned with perception and imperception, their basic experiment will provide them with information about the signals and not about the listener. While some progress has been made from data collected with this paradigm, correct inferences have been drawn in spite of and not because of the results obtained.

Another recurrent theme—that perhaps there is no information to be garnered from experiments that use one pure tone at a time—is relevant to the issue of auditory perception. Pure tones are basically uninteresting because they do not permit independent manipulation of the relevant variables, for example, place, periodicity, and envelope. To obtain interesting results one must use interesting signals.

B. Speech Perception

Our lack of good information about auditory perception and imperception is most serious in terms of understanding how speech is processed in the auditory system. Even if the lack of knowledge about imperception is blamed entirely on those trained as audiologists, the fact that the total of our current knowledge in audition is no help in understanding how speech is perceived must be shared by everyone who studies the auditory system. The fact that the most prevalent theory of speech perception (Liberman et al., 1967) has as a referent the articulators and not the auditory system is a reflection of failure of audiologists to present data that can be used in understanding how speech is perceived. Even if the so-called motor theory of speech perception is wrong, its development represents the best possible use of the data available in audiology. For those who sincerely doubt that the auditory system is necessary to speaking and to understanding speech and language, the plight of the congenitally deaf is cited as mute testimony to its significance.

For the field of audiology, in general, the major impediments to the acquisition of data relevant to understanding speech perception have been the assumptions that (1) pure tones are a sufficient stimulus and (2) the pathway between the sense organ and the cerebral cortex is just a pathway and not a system for processing the input into a more usable form. Although the auditory system implicit in a modern-day version of Ohm's Acoustic Law can, by brute force, be used to process speech, such a system locates all of the processing at the cortical level. The possibility that a feature analysis is performed on speech signals as they pass up the auditory system should be considered.

C. Nonperceptual Auditory Phenomena

The tacit assumption that audiology is properly defined as the study of hearing or even of auditory perception probably is the most significant impediment to real progress because it encourages researchers to ignore the role played by that system in processing, storage, and retrieval of the information entering the system. When Ramsdell (1947) discussed hearing at three levels (symbolic, signal, and background), he imputed to audiology a broader base than it would accept. Of the levels defined by him, audiology in essence accepts and works at only one level, the signal level. Since Ramsdell's list is not as broad as it should be to describe the role that the auditory system serves in establishing the "quality of life," it is unfortunate that more effort has not gone into broadening the basis of audiological experimentation.

D. Rehabilitation and Training

The most obvious consequence of limiting the scope of audiology to perceptual phenomena is seen in terms of the general lack of success experienced by those who are willing to try to educate the deaf and rehabilitate the hard-of-hearing. The only information our perceptually based audiology can offer to them is to suggest they make sounds louder. Audiological research probably could, by studying the role of audition in the context of memory, learning, decision making, etc., provide these educators with the information they need to do their work more effectively.

Another consequence of perceptual audiology is that the general scientific–clinical community and the community at large consider hearing to be one of the minor senses. Our society is much more willing to support research, rehabilitation, and prevention of the only recognized major sense (vision) than any one of the minor senses (taste, smell, audition, touch, etc.). For example, society will support legislation making the manufacture of shatterproof eyeglasses mandatory.

If the auditory sense is to be recognized as one of the two major senses, then audiologists must be the first to recognize its importance.

V. Significant Developments in Audiology

The works cited here as significant developments in audiology are primarily those readings out of which the present ideas evolved. They do not represent a systematic and critical review of the several bodies of literature, but instead reflect an individual pattern of searching and reading. Fortunately, there are relatively recent books summarizing or interpreting each of the three bodies of literature to be sampled. The reader, presumably a nonphysiologist, should be warned that this author is not a neurophysiologist. As a consequence, the interpretation of some results may reflect either bias or ignorance. In the areas labeled psychoacoustics and memory, the interpretations probably are less open to criticism. In any case, what is presented should not be blamed on the authors whose work is cited.

For each of the areas to be covered here, one or more comprehensive reviews are available. Whitfield (1967), Engebretson and Eldredge (1968), and Eldredge and Miller (1971) deal extensively with nonlinearities. The topic of single units and time encoding are treated in Whitfield (1967), Kiang (1965), and Plomp and Smoorenburg (1970). Whitfield (1967, 1970) and Erulkar et al. (1968) deal with signal processing and feature detection. The compendium edited by Plomp and Smoorenburg (1970) is the definitive treatment of the perception of complex tones. Finally, two excellent books on memory are available—Norman (1970) and Talland and Waugh (1969).

A. Nonlinearity in the Ear

The issue of nonlinearity is of interest here primarily because of the frequency with which distortion is invoked by audiologists as an explanation for the phenomena of normal or impaired hearing. It is of special interest because our own experience indicates that, while listeners with normal hearing and those with sensorineural loss are not different with respect to the higher harmonics of the primary (when sound pressure level is the intensive referent), they are very different from one another in terms of the "distortion" products that can occur in the frequency region below a complex (two or more) tonal signal (Bilger and Hopkinson, 1970). The difference is that this form of distortion appears to be absent for the listener with sensorineural loss.

In the literature on the neurophysiology of the auditory system, the issue of nonlinearity is considered primarily within the context of the cochlear microphonic (CM). The issues surrounding the interpretation of CM, however, are quite complex in themselves (Dallos, 1969; Whitfield, 1967) and, when the question of nonlinearity of the CM is assessed, the matter becomes even more complicated (Engebretson and Eldredge, 1968; Dallos and Sweetman, 1969; Sweetman and Dallos, 1969). To reduce these problems to manageable dimensions, only a selected part of that literature will be presented.

The first factor to consider is that combination tones, presumably the result of nonlinearity at the level of the cochlea, as a perceptual phenomena can be canceled by adjusting the phase and level of a bone-conducted tone corresponding in frequency to the perceived pitch of the combination tone. When Sweetman and Dallos (1969) tried to cancel the distortion components in CM in the guinea-pig cochlea by adjusting the phase and level of the bone-conducted tone, they found that "the combination tone components can never be canceled simultaneously throughout the cochlear [1969, p. 58]." The disparity between the auditory phenomena (complete cancellation) and the neurophysiological data can be resolved if one is willing to assume that CM includes aspects of the electrical activity in the cochlea that are not directly related to audition.

The fact is that even differential, intracochlear electrodes must be considered to be remote electrodes that average electrical activity of varying phase and amplitude across a wide population of hair cells (Dallos *et al.*, 1971). Thus, it cannot be assumed that CM represents the activity of any one hair cell under all circumstances (Whitfield, 1967, p. 67). This evidence is presumably sufficient for us as audiologists (but not for a neurophysiologist) to ignore the disparity between CM and perceptual data and proceed with a general consideration of nonlinearity.

Historically, three sources of distortion have been considered: in the middle ear, in mechanoelectrical conversion, and in the hydromechanical properties of the cochlear fluid. The possibility of the distortion products necessary to explain overtones and combination tones arising in the middle ear has been rejected repeatedly over the years. The mechano-electrical conversion process appears to be a major source of nonlinearity in that the transfer function (the relationship between the mechanical input and the electrical output) is generally recognized to be nonlinear. This transfer function takes the form of a polynomial power series that gives combination tones at the frequencies $mf_1 + nf_2$ (Eldredge and Miller, 1971). Dallos and his associates (Dallos and Sweetman, 1969; Sweetman and Dallos, 1969; Dallos et al., 1971) attribute distortion products at low and moderate sound pressure levels to such mechanoelectrical phenomena in the region of the primary tones, but they allow for the possibility that hydromechanical distortion products generated by a high-level input may be propagated from the region of direct stimulation of the basilar membrane to the region of the combination tone.

Goldstein and Kiang (1968) have reported the temporal aspect of the response of single units of the cat's auditory nerve in response to the cubic difference tone $2f_1 - f_2$, where $1 < f_2/f_1 < 2$ was approximately equal to the characteristic frequency of the neuron. They found synchronous firing related to the frequency of the cubic difference tone, even though no energy existed in the signal at that frequency, for signal levels of approximately 40 dB SPL. They conclude that their data represent essential nonlinearity, not overdriving, in the normal listening range.

Earlier in this chapter, the issue of linearity of the ear was treated as if it were a relatively simple issue. After looking at some of the relevant data, it should be obvious that nonlinearity of the ear is a complicated matter, even in the present simplified form. Audiologists should probably expect their data to reflect nonlinearity, when they give it a chance to, and should not assume too many linear mechanisms.

B. Single-Unit Response and Periodicity

Because data recorded from individual neurons in the auditory nerve reflect a strong phase-locked relationship with the signal, particularly for low frequencies, these data have generated considerable interest among those who study auditory perception (Plomp and Smoorenburg, 1970). Although even the earliest investigations of single units in the auditory system gave evidence of a time code (Rose et al., 1968), only recently has it become technologically practical to pursue the matter. With the advent of the digital computer as a laboratory device, it is now practical to time out and count several thousand events per second so that such data can be accumulated and processed on line.

The data of Rose *et al.* (1968) indicate that the quality or degree of phase-locked firings (time or periodicity code) is consistently high for frequencies up to about 1000 Hz. Beyond 1000 Hz the degree of synchrony decreases, first gradually to about 2000 Hz and then more rapidly, until for frequencies higher than 5000–6000 Hz evidence of synchronous firing is no longer present.

A further report by the same group (Brugge *et al.*, 1969) is on synchronous firing in the auditory nerve in response to complex tones. By ignoring periods of the fundamental for which no response occurs and plotting the histogram for only one period of the signal, a folded histogram, they are able to relate firing patterns to the waveform of the complex tone. Their results indicate that the folded histogram can be fitted with the negative going half-cycle of the complex waveform. This statement can be made in two other ways. The response of the neuron, over rather long time intervals, looks like a phase modulation of the input waveform. In other terms, this folded histogram could be used as a probability density function to describe the probability of the occurrence of a response at each point in the half-cycle.

Finally, it should be noted that this time code, in the form of phase-locked firings, is maintained in some cells at higher levels of the auditory nervous system (Lavine, 1971). Lavine found that the degree of synchrony was low to moderate for 16 cells in the dorsal cochlear nucleus but was consistently high for all 6 cells he observed in the anterior-ventral cochlear nucleus.

The more traditional single-unit data (Kiang, 1965) have been reported in terms of change in firing rate as a function of changes in frequency and level of the pure-tone probe, that is, a tuning curve. The frequency for which a change in firing rate occurs at the lowest intensity level is called the characteristic frequency (CF) of the neuron. Tuning curves for neurons are usually described as indicating that the neuron is highly (sharply) tuned to a narrow range of frequencies for low levels, but that, as signal level is increased, the neuron responds to a wider and wider range of frequencies and this range is progressively more skewed in the direction of low frequencies.

When tuning curves are considered from the point of view of a fixed rather than a variable frequency signal and of the population of neurons that is picked up by the traveling wave patterns for the specified signal at a specified level, the resultant pattern of activity in the auditory nerve as a whole corresponds quite closely to the masked audiogram for a noise of one critical bandwidth (Zwicker, 1970). The implication of this statement for the asymmetrical masking seen in the frequency region above a narrow-band masker is quite profound. The statement says that the so-called upward spread of masking (Bilger and Hirsh, 1956; Jerger et al., 1960) is not necessarily distortion but a reflection of the normal organization and function of the auditory nerve, organ of Corti, and cochlea.

Along this line, Schuknecht (1960) has argued that for signals about 40 dB above threshold, approximately 25% of the neural elements in the auditory nerve are active, with a change in percentage of fibers of about $\frac{1}{2}\%$ per decibel for changes in level. Given Schuknecht's interpretation of his data and Zwicker's (1970) interpretation of the significance of tuning curves for single units of the auditory neuron, one has a relatively large "window" into the auditory nerve. Add the time code that Rose and his associates (Rose et al., 1968; Brugge et al., 1969) report, and a theory similar to the volley theory (Wever, 1949) begins to look useful again.

The range of frequencies through which periodicity information can enter through the place window extends from between 100–200 Hz at the low end to between 5000–6000 Hz at the high-frequency end of the continuum. This lower limit is based on work reported by Flanagan and Guttman (1960) that showed that below 100 Hz a pure periodicity (pulse counting) mechanism governed pitch matching, while at 200 Hz pitch matches were related to the spectrum of a pulse train. The upper limit it based on the findings of Rose et al. (1968) that show 5000–6000 Hz to be the upper limit of synchronous firing, and on that of Ritsma (1962) whose work on the range of carrier frequencies through which residue pitch (presumably a periodicity phenomenon) could be created had an upper limit no higher than 5600 Hz. It must be remembered that once center frequency reaches the vicinity of 1000 Hz, the quality of this time code begins to limit the rate at which neurons can respond.

C. Signal Processing and Feature Detection

In 1959 Lettvin et al. published one of the most significant papers of the decade under the improbable but provocative title, "What the Frog's Eye Tells the Frog's Brain." Their initial argument was as follows:

"The assumption has always been that the eye mainly senses light, whose local distribution is transmitted to the brain in a kind of copy by a mosaic of impulses. Suppose we held otherwise, that the nervous apparatus in the eye is itself devoted to detecting certain lights and their changes, corresponding to particular relations in the visible world.

If this should be the case, the laws found by using small spots of light on the retina may be true and yet, in a sense be misleading [Lettvin et al., 1959, p. 1942]."

To implement their approach, they suggest using the widest possible range of stimuli in an attempt to extract what common "features" can be detected from single-unit recordings in the optic nerve. Once having identified such features, they then suggest looking for an anatomical basis for such "feature detectors."

As a result of the impetus provided by Lettvin et al. (1959), the organization of the visual system, in terms of receptive fields, has been completely reexamined along the lines they suggested. As predicted, the visual system can be considered in terms of "feature detectors." Feature detectors, however, are not found in the retina of all species (Micheal, 1969). Few mammals have the complex retinal organization to support feature detectors at that level, such as the rabbit and ground squirrel (chipmunk) whose retina is as complicated as the frog's. Primates quite typically have a simple retina and their feature detection occurs in the cortex (Micheal, 1969).

Analogies from the visual system to the auditory system are touchy ground. Since the visual system appears to function on the basis of extracting features from visual stimuli and since the major auditory stimulus (speech) is usually described in terms of its features, one is forced to ask if the auditory system also might not be organized in terms of feature detectors. Before considering the answer to that question, some attention should be given to the definition of a "feature" and to the nature of a "feature detector."

Lettvin et al. (1959) point out in their definition of features that even a spot of light has size, intensity, shape, contrast, etc. If we go ahead and assume some sort of interchangeability between space in the eye and time in the ear (in spite of good advice), then we can define auditory features in terms of onset and offset, abrupt changes in frequency or intensity, or the sudden addition or subtraction of components to a complex signal. For example, if we assume for the moment that rise and decay times of a tone burst are features, then even a gated pure tone has features. Surprisingly enough, there is strong evidence for the presence of feature detectors in the auditory system, but they are not called by that name.

Feature detectors must perform one of two basic functions. They must compare two or more aspects of the stimulus ensemble, or they must detect abrupt shifts (gradients) in that ensemble. To perform these functions, inhibition of some sort is necessary to minimize the competition between related features. Since there is no clear evidence concerning inhibition in the auditory system, it could be a hard requirement to meet.

In vision, binocularity is considered to be a feature and in the primate visual system the detector for that feature is located at the level of the cortex (Bishop, 1970). By analogy, then, the extraction of the relationship between the inputs to the two ears (binaurality) could be a feature. In their review article, Eldredge and Miller (1971) devote careful attention to experiments in which single-unit data on auditory nuclei were collected for binaural stimulation. In addition, they cite many researches that show that some cells in the medial superior olive, presumably of the cat, are differentially sensitive to interaural time and/or intensity difference. Perhaps most significant is their report (Eldredge and Miller, 1971) of a study by Watanabe et al. that they describe in some detail. Watanabe et al. (as cited by Eldredge and Miller) describe cells in the medial superior olive that exhibit an interesting phenomenon. When one ear led the other in time, these cells were "captured" by the leading ear in that they did not respond to the input from the ear lagging in time for as long as 50 msec after the leading ear was stimulated. The "capture" phenomenon seems closly related to the inhibition or suppression of related features that is necessary for feature detection.

Although the work cited in Eldredge and Miller (1971) related to feature detection seems pertinent, the major contributions of Whitfield (1967, 1970) and Erulkar et al. (1968) should be recalled to the reader's attention. Their work has dealt primarily with frequency-modulated tones. Frequency-modulated tones are less interesting than the signal discussed by Frishkopf et al. (1968), the mating call of the bullfrog, which is an appropriate signal in an appropriate species considering that feature detection began in the frog's retina.

As the literature on feature detectors in the central auditory pathways develops, great caution will be needed in evaluating such experiments with respect to human hearing because of the wide species variations known to exist in the structure of the auditory system (Eldredge and Miller, 1971). Variations in the location and nature of specific feature detectors can be expected to be even greater than anatomical variations (Micheal, 1969). In light of these variations, careful consideration should be given to feature detectors that might be associated with processing speech signals.

Although several systems of features have been proposed for analysis of speech (cf. Jakobson et al., 1969), those feature systems differ significantly from the kind of feature system proposed by Lettvin et al. (1959). The existing feature systems for speech are based in part on acoustical and perceptual data for speech and in part on insight and linguistic judgment. The feature system suggested by Lettvin *et al.* (1959) however, is posited in terms of the analysis performed by the sensory system itself as detected via microelectrode recordings from single cells. Obviously, no such study of processing of the speech signal can be performed on a human nervous system nor can it be done on a comparative basis. One must ask then if there is not some way to find a middle ground between existing systems of features for speech and the neurologically defined feature system.

If one is willing to accept some form of multidimensional scaling technique as being capable of revealing the feature system underlying an appropriate set of data, then one can find a middle ground between a neurologically defined and a speculative set of features for speech. One characteristic of the appropriate set of data is that it should be a sample of the behavioral responses of a single subject. If that subject has perfectly normal perceptual and nonperceptual auditory functioning, then the derived set of features might not tell anything about the underlying structures. On the other hand, if that subject has a speech discrimination loss, then the derived features may be informative. At least, the differences between the normal and impaired functioning cases will be interesting.

The appropriate data set has two more dimensions. One dimension involves the manner in which the speech is presented to the subject, acoustically or graphemically. The listener with poor speech discrimination might generate a normal set of derived features for visually presented speech material and still generate a different set of features for acoustically presented speech materials. The other dimension involves the task required of the subject. Perceptual confusions within a closed message set could be used with subjects who have a speech discrimination loss. Ratings of the similarity of pairs of sounds also could be used. Finally, estimates of perceptual distance based on triads of sounds could be utilized. In this case the subject would be required to name the pair of the triad that is most alike and the pair that is most different.

These procedures do not recognize quick data collection and analysis, but they provide direction in a difficult area. The quality of the results will depend primarily on how lucky one is in acquiring subjects who have hearing losses that will result in interesting data.

D. Perception of Complex Tones

In the past, two factors impeded research in the area of complex tones. First, generation and control of complex tones was technologically difficult until general-purpose digital computers became generally available. It should be noted, however, that Plomp (1964) solved the problem of generating a tonal complex without a computer. Perhaps a more significant impediment has been the so-called subjective nature of the listener's task in complex-tone experiments. Plomp (1964), Plomp and Levelt, (1965) and Plomp and Mimpen (1968) also have made significant contributions in testing procedures that move perception of complex tones from the subjective toward the objective. His procedures, in Tanner's terms (1961), minimize the load placed on the observer's memory.

Audiologists should be interested in using complex tones as stimuli for several reasons. Though most difficult to use, they are a vastly more interesting signal. It is reasonable to assume that pure tones are a minimal artificial signal on the continuum that runs from pure tones to natural complex sounds, that is, pure tones to speech. With a little ingenuity, the experimenter could use complex tones to move back and forth on any one of several continua. As noted several times previously, pure tones completely confound the place code with the time code; but perhaps a different approach can be used to demonstrate the desirability of using complex tonal stimuli in audiology.

The traditional experiment in audition, as noted earlier, deals with the very high correlation between the spectrum of the signal and the resultant perception. There is, however, a diverse class of perceptual phenomena in audition that can be characterized by the absence from the signal of the spectral components sufficient to explain the perception in terms of the direct correlation of spectrum and perception. This set includes combination tones (Dallos, 1970), the residue pitch phenomenon (Schouten, 1970; Schouten et al., 1962), and remote masking (Bilger and Hirsh, 1956). It may or may not include the masking of tones by tones of which the aural harmonic is a special case (Wegel and Lane, 1924) and the upward spread of masking (Jerger et al., 1960). The difference between the two classes of experiments is that in the second class of experiments, the ear is adding something to the perception that is not in the signal, rather than just mirroring it (Plomp, 1970).

Most of the results obtained recently in work concerning the perception of complex tones (Plomp and Smoorenburg, 1970) seem to be explainable in terms of the relationship of the tonal complex to the critical bandwidth (cf. Zwicker, 1970). This is particularly interesting, since Scharf et al. (1965) have reported that this critical bandwidth is widened in cases of sensorineural hearing loss. Thus, listeners with impaired hearing can be expected to perceive complex tones differently from normals. Since remote masking, that is, masking of low-frequency tones by complex signals of high frequency, is presumably the result of some kind of intermodulation distortion, it should be noted that both Keith and Anderson (1969) and Bilger and Hopkinson (1970) have reported that remote masking is reduced or absent in cases of sensorineural hearing loss. Although the more direct phenomena, combination tones and the residue pitch, have not been explored, it is reasonable to expect that they will be affected by sensorineural hearing loss.

E. Memory and Audition

In recent years, an area called "human information processing" has developed. Under the influence of mathematical models for learning, signal detection theory, and computer processes, a diverse group of scientists interested in perception, cognition, and learning have come together to study human memory. The resultant models of human memory emphasize the fact that information is processed in stages. On the input side, these stages include sensory buffers (auditory and visual) and short-term storage as initial steps; and, on the output side of information processing, these stages include the same short-term storage and response buffers as the final steps (cf. Morton, 1970).

One of the earlier findings from research in memory processes showed that when subjects were required to remember letters presented to them visually, their errors were related to auditory confusions rather than to the visual pattern of the letter (Conrad, 1964). Wickelgren (1965) has used this phenomenon to study encoding of speech patterns in the context of learning experiments. The explanation for the relationship of errors in memory experiments to the acoustic or auditory representation of the stimulus rather than to its visual representation is assumed to reflect the manner in which the input is encoded in short-term storage, that is, in semantic or phonological form (Baddeley, 1968; Morton, 1970). Sperling and Speelman (1970) have called this level of storage "auditory short-term memory." In one of the few articles on information processing that has been published in the audiological literature, Conrad and Rush (1965) confirmed Conrad (1964) on deaf children. They found that while the errors made by deaf children were relatively consistent, they did not follow any known system of classification. This result has broad implications in the education and psychology of the deaf. Blair (1957) has also reported differences between normally hearing and deaf children in terms of short-term storage of digits.

Although sensory input buffers were contemplated quite early in the development of information processing (Neisser, 1967), it probably is as a result of the auditory implication in short-term storage errors that the auditory buffer has received as much attention as it has. Murdock (1967) noted that rehearsing aloud allowed subjects to achieve better scores in a learning task than did silent rehearsal. Subsequent investigators noted that auditorily presented materials were learned more readily than visually presented materials and hypothesized that this difference might be attributed to an extra step in processing visual data to encode it for short-term storage (Posner, 1969). In their extensive treatment of what they call "precategorical acoustic storage" or PAS, Crowder and Morton (1969) suggest that the characteristics of the auditory buffer are sufficient to explain these differences between visual and auditory presentation, since the real differences occur in the last few items of a list. First, they note that the auditory buffer can apparently hold more information and hold it longer than the visual buffer. Next, they note that the auditory buffer holds information in sequence. That is, each item is shifted through the auditory buffer as new items are entered and when the buffer is full a new item pushes the oldest item out of the buffer.

On the output side of human information processing, the auditory characteristics of short-term storage again play a role. In searching new lists for familiar items, if the material fits the coding scheme of the short-term storage device, then the judgment that the item is the same as one on the earlier list can be made more readily than the different judgment. By the same token, if the items in the lists do not fit the code (pure tones, for example), then it is more difficult to judge sameness than difference. Search time is a function of the list (Sternberg, 1966) and of the complexity of the comparisons to be made (Posner and Mitchell, 1967). Searching generally has been found to be exhaustive rather than terminating on the correct item. Recently Swinney and Taylor (1971) have shown that in a nonverbal short-term memory experiment, aphasics have significantly longer search times but a self-terminating search. They suggest that memory search may be related to auditory and linguistic abilities.

Although these concepts of memory that derive from the literature on information processing obviously relate to audiological measurement, Schubert and West (1969) have observed that their application to psychophysical experiments is not always obvious. Recent work by Durlach and Braida (1969), however, offers the promise of making the relationship between the memory literature and psychophysics clear. In a series of experiments designed to resolve discrepancies within the literature on intensity resolution in terms of memory variables, they have demonstrated the existence of two different modes of memory. When they used a "jittered" standard tone (that is, varied through a narrow range of intensities), their data show no sensitivity to the temporal interval between the standard and comparison tone. When they varied the standard tone through a wide range (that is, 50 dB), on the other hand, there was a dependence of performance on the interval between the standard and comparison tone. They explained this difference by assuming that their subjects had to try to remember the sensory image or trace when the standard varied through a wide range. When the standard varied through a narrow range, however, their subjects were assumed to be categorizing the standard tones according to some rough scale. They called this latter mode of memory the "context mode."

Although there are obvious differences between the rough scaling of loudness presumably used by Durlach and Braida's (1969) subjects and the sophisticated semantic–phonological categories associated with short-term storage in verbal learning experiments, there are also obvious parallels. The correspondence between precategorical acoustic storage and the "trace" mode of memory is clearer. The problems encountered by Schubert and West (1969) in making the connection between memory and psychophysics is probably due, in large part, to the fact that they were studying pattern recognition of complex tonal patterns. The question of how the parameters necessary to categorize complex acoustic patterns can be established in memory should be one of the more interesting questions for future research.

The suggestion found in Swinney and Taylor (1971) that people differ in certain abilities related to memory and information processing should be explored further. In broad terms, the auditory memory buffer discussed here has to depend on the status of the individual's hearing, so that some hearing impairments could disrupt information processing. Further, both the auditory buffer and short-term memory seem to be implicated in refined skills that audiologists, so far, have been unable to assess with their standard tests. Finally, there is a clear implication that the relationship between audition and memory, if pursued by future audiological researchers, should give them something to say to the teachers of hearing-handicapped persons besides, "Make it louder."

VI. New Audiological Experiments

At the outset of this essay it was assumed that audiology is at a critical point in its history. It can continue to observe the grand traditions of the past and become an establishmental relic, or it can turn to the future. In hopes of facilitating a new turn, an attempt has been made to identify those assumptions about the auditory system and audiological experimentation that bind audiology to the past. Further, those aspects of the world around us that could be useful to maturing and expanding audiology have been reviewed, at least partially.

Three points should be reiterated in summary. First, audiological researchers should try to use interesting stimuli in their experimentation.

The technology will, as a matter of fact, support the use of complex tonal stimuli in a wide range of experimentation. These complex signals will in turn involve the pathological auditory system in the response to a much greater degree than pure-tone signals ever will.

The second point to be stressed in this summarization is that audiologists must recognize that their fundamental experimental paradigm was designed to study either the transmission of signals or the signals themselves and not to study the individual. To make audiology into a scientific study of the individual's auditory system, it is necessary to get a random sample of the individual's response behaviors in a particular context. While this will tend to increase the amount of time required in the laboratory, technology again can be utilized to solve otherwise tedious problems.

Finally, audiologists should recognize that, in addition to the obvious aspects of hearing, the auditory system mediates more subtle but equally important functions. The implications of the memory literature to problems in the habilitation and rehabilitation of the deaf and hard-of-hearing seem obvious. Further, the memory literature seems to point the way toward measuring skills and abilities relating to music, second languages, and other special auditory skills that have stubbornly resisted the audiologist's conventional battery of tests. That is to say, confronted with a shrinking world, perhaps audiologists should look to assessment of the more subtle auditory skills as a means of scientific and professional survival.

ACKNOWLEDGMENT

This work was supported by grants from the National Institute of Neurological Diseases and Stroke. The author would like to express his appreciation to those of his colleagues who suffered through the preparation of this manuscript with him, though they cannot be blamed for its shortcomings.

References

Baddeley, A. D. (1968). How does acoustic similarity influence short-term memory? *Quart. J. Exp. Psychol.* **20,** 249–264.

Békésy, G. von. (1960). "Experiments in Hearing." McGraw-Hill, New York.

Bilger, R. C., and Hirsh, I. J. (1956). Masking of pure tones by narrow bands of noise. *J. Acoust. Soc. Amer.* **28,** 623–630.

Bilger, R. C., and Hopkinson, N. T. (1970). Masking of low-frequency tones by high-frequency bands of noise and frequency-modulated tones. *J. Acoust. Soc. Amer.* **47,** 107(A).

Bishop, P. O. (1970). Neurophysiology of binocular single vision and stereopsis. *In* "Handbook of sensory physiology," (H. S. A. Datrnall, ed.). Verlag Chemie, Weinheim.

Blair, F. X. (1957). A study of the visual memory of deaf and hearing children, *Amer. Ann. Deaf* **102,** 254–263.

Boring, E. G. (1942). "Sensation and Perception in the History of Experimental Psychology." Appleton, New York.

Braithwaite, R. B. (1953). "Scientific Explanation." Cambridge Univ. Press, London and New York.

Brugge, J. F., Anderson, D. J., Hind, J. E., and Rose, J. E. (1969). Time structure of discharges in single auditory nerve fibers of the squirrel monkey in response to complex periodic sounds. *J. Neurophysiol.* **32**, 386–401.

Clarke, F. R., and Bilger, R. C. (1972). The theory of signal detectability and the measurement of hearing. *In* "Modern Developments in Audiology," (J. Jerger, ed.), 2nd ed., pp. 437–467.

Conrad, R. (1964). Acoustic confusions in immediate memory. *Brit. J. Psychol.* **55**, 75–84.

Conrad, R., and Rush, M. L. (1965). On the nature of short-term memory by the deaf. *J. Speech Hearing Dis.* **30**, 336–343.

Crowder, R. G., and Morton, J. Y. (1969). Precategorial acoustic storage (PAS). *Percept. Psychophys.* **5**, 365–373.

Dallos, P. (1969). Comments on the differential-electrode technique. *J. Acoust. Soc. Amer.* **45**, 999–1007.

Dallos, P. (1970). Combination tones in cochlear microphonic potentials. *In* "Frequency Analysis and Periodicity Detection in Hearing," (R. Plomp and G. F. Smoorenburg, eds.), pp. 218–226. Sijthoff, Leiden.

Dallos, P., and Sweetman, R. H. (1969). Distribution patterns of cochlear harmonics. *J. Acoust. Soc. Amer.* **45**, 37–46.

Dallos, P., Schoeny, Z. G., and Cheatham, M. A. (1971). On the limitations of cochlear-microphonic measurements. *J. Acoust. Soc. Amer.* **49**, 1114–1154.

Davis, H., Deatherage, B. H., Eldredge, D. H., and Smith, C. A. (1958). Summating potentials of the cochlea. *Amer. J. Physiol.* **195**, 251–261.

Diamond, I. T., and Neff, W. D. (1957). Ablation of temporal cortex and discrimination of auditory patterns. *J. Neurophysiol.* **20**, 300–315.

Durlach, N. I., and Braida, L. D. (1969). Intensity perception. I. Preliminary theory of intensity resolution. *J. Acoust. Soc. Amer.* **46**, 372–383.

Eldredge, D. H., and Miller, J. D. (1971). Physiology of hearing. *Ann. Rev. Physiol.* **33**, 281–310.

Engebretson, A. M., and Eldredge, D. H. (1968). Model for the nonlinear characteristics of cochlear potentials. *J. Acoust. Soc. Amer.* **44**, 548–554.

Erulkar, S. D., Nelson, P. G., and Bryan, J. S. (1968). Experimental and theoretical approaches to neural processing in the central auditory pathway. *In* "Contributions to Sensory Physiology," (W. D. Neff, ed.), Vol. III, pp. 150–184. Academic Press, New York.

Fechner, G .T. (1860). "Elemente der Psychophysik." Breitkopf und Hartel, Leipzig, 1860. English trans. of Vol. 1 by H. E. Adler (D. H. Howes, and E. G. Boring, eds.). Holt, New York, 1966.

Flanagan, J. L., and Guttman, N. (1960). On the pitch of periodic pulses. *J. Acoust. Soc. Amer.* **32**, 1308–1318.

Frishkopf, L. S., Capranica, R. R., and Goldstein; M. H., Jr. (1968). Neural coding in the bullfrog's auditory system—a teleological approach. *Proc. I.E.E.E.* **56**, 969–980.

Glorig, A., and Davis, H. (1961). Age, noise, and hearing loss. *Ann. Otol. Rhinol. Laryngol.* **70**, 556–571.

Goldstein, J. L., and Kiang, N. Y. S. (1968). Neural correlates of the aural combination tones $2f_1 - f_2$. Proc. I.E.E.E. **56**, 981–992.

Green, D. M., and Swets, J A. (1966). "Signal Detection Theory and Psychophysics." Wiley, New York.

Helmholtz, H. L. F. (1885). *"The Sensations of Tone,"* 2nd Eng. Ed. Longmans, Green, New York, 1885; Dover, New York, 1954.

Jakobson, R., Fant, C. G. M., Halle, M. (1969). "Preliminaries to Speech Analysis: The Distinctive Features and Their Correlates." M.I.T. Press, Cambridge, Massachusetts.

Jerger, J. Tillman, T. W., and Peterson, J. L. (1960). Masking by octave bands of noise in normal and impaired ears, J. Acoust. Soc. Amer. **32**, 385–390.

Keith, R. W., and Anderson, C. V. (1969). Remote masking for listeners with cochlear impairment. J. Acoust. Soc. Amer. **42**, 393–398.

Kiang, N. Y. S. (1965). "Discharge Patterns of Single Fibers in the Cat's Auditory Nerve." M.I.T. Press, Cambridge, Massachusetts.

Kiang, N. Y.-s., Sachs, M. B., and Peake, W. T. (1967). Shapes of tuning curves for single auditory-nerve fibers. J. Acoust. Soc. Amer. **28**, 852–858.

Lavine, R. A. (1971). Phase-locking in response of single neurons in cochlear nuclear complex of the cat to low-frequency tonal stimuli, J. Neurophysiol. **34**, 467–483.

Lawrence, M., and Yantis, P. A. (1956). Onset and growth of aural harmonics in the overloaded ear. J. Acoust. Soc. Amer. **29**, 852–858.

Lettvin, J. Y., Maturana, H. R., McCulloch, W. S., and Pitts, W. H. (1959). What the frog's eye tells the frog's brain. Proc. IRE. **47**, 1940–1951.

Liberman, A. M., Cooper, F. S., Shankweiler, D. R., and Studdert-Kennedy, M. (1967). Perception of the speech code. Psychol. Rev. **74**, 431–461.

Licklider, J. C. R. (1959). Three auditory theories. In "Psychology: A Study of a Science," (S. Koch, ed.), pp. 41–144. McGraw-Hill, New York.

Micheal, C. R. (1969). Retinal processing of visual images. Sci. Amer. **220** (No. 5), 104–114.

Morton, J. Y. (1970). A functional model for memory. In "Models of Human Memory, (D. A. Norman, ed.). Academic Press, New York.

Moushegian, G., Rupert, A., and Whitcomb, M. A. (1964). Medial superior-olivary-unit response patterns to monaural and binaural clicks. J. Acoust. Soc. Amer. **36**, 196–202.

Murdock, B. B., Jr. (1967). Visual and auditory stores in short term memory. Quart. J. Exp. Psychol. **18**, 206–211.

Neisser, U. (1967). "Cognitive Psychology." Appleton, New York.

Norman, D. A., ed. (1970). "Models of Human Memory." Academic Press, New York.

Plomp, R. (1964). The ear as a frequency analyzer. J. Acoust. Soc. Amer. **36**, 1628–1636.

Plomp, R. (1970). Timbre as a multidimensional attribute of complex tones. In "Frequency Analysis and Periodicity Detection in Hearing" (R. Plomp and G. F. Smoorenburg, eds.), pp. 397–411. Sijthoff, Leiden.

Plomp, R., and Levelt, W. J. M. (1965). Tonal consonance and critical bandwidth. J. Acoust. Soc. Amer. **38**, 548–560.

Plomp, R., and Mimpen, A. M. (1968). The ear as a frequency analyzer II. J. Acoust. Soc. Amer. **43**, 764–767.

Plomp, R., and Smoorenburg, G. F. (eds.). (1970). "Frequency Analysis and Periodicity Detection in Hearing." Sijthoff, Leiden.

Posner, M. I. (1969). Representational systems for storing information in memory. In "The Pathology of Memory," (G. A. Talland and N. C. Waugh, eds.). Academic Press, New York.

Posner, M. I., and Mitchell, R. F. (1967). Chronometric analysis of classification. Psychol. Rev. 74, 392–409.

Ramsdell, D. A. (1947). The psychology of the hard-of-hearing and deafened adult. In "Hearing and Deafness," (H. Davis, ed.), pp. 394–400. Holt, New York.

Rhode, W. S. (1971). Observations of the vibration of the basilar membrane in squirrel monkeys using the mossbauer technique. J. Acoust. Soc. Amer. 49, 1218–1231.

Ritsma, R. J. (1962). Existence region of the tonal residue. J. Acoust. Soc. Amer. 34, 1224–1229.

Rose, J. E., Brugge, J. F., Anderson, D. J., and Hird, J. E. (1968). Patterns of activity in single auditory nerve fibers of the squirrel monkey. In "Hearing Mechanisms in Vertebrates," (De Reuck and Knight, eds.), pp. 144–157. Little, Brown and Co., Boston, Massachusetts.

Scharf, B., Holohan, C. M., and Hellman, R. P. (1965). Loudness summation in cochlear deafness. In "Proceedings of the Fifth International Congress on Acoustics," (D. E. Commins, ed.), Vol. la, paper B35. Imprimerie George Thone, Liege.

Schouten, J. F. (1970). The residue revisited. In "Frequency Analysis and Periodicity Detection in Hearing," (R. Plomp and G. F. Smoorenburg, eds.), pp. 41–54. Sijthoff, Leiden.

Schouten, J. F., Ritsma, R. J., and Cardoza, B. L. (1962). Pitch of the residue. J. Acoust. Soc. Amer. 34, 1418–1424.

Schubert, E. D., and West, R. A. (1969). Recognition of repeated patterns: A study of short-term auditory storage. J. Acoust. Soc. Amer. 46, 1493–1501.

Schuknecht, H. F. (1960). Neuroanatomical correlates of auditory sensitivity and pitch discrimination in cats. In "Neural Mechanisms of the Auditory and Vestibular Systems." (G. L. Rasmussen, and W. F. Windle, eds.).

Sekey, A. (1963). Short-term auditory frequency discrimination. J. Acoust. Soc. Amer. 35, 682–690.

Shower, E. G., and Biddulph, R. (1931). Differential pitch sensitivity of the ear. J. Acoust. Soc. Amer. 3, 275–287.

Sperling, G., and Speelman, R. (1970). Acoustic similarity and auditory short-term memory: Experiments and a model. In "Models of Human Memory," (D. A. Norman, ed.), Academic Press, New York.

Spoendlin, H. (1970). Structural basis of peripheral frequency analysis. In "Frequency Analysis and Periodicity Detection in Hearing," (R. Plomp and G. F. Smoorenburg, eds.), pp. 2–36. Sijthoff, Leiden.

Sternberg, S. (1966). Highspeed scanning in human memory. Science, 153, 652–654.

Stevens, S. S. (1934a). The attributes of tones. Proc. Nat. Acad. Sci. 20, 457–459.

Stevens, S. S. (1934b). Volume and intensity of tones. Amer. J. Psychol. 46, 397–408.

Sweetman, R. H., and Dallos, P. (1969). Distribution pattern of cochlear combination tones. J. Acoust. Soc. Amer. 45, 58–71.

Swets, J. A. (1961). Is there a sensory threshold? Science 134, 168–177.

Swinney, D. A., and Taylor, O. L. (1971). Short-term memory recognition search in aphasics. J. Speech Hearing Res. (in press).

Talland, G. A., and Waugh, N. C. (eds.) (1969). "The Pathology of Memory." Academic Press, New York.

Tanner, W. P. Jr. (1961). Physiological implications of psychophysical procedures. *Ann. N.Y. Acad. Sci.* **89**, 752–765.

Tonndorf, J. (1962). Time/frequency analysis in cochlear models. *J. Acoust. Soc. Amer.* **34**, 1337–1350.

Wegel, R. L., and Lane, C. E. (1924). The auditory masking of one pure tone by another and its relation to the dynamics of the inner ear. *Phys. Rev.* **23**, 226–285.

Wever, E. G. (1949). "Theory of Hearing." Wiley, New York.

Whitfield, I. C. (1967). "The Auditory Pathway." Williams and Wilkins. Baltimore, Maryland.

Whitfield, I. C. (1970). Central nervous processing in relation to spatio-temporal discrimination of auditory patterns. *In* "Frequency Analysis and Periodicity Detection in Hearing," (R. Plomp and G. F. Smoorenburg, eds.), pp. 136–147. Sijthoff, Leiden.

Wickelgren, W. A. (1965). Distinctive features and error in short-term memory for English vowels. *J. Acoust. Soc. Amer.* **38**, 583–588.

Zwicker, E. (1970). Masking and psychological excitation as consequences of the ear's frequency analysis. *In* "Frequency Analysis and Periodicity Detection in Hearing," (R. Plomp and G. F. Smoorenburg, eds.), pp. 376–394. Sijthoff, Leiden.

Zwislocki, J. (1969). Temporal summation of loudness: An analysis. *J. Acoust. Soc. Amer.* **46**, 431–441.

Author Index

Numbers in italics refer to the pages on which the complete reference are listed.

Subject Index